PHARMACEUTICAL CARE PRACTICE
THE CLINICIAN'S GUIDE

Notice

Medicine is an ever-changing science. As new research and clinical experience broaden our knowledge, changes in treatment and drug therapy are required. The authors and the publisher of this work have checked with sources believed to be reliable in their efforts to provide information that is complete and generally in accord with the standards accepted at the time of publication. However, in view of the possibility of human error or changes in medical sciences, neither the authors nor the publisher nor any other party who has been involved in the preparation or publication of this work warrants that the information contained herein is in every respect accurate or complete, and they disclaim all responsibility for any errors or omissions or for the results obtained from use of the information contained in this work. Readers are encouraged to confirm the information contained herein with other sources. For example and in particular, readers are advised to check the product information sheet included in the package of each drug they plan to administer to be certain that the information contained in this work is accurate and that changes have not been made in the recommended dose or in the contraindications for administration. This recommendation is of particular importance in connection with new or infrequently used drugs.

PHARMACEUTICAL CARE PRACTICE

THE CLINICIAN'S GUIDE

Second Edition

Robert J. Cipolle, PharmD

Linda M. Strand, PharmD, PhD, DSc (Hon)

Peter C. Morley, PhD

Peters Institute of Pharmaceutical Care
College of Pharmacy
University of Minnesota
Minneapolis, Minnesota

McGraw-Hill
Medical Publishing Division

New York   Chicago   San Francisco   Lisbon   London
Madrid   Mexico City   Milan   New Delhi
San Juan   Seoul   Singapore   Sydney   Toronto

The McGraw·Hill Companies

Pharmaceutical Care Practice: The Clinician's Guide, Second Edition

2 3 4 5 6 7 8 9 0   DOC/DOC   0 9 8 7 6 5 4

ISBN 0-07-136259-2

This book was set in Times Roman by International Typesetting and Composition.
The editors were Michael Brown and Christie Naglieri.
The production supervisor was Richard Ruzycka.
Project management was provided by International Typesetting and Composition.
RR Donnelley was printer and binder.

This book was printed on acid-free paper.

Library of Congress Cataloging-in-Publication Data

Cipolle, Robert J.
    Pharmaceutical care practice : the clinician's guide / Robert J. Cipolle, Linda M. Strand, Peter C. Morley.—2nd ed.
        p. ; cm.
    Includes bibliographical references and index.
    ISBN 0-07-136259-2 (hardcover : alk. paper)
    1. Pharmacy—Practice. I. Strand, Linda M. II. Morley, Peter C. III. Title.
    [DNLM: 1. Pharmacology. 2. Professional Practice. 3. Drug Therapy. 4. Pharmaceutical Services. QV 21 C577p 2004]
    RS122.5.C56 2004
    615'.1'068—dc22
                                                                                            2003062071

We wish to dedicate this volume
to the next generation of pharmaceutical care practitioners;
to those who will use the ideas contained herein to make life better for others.

We dedicate this volume
to one special practitioner, who did just that, Kevin Coit (1957–2003).

CONTENTS

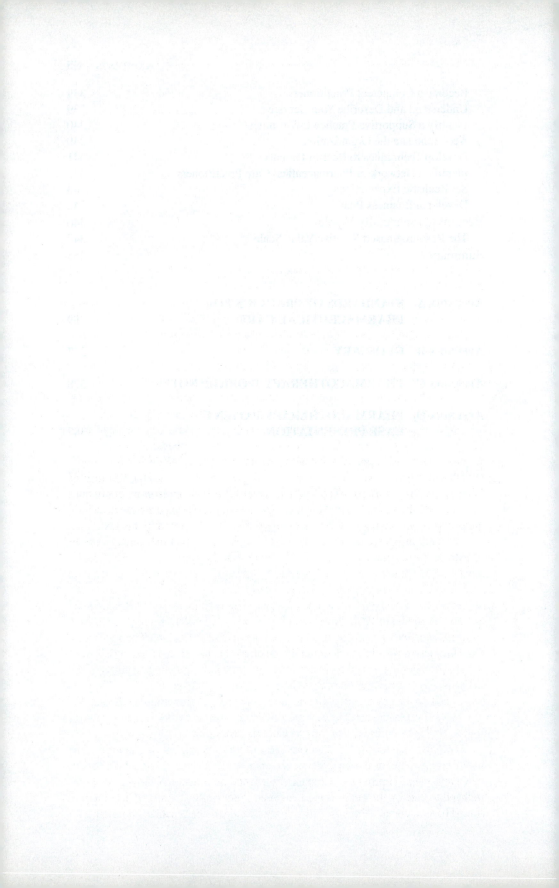

PREFACE

This text builds upon the original concepts presented in the first edition and adds sufficient detail for pharmaceutical care to be learned, taught, and practiced. We have attempted to describe not only the entire scope of practice, but to detail how each component relates to and influences the others. This book is intended to be used as a textbook or guide to the knowledge and skills required in clinical practice. It is our hope that we have met this challenge.

We now have extensive experience with this practice in a number of different settings. The service has been provided to over 20,000 patients during more than 60,000 patient encounters with pharmaceutical care practitioners. Therefore, we can describe, from experience, how to provide pharmaceutical care to patients.

We first conceptualized the original ideas that are described here as pharmaceutical care practice over 25 years ago. At that time we began searching for a rational, systematic approach to making decisions in drug use. When we discovered that one did not exist in the literature or in practice, we created the Pharmacists Workup of Drug Therapy. The Pharmacists Workup has undergone continuous revision over the years, has proven to be effective in structuring drug use decisions, and eventually became the Pharmacotherapy Workup described in this text.

We certainly were not the first ones to use the term "pharmaceutical care" or even to define it. After Dr. Charles D. Hepler clearly defined the philosophy of clinical pharmacy practice, it became obvious that the work we were doing and the term *pharmaceutical care* made a constructive match. It was then time to define and develop the practice itself, one that was consistent with the concepts described by Hepler and Strand in 1990. We accomplished this as a result of research conducted from 1992 to 1997 in a project that became known as the Minnesota Pharmaceutical Care Project. In addition to defining the practice, this project resulted in the development of a computerized software program to support the practice and the data generated from practice, as well as the application of the resource-based relative value scale to the practice of pharmaceutical care for reimbursement purposes. We have been fortunate to conduct the research that interested us these many years, and it is a privilege to present it to you now in this textbook.

The first chapter provides an overview of pharmaceutical care practice. The major components of the practice are described, and a short historical account of its development is provided. Chapter 2 presents the practice-based results accumulated to date by the authors and their practitioner colleagues. The data are presented here to create a "picture" of a pharmaceutical care practice, complete with the types of patients, types of medical problems, and types of drug therapy problems seen in practice. In addition, these data are meant to help the reader visualize the work that is involved in the practice and the patient outcomes practitioners can expect from the interventions they make.

Chapters 3 and 4 discuss the responsibilities of both the practitioner and the patient in this practice. Chapter 5 introduces a new concept in health care—that of the patient's medication experience. Because pharmaceutical care practice was developed to identify and meet the drug-related needs of patients, this chapter explains how the pharmaceutical care practitioner can accomplish these objectives through an understanding of the patient's medication experience.

Chapters 6, 7, 8, and 9 form the core of this text in that they describe the essence of the practice—the patient care process used to provide pharmaceutical care. These chapters explain, in detail, how to assess a patient's drug-related needs, determine which drug therapy problems exist, construct a care plan, and conduct a follow-up evaluation of the outcomes of drug therapy for each patient.

Whenever patients and practitioners interact, there is a need to attend to the ethical considerations of practice. Chapter 10 focuses on these ethical issues. Chapters 11 and 12 continue by describing the knowledge and skills that are required to practice at a level that meets the established standards. Chapter 13 continues the skills discussion by describing the Pharmacotherapy Patient Case Presentation Format that is used by pharmaceutical care practitioners. Finally, chapter 14 reviews the basic issues that must be addressed if the practitioner is interested in establishing a new pharmaceutical care practice.

Each chapter of this edition begins with a list of its key concepts. This is meant to serve as a resource for quick reference to a specific topic area. At the end of each chapter are exercises designed to allow the reader to "practice" each key concept. Learning a new practice takes time, commitment, and repetition. These exercises are important to determine if the concepts are understood and progress is being made in learning the practice.

It is our intention that at the completion of this text, the reader will be able to determine if pharmaceutical care practice is an appropriate career and will understand the practice well enough to begin caring for patients.

ACKNOWLEDGMENTS

The practice of pharmaceutical care as described here has been under development since 1978. It would be virtually impossible to thank all of the individuals who have helped to create the ideas described in this book. There have been practitioner colleagues, professional students, and graduate students, as well as thousands of patients who have contributed significantly to the development of this practice. There have been those who have supported our research financially and those who have constructively disagreed with us. We owe a tremendous amount of gratitude to all of them.

This text could not have been prepared without the efforts of Karen E. Meyers and Jenny Gordon. The constructive reviews provided by Brian Isetts, PhD, and Sarah Westberg, PharmD, are also greatly appreciated.

The authors want to recognize the support, contributions, and friendship of Mike Frakes, PharmD. Dr. Frakes has led the efforts to develop and continually improve the computerized documentation system that supports our pharmaceutical care practitioners. All of the clinical evidence describing the impact of pharmaceutical care in this text was made possible through his work and the work of our pharmaceutical care practitioner colleagues within Fairview Health Services. These practitioners provide the evidence of the value of this practice on a daily basis.

We are forever indebted to Dean Emeritus Lawrence C. Weaver, PhD, of the College of Pharmacy at the University of Minnesota, who is the greatest mentor any group with ideas could ever have. His moral support, wonderful vision, and constant enthusiasm have kept us focused for over two decades.

Finally, the three of us would like to thank each other for a quarter of a century of productive work. It is indeed an honor when in the course of a lifetime even *one* individual can be found who strengthens another's weaknesses. Each of us has found *two* such individuals. Through it all, we have learned to respect one another, and have been able to develop the practice described here; it has been a pleasure, a privilege, and a dream realized. To the others, thank you.

Robert J. Cipolle   Dr. Cipolle is a pharmacist and educator. He received his Bachelor of Pharmacy Degree (Honors) from the College of Pharmacy at the University of Illinois Medical Center, and the Doctor of Pharmacy Degree from the University of Minnesota College of Pharmacy. He has held faculty and administrative positions at the University of Minnesota that included Department Chair, Associate Dean for Academic Affairs, and Dean of the College of Pharmacy.

Dr. Cipolle has practiced in the areas of clinical pharmacokinetics, ambulatory care, and long-term care. He has developed educational programs for pharmacy students, residents, fellows, and graduate students in therapeutic drug monitoring, specialty areas of pharmacotherapy and pharmaceutical care. Dr. Cipolle joined Dr. Strand in 1978 to begin the work that eventually resulted in the development of the practice of pharmaceutical care and a documentation system to support practitioners.

Dr. Cipolle was one of the first clinical pharmacists to be recognized as a fellow by both the American College of Clinical Pharmacy (FCCP—1985) and the American Society of Health System Pharmacists (FASHP—1991). He has received a number of awards to recognize his contribution to pharmacy practice. These include the Hallie Bruce Award from the Minnesota Society of Hospital Pharmacists, and the Larry and Dee Weaver Medal for sustained contributions to the University of Minnesota College of Pharmacy.

Dr. Cipolle presently holds the position of Professor and Director of the Peters Institute of Pharmaceutical Care in the College of Pharmacy at the University of Minnesota in Minneapolis, Minnesota. In 1998, the Peters Institute was recognized with the Innovative Pharmacy Practice Award by the Minnesota Pharmacists Association. His most recent research focuses on the development of educational programs to prepare pharmaceutical care practitioners.

Linda M. Strand   Dr. Strand is a pharmacist and an educator. She received her Bachelor of Science Degree, Doctor of Pharmacy Degree, and Doctor of Philosophy Degree in Pharmacy Administration from the University of Minnesota. In 2001, Dr. Strand was presented an honorary Doctor of Science Degree from Robert Gordon University in Aberdeen, Scotland.

Dr. Strand held faculty positions in the colleges of pharmacy at the University of Utah and the University of Florida before returning to the University of

Minnesota. Throughout her career, she practiced in community, hospital, and clinical pharmacy settings. Dr. Strand has taught the practice of pharmaceutical care at the professional student level as well as the graduate level.

Dr. Strand began working with the ideas that eventually became the practice of pharmaceutical care in 1978. She began working with Dr. Cipolle at that time and in 1983 Dr. Peter Morley joined the research team. In 1990, her work was integrated with the work of Dr. Charles D. Hepler in the landmark paper entitled "Opportunities and Responsibilities in Pharmaceutical Care." Since then she has worked to further develop and teach the practice of pharmaceutical care.

Dr. Strand received the Remington Medal in 1997 from the American Pharmacists Association. This medal is the highest recognition given to an individual working in the profession of pharmacy.

Dr. Strand's work is internationally recognized. She has lectured throughout the world and conducted pharmaceutical care training programs for practitioners from over 12 nations.

Dr. Strand presently holds the position of Distinguished Professor in the College of Pharmacy at the University of Minnesota in Minneapolis, Minnesota. Her most recent research involves the development of an international educational program that will prepare pharmaceutical care practitioners.

Peter C. Morley Dr. Morley is a medical anthropologist and an educator. He received his Bachelor of Arts Degree (Honors) in politics, sociology, and anthropology and the Master of Arts Degree in Political Science from Simon Fraser University in British Columbia, Canada. He continued his education at Stirling University in Stirling, Scotland, where he received the Doctor of Philosophy Degree in Anthropology.

Dr. Morley held faculty positions at Stirling University in Scotland and Memorial University Medical School of Newfoundland, Canada, the School of Nursing and College of Pharmacy at the University of Utah, the College of Pharmacy at the University of Florida and the College of Pharmacy at the University of Minnesota. He served as the Director of the Transcultural Nursing program while at the University of Utah. Dr. Morley's work has taken him to many countries and involved him in many different cultures around the world.

Dr. Morley has advised over 100 graduate students from every discipline in the health and social sciences. He has been elected a fellow of the Royal Anthropological Institute of Great Britain and a fellow of the Society for Applied Anthropology of the United States.

Dr. Morley joined the research team of Drs. Cipolle and Strand in 1983 and has been working to further develop and teach the practice of pharmaceutical care since then. His work focuses on the ethical, and sociocultural aspects of pharmaceutical care practice. He has been instrumental in making the patient's perspective central to the practice of pharmaceutical care and understanding the process of change and development in a health profession.

Dr. Morley presently holds the position of Professor in the College of Pharmacy at the University of Minnesota in Minneapolis, Minnesota.

PHARMACEUTICAL CARE PRACTICE
THE CLINICIAN'S GUIDE

CHAPTER ONE

AN OVERVIEW OF PHARMACEUTICAL CARE PRACTICE

Key Concepts

1. *Pharmaceutical care is a new patient care practice.*

2. *The pharmaceutical care practitioner takes responsibility for optimizing all of a patient's drug therapy.*

3. *The pharmaceutical care practitioner assures that (a) all of a patient's drug therapy is used appropriately for each medical condition; (b) the most effective drug therapy available is used; (c) the safest drug therapy possible is used, and (d) the patient is able and willing to take the medication as intended.*

4 *The pharmaceutical care practitioner identifies, resolves, and prevents drug therapy problems.*

5 *Pharmaceutical care is a generalist practice that can be applied in all settings: community, hospital, long-term care, and the clinic. It can be used to care for all types of patients with all types of diseases taking any type of drug therapy.*

6 *Pharmaceutical care practitioners use a common vocabulary with medicine, nursing, and other patient care practices.*

7 *The requirements to become a pharmaceutical care practitioner are to (a) understand and execute the practitioner's responsibilities; (b) learn how to establish a therapeutic relationship with each patient; (c) internalize the rational thought process used for making clinical decisions; (d) acquire a unique and specific knowledge base; (e) develop clinical skills; (f) understand and apply the standards of care, standards of professional behavior, and ethical principles involved in practice.*

8 *The Pharmacotherapy Workup is the rational thought process that is used by pharmaceutical care practitioners to make drug therapy decisions.*

9 *The patient care process is used to provide direct care to patients and includes the assessment of the patient's drug-related needs to identify drug therapy problems and their causes, the development of care plans that include goals of therapy, and the follow-up evaluation of outcomes.*

10 *All decisions made in pharmaceutical care practice are documented in a pharmaceutical care patient chart.*

PHARMACEUTICAL CARE DEFINED

The goal of this text is to provide a guide for those who want to understand pharmaceutical care practice and gain the knowledge and skills necessary to deliver this level of care to patients.

> **Definition**   Pharmaceutical care is a patient-centered practice in which the practitioner assumes responsibility for a patient's drug-related needs and is held accountable for this commitment.[1]

Pharmaceutical care practitioners accept responsibility for optimizing all of a patient's drug therapy, regardless of the source (prescription, nonprescription, alternative, or traditional medicines), to achieve better patient outcomes and to improve the quality of each patient's life. This occurs with the patient's cooperation and in coordination with the patient's other health care providers.

The practitioner uses a rational decision-making process called the Pharmacotherapy Workup to make an assessment of the patient's drug-related needs, identify drug therapy problems, develop a care plan, and conduct follow-up evaluations to ensure that all drug therapies are effective and safe. Together, these steps are the patient care process.

All patients have drug-related needs, and it is the pharmaceutical care practitioner's responsibility to determine whether or not a patient's drug-related needs are being met. These drug-related needs are described in Table 1-1.

If all of these criteria are met, then the patient's drug-related needs are also being met at this time, and no drug therapy problems exist. In this case, it is the pharmaceutical care practitioner's responsibility to do what is necessary in the care plan to ensure that the goals of therapy for each medical condition continue to be achieved.

When the practitioner's assessment reveals that the above criteria are not met, a drug therapy problem exists. It is then the pharmaceutical care practitioner's responsibility to resolve drug therapy problems with and for the patient.

It is also this practitioner's responsibility to assure that the goals of therapy are achieved by developing a care plan for each medical condition and by conducting follow-up evaluations at appropriate times. The pharmaceutical care practitioner also works to *prevent* drug therapy problems whenever possible.

Pharmaceutical care is a professional practice that has evolved from many years of research and development in the profession of pharmacy.[1-7]

Table 1-1 The patient's drug-related needs

During a pharmaceutical care encounter, the patient, his/her medical conditions, and all of the drug therapies are assessed to determine if the following drug-related needs are being met:

The medication is appropriate
  There is a clinical indication for each medication being taken.
  All of the patient's medical conditions that can benefit from drug therapy have been
    identified.
The medication is effective
  The most effective drug product is being used.
  The dosage of the medication is sufficient to achieve the goals of therapy.
The medication is safe
  There are no adverse drug reactions being experienced.
  There are no signs of toxicity.
The patient is compliant
  The patient is willing and able to take the medications as intended.

The practice was defined after a rational decision-making process was developed for drug therapy selection, dosing, and follow-up evaluation. Pharmaceutical care is designed to complement existing patient care practices to make drug therapy more effective and safe. This practitioner is not intended to replace the physician, the dispensing pharmacist, or any other health care practitioner. Rather, the pharmaceutical care practitioner is a new patient care provider within the health care system.

The responsibilities associated with drug therapy have become so numerous and complex that the need for a practitioner with this focus has become urgent.

The need for this practitioner results from

- multiple practitioners writing prescriptions for a single patient, often without coordination and communication;
- the large number of medications and overwhelming amount of drug information presently available to patients;
- patients playing a more active role in the selection and use of medications;
- an increase in the complexity of drug therapy;
- an increase in self-care through alternative and complementary medicine;
- a high level of drug-related morbidity and mortality which results in significant human and financial costs.

Pharmaceutical care must be understood by all patient care providers making decisions about drug therapy including physicians, nurses, and all other prescribers. However, it is expected that the practitioner who will practice pharmaceutical care as a primary role and full-time career is the pharmacist. The pharmacist is equipped with a minimum of 6 years of academic preparation that focuses on pharmacology, pharmacotherapy, and pharmaceutical care practice. New curricula in colleges of pharmacy must be developed to prepare practitioners capable of providing pharmaceutical care to patients. The goal of this text is to provide a guide for those who want to understand pharmaceutical care practice and gain the knowledge and skills necessary to deliver this level of care to patients.

PHARMACEUTICAL CARE AS A GENERALIST PRACTICE

Definition   A generalist practitioner is one who provides continuing, comprehensive, and coordinated care to a population undifferentiated by gender, disease, drug treatment category, or organ system (adapted from American Boards of Family Practice and Internal Medicine).[8]

The pharmaceutical care practitioner assesses all of a patient's medications, medical conditions, and outcome parameters, not just those chosen by disease state, drug action, or quantity of medications consumed. The generalist identifies, resolves, and prevents drug therapy problems up to a level of complexity that represents a standard of care for practice.

The generalist practice described here is applicable in all patient care practice settings including ambulatory, long-term care, hospital, and clinic settings. The practice of pharmaceutical care does not change depending upon setting because the practice can accommodate all types of patients and medical conditions, as well as all types of drug therapies.

Patient care specialists in health care disciplines are defined relative to the generalist. Therefore, only when pharmaceutical care is practiced widely, and practitioners become familiar with the practice process, can specialists develop practice areas. The generalist and the specialist must use the same patient care process, have a common vocabulary, and refer patients back and forth between themselves for the practice to work efficiently and cost effectively.

In pharmaceutical care, the complexity of the drug therapy problem will dictate whether the patient's pharmacotherapy is best managed by a generalist or a specialist.

Pharmaceutical care has been expressly defined to allow the pharmaceutical care practitioner to work alongside physicians, nurses, and other patient care providers to optimize care. This collaborative effort requires a common vocabulary.

THE LANGUAGE OF PRACTICE

The ability to use precise language appropriately in practice will directly reflect upon your level of competency and confidence.

Pharmaceutical care practitioners use the same practice vocabulary as the other health sciences (medicine, nursing, and dentistry) because common meanings facilitate communication between practitioners. Terms such as *assessment, care plan*, and *follow-up evaluation* are used by all health care practitioners in the same way. It is important to be specific, concise, and consistent in the use of terminology—a patient's life may depend on it.

However, because pharmaceutical care is a unique practice wherein the practitioner focuses his/her attention on the patient's drug-related needs, it is necessary to introduce terminology not currently used in medicine and nursing. This includes *drug therapy problem, medication experience*, and *drug-related needs* to name just a few. Specific meanings have been given to these terms to ensure that they conform to the language of patient care in a way that other practitioners will understand. In other words, pharmaceutical care practice does not introduce a new language into health care; it expands the vocabulary that currently exists.

Throughout this text we use the terms *practitioner* and *clinician* synonymously. Similarly, the terms *drug therapy* and *pharmacotherapy* are used interchangeably, and both terms include the drug, product, dose, dosing interval, and duration of treatment.

We have constructed a glossary which can be found at the end of this book to facilitate the use of a common vocabulary including those terms most directly related to pharmaceutical care practice. It will be helpful to take the time to learn the meaning of these terms when you encounter them.

THE PRACTITIONER AND THE PATIENT FORM A PRACTICE

Pharmaceutical care practice, like all other patient care practices, includes a qualified practitioner, a patient in need, and the work that occurs between them. All of the work focuses on the patient. Although you will collaborate with the patient's other providers and care-givers to ensure that he/she receives coordinated care in an efficient manner, your responsibility is to the patient.

Your primary and unique responsibility on the health care team is to manage all of the patient's pharmacotherapy. In the context of practice, a drug is defined as any substance or product used by or administered to a patient for preventive or therapeutic purposes.[9] Therefore, your responsibility includes all of the patient's prescription medications, over-the-counter products, herbal remedies, nutritional supplements, traditional medicines, and any other products the patient may take for therapeutic purposes. Your responsibility includes products being used to treat medical conditions, to prevent illnesses, and to improve the quality of the patient's life.

Because no other health care practitioner focuses attention on all of a patient's medications, your role is both unique and important. A number of patient care providers manage a portion of drug therapy for a finite amount of time, and you must work with all of them to create a coordinated plan for the patient's medications in order to achieve the desired goals of therapy in all cases.

Care occurs one-on-one with a patient in the context of what is called the *therapeutic relationship*. The relationship you develop with the patient determines the quality and the quantity of care that can be delivered. This relationship can be quite personal as private information is exchanged in order to provide the care patients need. The level of trust is extraordinary because clinicians will help the patient to make decisions that can have life-threatening or life-saving consequences. In order to help the patient as much as possible you will need a structured thought process that helps you to be thorough and consistent in the care you provide. This rational thought process is called the Pharmacotherapy Workup.[2]

THE PHARMACOTHERAPY WORKUP

All patient care practitioners, be they physicians, nurses, dentists, or pharmaceutical care practitioners, need a structured, rational thought process for making clinical decisions. What makes a practitioner qualified to do his or her work is the application of a unique knowledge base and set of clinical skills using a systematic thought process to assess the needs of a patient, identify and resolve problems, and prevent problems from occurring. In the case of the pharmaceutical care practitioner, this unique knowledge base is focused on pharmacology, pharmacotherapy, and pharmaceutical care practice, and the practitioner identifies, resolves, and prevents drug therapy problems. The systematic thought process is the Pharmacotherapy Workup. The Pharmacotherapy Workup is described in detail in Chapter 6 and is illustrated in Figures 6-3 to 6-7. Because it is central to your activities as a pharmaceutical care practitioner, a significant portion of this text is devoted to learning the Pharmacotherapy Workup.

The Pharmacotherapy Workup is a logical thought process that guides work and decisions as the clinician assesses the patient's drug-related needs and identifies drug therapy problems. The Pharmacotherapy Workup also organizes the interventions that need to be made on the patient's behalf. Lastly, the Pharmacotherapy Workup establishes appropriate parameters to evaluate at follow-up and allows the practitioner to contribute uniquely to the patient's care.

The Pharmacotherapy Workup helps to fulfill the practitioner's primary responsibility to determine if a patient's drug therapy is appropriately indicated, effective, and safe and to determine if the patient is being compliant. This is accomplished through the rational thought process of problem solving, which consists of an ordered series of decisions that allow the practitioner to determine whether drug therapy problems exist in any category: indication, effectiveness, safety, or compliance.

Practitioners use a scientifically-based, patient-focused set of knowledge and skills to identify drug therapy problems, determine the best solution, and evaluate the patient to determine if all of their drug therapies are producing optimal results.

This systematic thought process allows practitioners to use knowledge already learned and apply it to a new patient. It is the process that allows the practitioner to apply the knowledge learned from textbooks and research results to a specific patient in practice. The Pharmacotherapy Workup involves asking a standard series of questions, constantly generating a set of hypotheses, continuously searching for cues that reject or accept these hypotheses, and eliciting more information, while integrating all of this with existing knowledge to decide on the best pharmacotherapy for the patient.

The Pharmacotherapy Workup is the framework both for learning the practice and for doing the practice. The process makes it possible to learn and recall vast amounts of patient-specific information, pharmacological data, and optimal therapeutic approaches as needed. It helps accomplish this because it is simple and straightforward yet comprehensive and logical.

> **Note** Practitioners meet thousands of patients during a career. They will all have different needs. The Pharmacotherapy Workup can be applied to help all types of patients, with all types of diseases, with any type of drug therapy. Hospitalized patients can benefit from pharmaceutical care as can ambulatory patients.

Although all of this can *sound* overwhelming, the Pharmacotherapy Workup is what keeps your responsibilities from *becoming* overwhelming. The Pharmacotherapy Workup is orderly in that there is a systematic way of performing your responsibilities. Perhaps most helpful of all, you will always be working toward the same goal—to optimize the patient's medication experience.

The questions, hypotheses, and cues of the Pharmacotherapy Workup are always generated as a response to two basic questions

- Is the patient's problem caused by drug therapy?
- Can the patient's problem be treated with drug therapy?

No other practitioner approaches the patient with these two primary questions in mind, making your contribution unique. A surgeon has the clinical approach that surgery can either cure or is the cause of each problem he/she sees. The pharmaceutical care practitioner's clinical approach is that drug therapy is the cause of or cure for the problem. Using this approach will allow you to find problems that other practitioners are not looking for, and it allows you to solve problems in ways that other practitioners would not consider. This approach to the patient addresses a void in the health care system that has allowed drug-related morbidity and mortality to expand exponentially in the past 10 years.[10-12] Pharmaceutical care will fill this void.

The Pharmacotherapy Workup is the cognitive work occurring in the mind of the practitioner while caring for the patient. In contrast, the patient care process, is what the patient experiences when he/she receives pharmaceutical care. This process is a series of interactions between patient and pharmaceutical care practitioner. The patient care process is where the practitioner's unique knowledge and clinical skills are applied to solve health care problems for patients.

THE PATIENT CARE PROCESS

The three major steps in the patient care process are the *assessment* of the patient, his/her medical problems, and drug therapies leading to drug therapy problem identification, *care plan* development, and follow-up *evaluation*. These steps are all highly dependent upon each other. The completion of all steps is necessary to have a positive impact on your patient's medication experience. The process is continuous and occurs over multiple patient visits. Your initial assessment, drug therapy problem identification, and care planning occur at your first encounter with each patient, and follow-up evaluations and additional adjustments to drug therapy occur at subsequent patient encounters.

> **Note** Learning the entire patient care process takes time and energy. You will focus on various portions of each step to learn them well, but keep in mind that all steps must be completed to provide pharmaceutical care to patients.

Each step of the process depends on the previous step having been completed well. The quality of your assessment, for example, depends on the quality of the relationship you have established. Similarly, the success of the care plan that you create with your patient will be a direct result of how well you have performed the assessment. Finally, the outcomes your patient achieves are the direct result of the decisions you made when you developed the care plan.

The best way to think about pharmaceutical care practice is in terms of the work that occurs between the patient and the practitioner. This work is described as the patient care process. The three steps of the patient care process, the activities and responsibilities of each step, are summarized in Table 1-2 and will be described in detail in Chapters 6–9.

Because the identification, statement of cause, prioritization, resolution, and prevention of drug therapy problems represent the unique contribution of the pharmaceutical care practitioner, a separate chapter has been devoted to this portion of the assessment (refer to Chapter 7).

Remember that the patient care process describes the interaction between the patient and the practitioner. It is that portion of practice that is actually *seen* and *experienced* by both patients and practitioners. All practitioners use the same patient care process and structured decision-making process regardless of the patient's characteristics or the practitioner's expertise. However, the Pharmacotherapy Workup describes the rational thought processes, decision-making and problem solving that the practitioner is engaged in throughout the patient care process, and this should be a major focus as you study. The Pharmacotherapy Workup describes all the work that you do mentally while the patient care process describes the work that you do physically.

Table 1-2 integrates both the cognitive and physical work of the pharmaceutical care practitioner.

Each of these steps will be briefly presented here to describe the entire patient care process.

Assessment

The purpose of the assessment is threefold: (1) to understand the patient well enough to make rational drug therapy decisions with and for him/her; (2) to determine if the patient's drug therapy is appropriate, effective, and safe, and to determine if the patient is compliant with his/her medications; (3) to identify drug therapy problems.

The information required to make clinical decisions with your patient includes *patient data* (demographic information, medication experience), *disease data* (current medical conditions, medical history, nutritional status, review of systems), and *drug data* (current medications, past medication use, social drug use, immunizations, allergies, and alerts).

The two major activities that occur during the assessment are:

- Eliciting information from the patient, and
- Making clinical decisions about the patient's medications and meeting his/her drug-related needs or drug therapy problems.

The assessment begins by getting to know your patient and starting to establish a therapeutic relationship with him/her. This is done by discussing the patient's *medication experience.*

Table 1-2 Activities and responsibilities in the patient care process

	Activities	Responsibilities
Assessment	Meet the patient	Establish the therapeutic relationship
	Elicit relevant information from the patient	Determine who your patient is as an individual by learning about the reason for the encounter, the patient's demographics, medication experience, and other clinical information
	Make rational drug therapy decisions using the Pharmacotherapy Workup	Determine whether the patient's drug-related needs are being met (indication, effectiveness, safety, compliance), identify drug therapy problems
Care plan	Establish goals of therapy	Negotiate and agree upon endpoints and timeframe for pharmacotherapies with the patient
	Select appropriate interventions for: resolution of drug therapy problems achievement of goals of therapy prevention of drug therapy problems.	Consider therapeutic alternatives Select patient-specific pharmacotherapy Consider nondrug interventions Educate patient
	Schedule a follow-up evaluation	Establish a schedule that is clinically appropriate and convenient for the patient
Follow-up evaluation	Elicit clinical and/or lab evidence of actual patient outcomes and compare them to the goals of therapy to determine the effectiveness of drug therapy	Evaluate effectiveness of pharmacotherapy
	Elicit clinical and/or lab evidence of adverse effects to determine safety of drug therapy	Evaluate safety of pharmacotherapy Determine patient compliance
	Document clinical status and any changes in pharmacotherapy that are required	Make a judgment as to the clinical status of the patient's condition being managed with drug therapy
	Assess patient for any new drug therapy problems	Identify any new drug therapy problems and their cause
	Schedule the next follow-up evaluation	Provide continuous care

The medication experience is a new and important concept in health care (refer to Chapter 5). Patients relate to the impact that taking medications has on their every day lives as their medication experience.

The medication experience is the patient's personal approach to taking medication. It is the sum of all the events in a patient's life that involve medication use. The medication experience is first and foremost the patient's beliefs, perceptions, understandings, attitudes, and behaviors about drug therapy. It is these factors that will most directly influence the patient's decisions about whether to take a medication or not, how much of the medication to take, and how to take the medication. Patients come with their own medication experience. Our responsibility is to positively influence it. Therefore, the more you know about the patient's medication experience, the more likely you are to have a lasting and positive influence on it.

The medication experience includes more technical aspects as well; the patient's current medications, social drug use, immunizations, allergies, alerts, and medication history. It is usually easier to deal with this aspect of the medication experience; however, your ability to influence these technical dimensions depends upon how well you understand the patient's personal approach to taking medication. Take the time and learn the skills to effectively elicit the patient's description of his/her medication experience—it will always be worth your effort. The quality of the care you can provide depends upon it.

The pharmaceutical care practitioner has a responsibility to understand the patient's medication experience because it directly impacts the decisions a patient makes about his/her drug therapy. Although physicians, nurses, and pharmaceutical care practitioners can make suggestions to a patient, it is the patient who ultimately decides what he/she will do about taking the medication.

The major decisions that the pharmaceutical care practitioner makes are that the patient's drug-related needs are being met at this time or that the patient is experiencing drug therapy problems. Therefore, an understanding of drug therapy problems is important.

Identifying Drug Therapy Problems

Definition   Drug therapy problems are undesirable events or risks experienced by the patient that involve or are suspected to involve drug therapy and that inhibit or delay him/her from achieving the desired goals of therapy. These problems are identified during the assessment process, so that they can be resolved through individualized changes in the patient's drug therapy regimens.

Drug therapy problems are identified by analyzing sociological, patho-physiological, and pharmacological knowledge of the patient, disease, and drug therapy information collected during the assessment step. The synthesis and application of this knowledge occurs in a logical, systematic manner using the Pharmacotherapy Workup.

The process used to identify whether or not the patient is experiencing a drug therapy problem requires a continuous assessment of four logical questions

- Does the patient have an indication for each of his/her drug therapies, and is each of the patient's indications being treated with drug therapy?
- Are these drug therapies effective for his/her medical condition?
- Are the drug therapies as safe as possible?
- Is the patient able and willing to comply with the drug therapies as instructed?

When clinicians apply knowledge of patient, diseases, and drugs to this set of inquires, they can make clinical decisions as to whether or not a drug therapy problem exists. If the patient is experiencing a drug therapy problem, it can be classified into one of the seven categories described in Table 1-3.

Table 1-3 Categories of drug therapy problems

Drug Therapy Problem	Description of the Drug Therapy Problem
Unnecessary drug therapy	The drug therapy is unnecessary because the patient does not have a clinical indication at this time.
Needs additional drug therapy	Additional drug therapy is required to treat or prevent a medical condition.
Ineffective drug	The drug product is not effective at producing the desired response.
Dosage too low	The dosage is too low to produce the desired response.
Adverse drug reaction	The drug is causing an adverse reaction.
Dosage too high	The dosage is too high resulting in undesirable effects.
Noncompliance	The patient is not able or willing to take the drug regimen appropriately.

Once categorized, it is then necessary to identify the cause for each drug therapy problem. Knowing the cause of the problem leads to the best solution for the patient. These three components are necessary to be able to adequately describe the patient's drug therapy problem. This process includes identifying the medical condition involved in the problem, the drug therapy associated with the problem, and the cause of the problem.

When multiple drug therapy problems are present, they need to be prioritized to determine which should be addressed first. The order of priority of drug therapy problems is based on the patient's views regarding which one is causing the most concern, and the preferences he/she has toward addressing the problem(s).

The result of the assessment of a patient's drug-related needs is the description and prioritization of the drug therapy problem(s) to be resolved through specific interventions in the care plan. The identification and resolution of drug therapy problems represents the unique contribution made to the patient's care by the pharmaceutical care practitioner.

Care Plan Development

The purpose of the care plan is to organize all of the work agreed upon by the practitioner and the patient to achieve the goals of therapy. This requires interventions to resolve drug therapy problems, to meet these goals, and to prevent new drug therapy problems from developing, thereby optimizing the patient's medication experience.

Care plans are developed primarily to help the patient achieve the established goals of therapy for each of his/her medical conditions or illnesses. Constructing care plans is done in collaboration with the patient and, when appropriate, other health care practitioners providing care to the patient.

Care plans are organized by medical condition, and a separate care plan is constructed for each condition or illness. Constructing a care plan involves three steps: establishing goals of therapy, selecting appropriate individualized interventions, and scheduling the next follow-up evaluation.

The first and most important step in the care planning process is to establish goals of therapy for each medical condition. Goals of therapy consist of a parameter, a value, and a timeframe. Throughout the text, goals of therapy are used to describe the future desired endpoints. The term *outcomes* is used to describe the actual results from drug therapies. The goals of therapy guide all subsequent decisions, actions, interventions, and patient education. Therefore, goals of therapy must be explicitly stated, consistent with the patient's preferences and desires, clinically sound, and observable or measurable in a stated timeframe. Perhaps most importantly, the goals of therapy must be understood and agreed upon by practitioner and patient. It should be noted that the term "outcomes" is used in pharmaceutical care to describe the actual results and should not be confused with goals of therapy.

Each care plan contains a plan of action to be taken on behalf of the patient. The specific actions are called *interventions*.

Care plans contain interventions designed to:

- resolve drug therapy problems;
- achieve the stated goals of therapy;
- prevent new drug therapy problems from developing.

The first interventions in a care plan should be those intended to resolve identified drug therapy problems. Resolving drug therapy problems takes precedence within the care planning process because goals of therapy cannot be achieved until and unless the patient's drug therapy problems are successfully resolved.

A second type of intervention in care plan development ensures that the patient achieves the goals of therapy. Interventions to achieve goals of therapy most often include changes in drug therapy regimens and individualized patient instructions. These interventions include relevant patient education or instructions as to the optimal use of medications, related technology, and/or diet and exercise to increase the probability of success with the medication regimen.

Interventions made to prevent the development of drug therapy problems are necessary to complete a care plan. These interventions are especially important for patients who have a higher than normal probability of developing a drug therapy problem due to some identified risk factor(s).

The final step in every care plan is to schedule the follow-up evaluation to determine the outcomes of drug therapy. During the follow-up evaluation, the results of care plan actions are judged as to their positive or negative impact on the patient. Therefore, the decision regarding when to schedule the next follow-up evaluation needs to incorporate the timing of the expected positive outcomes, achievement of the goals of therapy, and the probable timing of any negative outcomes including side effects and/or adverse reactions from the medication. If there are multiple care plans, the schedules for the follow-up evaluations must be coordinated.

The patient and the practitioner always negotiate the components of the care plan including goals of therapy, interventions, and the schedule for the next evaluation.

Follow-up Evaluation

The purpose of the follow-up evaluation is to determine the actual outcomes of drug therapy for the patient, compare these results with the intended goals of therapy, determine the effectiveness and safety of pharmacotherapy, evaluate patient compliance, and establish the current status of the patient.

The evaluation step is where clinical experience and new knowledge are gained. In fact, most learning occurs during follow-up evaluations. The follow-up evaluation is the step in the process when the practitioner sees which medications and doses were most effective or caused the most harm. In a well-conducted follow-up evaluation, the practitioner evaluates the patient's response to drug therapies in terms of effectiveness, safety, and compliance and also determines if any new problems have developed.

The specific activities performed at a follow-up evaluation are described as follows:

- Observe or measure the positive results the patient has experienced from drug therapies (effectiveness).
- Observe or measure any undesirable effects the patient has experienced that were caused by a drug therapy (safety).
- Determine the actual dosage of medication the patient is taking that is producing the results observed (compliance).
- Make a clinical judgement of the status of the patient's medical condition or illness being managed with drug therapy (outcomes).
- Reassess the patient to determine if he/she developed any new drug therapy problems.

The practitioner must gather data to evaluate the effectiveness of the drug therapies. These data often include the improvement or reduction of the signs or symptoms of the patient's medical condition or illness. Effectiveness is also evaluated using data to demonstrate the extent to which abnormal laboratory test results have returned to within the desired or normal range. The practitioner must also gather data to evaluate the *safety* of the drug therapies instituted in the care plan. Safety data include the evaluation of unintended pharmacological effects (side effects) of the patient's drug therapy. Evaluation of safety data also includes whether laboratory tests have become dangerously abnormal due to the drug therapy. Because both effectiveness and safety are evaluated based upon the drug dosages that the patient has actually taken, it is important to determine patient compliance at each follow-up evaluation.

The practitioner makes a clinical judgment about the outcomes of drug therapy at the follow-up evaluation. A clinical judgment is made as to the outcome status of each medical condition being treated with drug therapies. At each evaluation the status might be resolved, stable, improved, partially improved, unimproved, worsened, or failed. Each term has a specific meaning in practice and contains two items of important information: the patient's present condition and what was done to the drug therapy in response to the patient's condition. This clinical judgment is recorded and compared to the status at each subsequent evaluation to determine if the individualized drug therapies are helping the patient meet the desired goals of therapy.

At each follow-up evaluation, the practitioner must also determine if the patient has developed any new drug therapy problems or illnesses since the last encounter. If so, a care plan is developed to address them.

Documentation in Practice

Documentation of the care provided is required for all practitioners. As pharmacotherapy and medical services become more complex, creating an effective record of all decisions made concerning the patient's drug therapies and the outcomes of those decisions is essential. Comprehensive documentation is required and includes the patient's clinical information, drug therapy problems, a comprehensive medication record, goals of therapy, and evidence of effectiveness and safety of pharmacotherapies at every follow-up visit. The specific requirements of documentation in practice are described in Chapters 6–9. Documentation is also required to facilitate collaboration between members of the health care team.

THE PHARMACEUTICAL CARE PRACTITIONER AS A MEMBER OF THE HEALTH CARE TEAM

Much has been said and written about working as a member of the health care team. However, to participate in caring for patients as a team, a practitioner must reflect on his/her role, responsibilities, and relationship to each member of the team. To be successful, each team member must contribute something unique, and he/she must be able to articulate this contribution clearly to other team members and demonstrate that he/she can execute it effectively.

Pharmaceutical care practice was designed for a practitioner who participates in a clearly defined and equal manner on the patient care team. The practice was developed so that the pharmaceutical care practitioner could share a common vocabulary, patient care process, and orientation to the patient with the members of the health care team. Specifically, the practice was designed to facilitate the set of competencies that have been identified and articulated in a report prepared by the Academic Health Center Task Force on Interdisciplinary Health Team Development at the University of Minnesota in 1996. These competencies must be mastered before constructive participation on a health care team can be achieved. These competencies are so clearly stated and well developed that they warrant inclusion here.

1. Patient-centered focus   A good team's first priority must be to meet the patient's needs. A team with a patient-centered focus will consider and respect the patient's values and preferences when making care decisions.

2. Establishment of a common goal   If the patient's needs are the focus, it is critical that all team members know what a successful outcome or goal of therapy will be.[13] At times, the goals of therapy are straightforward (i.e., resolving an infection). However, in some instances, a successful outcome may not be self-evident. For example, health care professionals may work at cross purposes if some feel the patient should be treated aggressively while others feel that the patient should only receive palliative care. Such confusion may be avoided only through an explicit process for goal definition. If choices are to be made between competing outcomes, the patient (or the patient's family) must, of course, be involved.

3. Understanding of the other members' roles   Each team member must be familiar with the professional capabilities of the other members and must be willing to acknowledge greater expertise and, in some instances, defer to other team members.

4. Confidence in other team members   Confidence in other team members develops with time and most certainly requires an understanding of the other members' roles. Each member must be able to trust the work of others. If professionals do not have trust in each other's work, duplication of services may occur. For example, a specialist practitioner who is not confident in the care provided by the primary care practitioner may order extra or unnecessary tests for the patient.

5. Flexibility in roles   While understanding and respect for each person's specific role is important, flexibility in assignments is also important. It is undesirable for each team member to duplicate efforts made by others, but, if meeting the agreed upon objective calls for changes or flexibility in roles, team members must be prepared to act accordingly and with respect to professional standards of practice.

6. Joint understanding of group norms   Members of successful teams will be aware of the expectations of others in the group. These expectations are often behavioral such as punctuality or willingness to stay current in one's field.

7. Mechanism for conflict resolution   Every health care team will experience instances of conflict. However, a successful health care team will identify a specific mechanism, clearly understood by all, for resolving conflict, through a team leader, outside leader, or other process.

8. Development of effective communications   Good health care team communication involves at least two components: a shared efficient and effective record keeping mechanism, electronic or other, and a common vocabulary. While wholesale reform of medical record keeping is beyond the reach of individual practitioners, development of common language among professionals is not, nor is instilling in students the need for shared, clear patient records.

9. Shared responsibility for team actions   Effective team functioning can occur only if each team member fully shares the responsibility for those actions. Undertaking of such responsibility requires confidence in the abilities of the other team members, good communication, and agreement upon a common goal. Thus, these team *competencies* must reinforce each other.

10. Evaluation and feedback   Team design must be dynamic and open for evaluation and revision on a continuing basis. A model that worked previously may no longer be optimal as there can be change in the patient's needs, the health care delivery system, or the expertise of team members. A specific mechanism must be developed for ongoing evaluation of a team's effectiveness and redesign where needed.

Ultimately, the test of a valuable patient care provider is his/her ability to improve the patient's health. This can only occur with the coordinated efforts of a health care team. The pharmaceutical care practitioner's expertise is an important and unique contribution to this team's efforts.

SUMMARY AND OVERVIEW OF THE BOOK

Perhaps the greatest justification for the practice of pharmaceutical care came from Nies and Spielberg in *Goodman & Gilman's: The Pharmacological Basis of Therapeutics*[14] when they explained that:

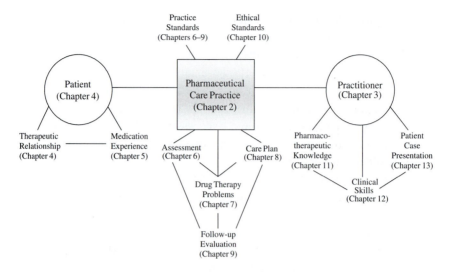

Figure 1-1 Overview of book content.

Over the past three decades, the principles of human experimentation have been defined, and the techniques for evaluation of therapeutic interventions have progressed to the point that it should now be considered absolutely unethical to apply the art, as opposed to the science, of therapeutics to any patient who directly (the adult or child) or indirectly (the fetus) receives drugs for therapeutic purposes. Therapeutics must now be dominated by objective evaluation of an adequate base of factual knowledge.[14]

The purpose of this book is to prepare those who want to become pharmaceutical care practitioners. Figure 1-1 illustrates the content of the book.

We will take each step of the process in a logical order. First, you will need to understand your responsibilities as a pharmaceutical care practitioner. Then you must understand the patient's role in care and the necessity of optimizing his/her medication experience.

Next you will learn to think as a pharmaceutical care practitioner in order to assess a patient's drug-related needs. This thought process is the Pharmacotherapy Workup and is the key to your success. The Pharmacotherapy Workup, which integrates knowledge about patient, diseases, and drug therapy with your clinical skills, is applied in practice using the patient care process.

Finally, in this book we will describe a number of clinical skills to advance your clinical experience. Eliciting information from patients and the literature, integrating patient-specific information with accumulated knowledge, documenting care, presenting patient cases, and being reflective in practice are all necessary to expand your knowledge and skill levels as quickly as possible.

Requirements for the pharmaceutical care practitioner

- Understand your responsibilities.
- Develop a therapeutic relationship with each patient.
- Apply the Pharmacotherapy Workup to make rational drug therapy decisions.
- Learn the patient care process.
- Acquire an appropriate pharmacotherapeutic knowledge base.
- Develop clinical skills.
- Understand practice standards and ethical considerations.
- Document all care provided.

Pharmaceutical care practice has an important role to play in the alleviation of pain and suffering. Practicing pharmaceutical care requires responsiveness and sensitivity to the needs of others and a fundamental commitment to an ethic of care. As we will demonstrate, the practice of pharmaceutical care can make a difference in the lives of individuals experiencing drug therapy problems. The problems are enormous, the challenges great, the opportunities exciting. The practice of pharmaceutical care has been developed to meet a unique and growing health care need. Along with medical care, nursing care, dental care, surgical care, and others, pharmaceutical care can improve patient health and even save lives (Fig. 1-2). Imagine it—and create a vision of the possibilities.

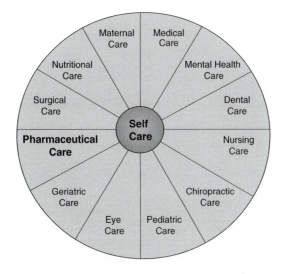

Figure 1-2   Meeting the health care needs of a patient.

Before we begin the process of preparing the pharmaceutical care practitioner, Chapter 2 describes the impact that practitioners can have on the drug-related needs of patients. This chapter is meant to present a picture of practice to provide a meaningful context for the remaining material in the book.

EXERCISES

1-1 Select an acquaintance (friend or family) with whom you are comfortable carrying on a discussion. Be sure he/she is taking at least one prescription medication, nonprescription product, alternative therapy, or nutritional supplement. Set aside approximately 20 minutes to talk with him/her about the medication. You might begin by asking the individual to describe why the medication is being taken, how well it is working, and what changes would he/she make to improve the experience. Ask the individual anything else you might like to know and are comfortable asking related to medication use. Try to understand the individual's perspective on taking medications.

After you are finished, reflect on what you learned from the individual. Think about what surprised you, what was different from, and what was similar to what you expected.

1-2 Select a colleague and discuss the similarities and differences between the responsibilities of the pharmaceutical care practitioner, the physician, and the nurse.

1-3 What is meant when a medication is said to be
(a) indicated
(b) effective
(c) safe

1-4 What are some common reasons why a patient would be
(a) unable to comply with the instructions as to when and how to take a medication;
(b) unwilling to comply with the instructions given.

REFERENCES

1. Cipolle, R., Strand, L.M., Morley, P.C. *Pharmaceutical Care Practice*. New York: McGraw Hill; 1998.
2. Strand, L.M., Cipolle, R.J., Morley, P.C. Documenting the clinical pharmacist's activities: back to basics. *Drug Intell Clin Pharm* 1988; 22:63–67.

3. Hepler, C.D., Strand, L.M., Opportunities and responsibilities in pharmaceutical care. *Am J Hosp Pharm* 1990; 47:533–43.
4. Strand, L.M., Cipolle, R.J., Morley, P.C. *Pharmaceutical Care: An Introduction, in Current Concepts.* Kalamazoo, MI: The Upjohn Company;1992.
5. Strand, L.M., Cipolle, R.J., Morley, P.C., Perrier, D.G. Levels of pharmaceutical care: a needs-based approach. *Am J Hosp Pharm* 1991; 48:547–550.
6. Strand, L.M., Cipolle, R.J., Morley, P.C., Ramsey, R., Lamsam, G.D. Drug-related problems: their structure and function. *DICP Ann Pharmother* 1990; 24:1093–1097.
7. Cipolle, R.J., Strand, L.M., Morley, P.C., Frakes, M.J. Resultados del Ejercicio de la Atencion Farmaceutica. *Pharm Care Espana* 2000; 2(2):94–106.
8. Glassman, P.A., Garcia, D., Delafiel, J.P., *Outpatient Care Handbook*, 2nd ed. Philadelphia: Hanley & Belfus, Inc.; 1999.
9. *Dorland's Illustrated Medical Dictionary*, 30th ed. Philadelphia, PA: WB Saunders; 2003, p. 565.
10. Johnson, J., Bootman, J.L. Drug-related morbidity and mortality. *Arch Intern Med* 1995; 155(18):1949–1956.
11. Johnson, J.A., Bootman, J.L. Drug-related morbidity and mortality. *Am J Health Syst Pharm* 1997; 54(5):554–558.
12. Ernst, F.R., Grizzle, A.J. Drug-related morbidity and mortality: updating the cost-of-illness model. *J Am Pharm Assoc* 2001; 41(2):192–199.
13. Pronovost, P., Berenholtz, S., Dorman, T., Lipsett, P.A., Simmonds, T., Haraden, C. Improving communication in the ICU using daily goals. *J Crit Care* 2003; 18(2):71–75.
14. Nies, A.S., Speilberg, S.P. Principles of Therapeutics, *Goodman & Gilman's: The Pharmacological Basis of Therapeutics*, McGraw Hill; 1996, p. 43.

CHAPTER TWO

CLINICAL & ECONOMIC IMPACT OF PHARMACEUTICAL CARE PRACTICE

Key Concepts

[1] *A database of 20,761 patients who received pharmaceutical care during 59,361 patient encounters has been established over the past 10 years. A sample of 5136 patients was selected and evaluated from this population, and the outcomes are described here.*

2 *Younger patients, those less than 65 years old (n = 3064), had an average of three medical conditions with an average of five drug therapies. Older patients, those 65 years and older (n = 2072), had an average of five medical conditions being treated with seven medications.*

3 *Thirty-four percent of the younger patients experienced a drug therapy problem, while 54% of the older patients had one or more drug therapy problems identified by the clinician at the first pharmaceutical care visit.*

4 *The most common drug therapy problem, in both groups of patients, was the need for additional drug therapy, followed by dosages too low and then patient compliance problems. The distribution of the types of drug therapy problems experienced was similar for the two groups.*

5 *The decisions made by pharmaceutical care practitioners have been found to be clinically credible based on the evaluations and comments of peer-reviewed panels.*

6 *Pharmaceutical care practitioners resolve almost 80% of drug therapy problems directly with the patient.*

7 *Practitioners were able to produce positive patient outcomes in 90% of patients, regardless of the patient's age, medical conditions, or type of drug therapy problem.*

8 *Pharmaceutical care practice saves patients and the health care system a significant amount of money and produces a positive savings to cost ratio.*

INTRODUCTION

Chapter 1 presented an overview of pharmaceutical care practice. Chapter 2 describes practice-based results achieved with pharmaceutical care. This chapter presents a graphic *picture* of pharmaceutical care at work. In essence, the data presented here represent the systematic application of pharmaceutical care knowledge, both technical and clinical, to drug-related morbidity and mortality. Moreover, these data demonstrate the legitimacy and value of a serious therapeutic undertaking on the part of committed practitioners. This book is about becoming a pharmaceutical care practitioner. It shows you how this can become a reality. By any measure, a reading of this chapter will convince the reader that the journey will be worthwhile, and that pharmaceutical care can and does make a difference in the lives of patients who have drug-related needs that must be met.

Understanding a patient care practice includes knowing the impact the practice has on patients and the health care system as a whole. However, research reported in the literature has confused this issue somewhat. A number of studies claiming to report the impact of pharmaceutical care on patient outcomes either vaguely describe the care provided or describe activities that only partially resemble the practice described in this book. Practitioners should be aware of this when reading and interpreting the literature on this subject.

This chapter describes the impact pharmaceutical care practice can have on patients and the health care system. Since November 1994 when pharmaceutical care was defined as a practice, practitioners have cared for over 20,000 patients. These practitioners were trained by personnel in the Peters Institute of Pharmaceutical Care at the University of Minnesota. The patients were seen during 59,361 documented patient encounters with pharmaceutical care practitioners. All care was provided by pharmaceutical care practitioners whose practices were independent of the Peters Institute of Pharmaceutical Care. Patient identifiers were removed from the data before the patient data were consolidated, audited, and analyzed by personnel at the Peters Institute of Pharmaceutical Care. These patient cases were documented in the Assurance Pharmaceutical Care electronic documentation system. A description of this database follows.

ASSURANCE PHARMACEUTICAL CARE DOCUMENTATION SYSTEM

Soon after the development of the practice in 1994, it became obvious that an electronic documentation system was necessary. The structure for the database was established in collaboration with Michael J. Frakes, Pharm. D. at the Peters Institute of Pharmaceutical Care in the College of Pharmacy at the University of Minnesota, Minneapolis, Minnesota.

Assurance Pharmaceutical Care (copyright: 2001–2003. Regents of the University of Minnesota) is an electronic charting system specifically designed to help provide and document pharmaceutical care practice. It allows for the collection of patient demographics, patient-specific care planning, medication documentation, drug interaction checking, drug therapy problem identification, follow-up evaluations, physician and patient reporting, billing, workload tracking, clinical outcome tracking, and data consolidation among numerous practitioners. This system supports the provision of services on a continuous basis, over repeated patient encounters, at multiple practice sites, by multiple practitioners. The Assurance Pharmaceutical Care Documentation system presently supports practices in community pharmacies, clinics, universities, and managed care organizations. Inquiries about the program should be directed to pipc@umn.edu. The results presented below were all generated by the Assurance Pharmaceutical Care system.

THE PATIENT SAMPLE

The sample of patients selected for this evaluation is part of the database of 20,761 patients and 59,361 encounters. This is not the first sample to be evaluated from this database. In 1998, a sample was selected, evaluated, and described in *Pharmaceutical Care Practice.*[1] That sample represented 5480 patients cared for between November 1994 and October 1995. The sample reported here includes different patients.

The sample of patients selected for discussion in this chapter was cared for between January 1, 1996 and December 31, 2002. The patients were selected from the database if they received an initial assessment and at least one follow-up evaluation by a pharmaceutical care practitioner. For a patient to be included in this analysis, he/she must have had his or her drug-related needs assessed by a pharmaceutical care practitioner, who constructed care plans including goals of therapy, and who conducted at least one follow-up evaluation to determine the clinical and economic impact of pharmaceutical care. The sample consisted of 5136 patients who participated in over 26,238 documented encounters with 95 different pharmaceutical care practitioners providing the care. Patients presented themselves to these practitioners in their community pharmacy, ambulatory clinic, or were referred by a physician for pharmaceutical care services. All the practitioners earned a certificate in pharmaceutical care practice in addition to having a Bachelor of Science Degree in Pharmacy or the Doctor of Pharmacy Degree.

All patients in the sample received pharmaceutical care as described in this book. The practitioners evaluated all of each patient's drug therapy and completed an assessment, a care plan, and a follow-up evaluation(s). The documentation system established that the same standard of care was delivered to each patient.

The patients were seen in two different settings: clinic and community pharmacy. These pharmaceutical care practices were established separately from the dispensing business. The data from all practice settings and practitioners were combined and analyzed together because neither practice setting nor specific practitioner were shown to have an effect on the outcome measures.

The only variable shown to significantly differentiate groups of patients was the age of the patient. It became clear from the data analysis that two different groups of patients were cared for: patients less than 65 years old ($n = 3064$) and patients 65 years old or older ($n = 2072$) at their initial assessment. These groups differentiated themselves on most variables measured. Therefore, the data will be presented for each of the two age groups and will be referred to as the younger group and the older group. All the data reported, exempting outcomes and economic impact, were collected at the initial assessment performed by the pharmaceutical care provider. The data describing outcomes and economic impact were collected throughout the care of the patient and included all 26,238 encounters.

Demographic Information

Age The demographic information describing the two groups is summarized in Table 2-1.

The ages in the younger group varied from 7 days to 64 years old. The average age of the younger group was 48.3 years (SD = 15.2 years). The older group had an average age of 77.2 years (SD = 6.4 years). The ages in this group varied from 65 to 99 years old. Figure 2-1 provides a frequency distribution of the ages for the two groups.

The gender distribution in the two age groups was almost identical. Men represented approximately one-third and women represented approximately two-thirds of these patients. The undocumented portion of the sample results from the practitioner failing to record the patient's gender. This sample primarily represents employed adults, their family members, and retirees. There were 593 (11.6%) patients who had no health insurance coverage and were seen as private pay patients. The remaining 4543 (88.4%) patients had some form of third party health insurance.

Table 2-1 Descriptive demographic information

Variable	Patients < 65 yrs old	Patients ≥ 65 yrs old	Total
No. of patients	3064	2072	5136
Age (yrs)[a]	48.3 ± 15.2	77.2 ± 6.4	59.8 ± 18.3
Gender			
Male	1091 (35.6%)	699 (33.7%)	1790 (34.9%)
Female	1770 (57.8%)	1208 (58.3%)	2978 (58.0%)
Undocumented	203 (6.6%)	165 (8.0%)	368 (7.2%)

[a]Average ± S/D.

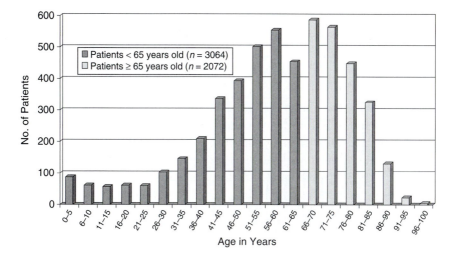

Figure 2-1 Frequency of patients by age.

Number of Medication Conditions

While the younger group had an average of three medical conditions (SD = 2), the mode for the group was one and the median was two. The number of medical conditions varied from 0 to 19. A major difference between the two groups is illustrated by the mean number of medical conditions in the older group of five (SD = 3) with a mode of four and a median of five medical conditions per patient (Table 2-2). The number of medical conditions in this group also varied from 0 to 19. These data are displayed in Fig. 2-2.

The vast majority (69.4%) of patients had multiple medical conditions that required treatment or prevention with drug therapies. Over 56% of patients had three or more medical conditions, and 36% of these patients

Table 2-2 Number of medical conditions experienced by patients

Variable	Patients < 65 yrs old (n = 3064)	Patients ≥ 65 yrs old (n = 2072)
Number of medical conditions	9461	10,471
Average ± SD	3 ± 2	5 ± 3
Mode	1	4
Median	2	5

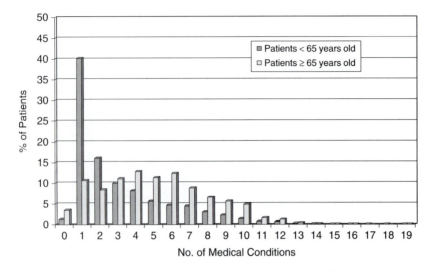

Figure 2-2 Frequency of patients by number of medical conditions.

had five or more active medical conditions requiring pharmacotherapy. The frequency of patients with multiple medical conditions, or comorbidities, requires that the pharmaceutical care practitioner conduct a comprehensive assessment of each patient and not simply focus on a single disease state.

The differences in the number of medical conditions in the younger and older groups carried over to the analysis of medication use. This difference was consistent when reviewing the number of associated medications taken for the medical conditions. The younger group was taking an average of five (SD = 4) medications at the time of the initial assessment. The mode was one medication per patient in this group and the median was three medications. The number of medications ranged from 0 to 28 in the younger group.

The older group of patients was taking an average of seven (SD = 4) medications, with a variation from 0 to 28. The mode and the median were six medications per patient at the initial assessment (Table 2-3). Especially interesting is the 4% of patients who received pharmaceutical care but were not taking any medications at the time of the initial assessment. It is highly likely that these patients needed to be treated for a new medical condition or illness or required preventive pharmacotherapy at the time of the encounter. Figure 2-3 displays the distribution for the two groups.

Again, these practice-based results clearly demonstrate that the majority of patients take numerous medications on a daily basis. This requires a systematic and comprehensive assessment of their drug-related needs. The typical adult patient seen by the pharmaceutical care practitioner has three to six medical conditions and is taking four to eight drug products each day.

Table 2-3 Number of drug therapies taken by patients

Variable	Patients < 65 yrs old (n = 3064)	Patients ≥ 65 yrs old (n = 2072)
Number of drug therapies per patient	14,489	14,355
Average ± SD	5 ± 4	7 ± 4
Mode	1	6
Median	3	6

A closer assessment of the type of medications taken by these patients is displayed in Table 2-4. Although the majority of medications is represented by prescription products (77 and 73%, respectively), a significant number of nonprescription items were being taken by the patients in this sample (18 and 22%, respectively). Because the number of medications consumed by these two groups of patients is relatively high (average of five and seven), the number of medications received from friends or family members and the number of physician samples should be noted.

These patients were taking 1067 drug products obtained directly from friends or family members. These products included prescription and nonprescription

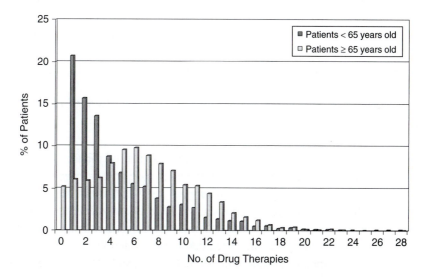

Figure 2-3 Frequency of patients by number of drug therapies.

Table 2-4   Sources of medications taken by patients

Sources of drug products	Patients < 65 yrs old (%)	Patients ≥ 65 yrs old (%)	Total (%)
Physician prescription	77.3	73.4	75.3
Nonprescription purchase	17.5	21.7	19.7
Friends or family members	3.8	3.6	3.7
Physician samples	0.7	0.9	0.8
Nonphysician prescription	0.2	0.4	0.3

medications and were being used by patients to treat conditions including arthritis, hyperlipidemia, diabetes, pain, constipation, hypertension, ischemic heart disease, and anemia. Of interest is the observation that compliance problems associated with medications obtained from friends or family members are quite rare (<6%). One interpretation of these findings is that when patients obtain drug products from individuls who they trust, compliance rates are very high. Friends or family members can and do have a strong influence on patient compliance behavior and their medication experience. These are medications that go unrecognized in most practice settings and most record systems. The nonphysician prescriptions in this table represent prescriptions written by nurse practitioners, dentists, and other health-related practitioners other than physicians.

These findings are consistent with other reports that describe an underreporting of dietary supplement and nonprescription product use by patients responding to written questionnaires compared to information gained through a structured interview process.[2] Additionally, individuals who report using herbal remedies also report taking more prescription products than those not using herbal products compared to nonusers.[3] A comprehensive assessment is required to assemble an accurate description of a patient's medication use.

Social drug use   Information about the social use of tobacco, alcohol, and caffeine is also collected in pharmaceutical care practice because each of these products has the potential to impact decisions about the patient's other drug therapies. As Table 2-5 indicates, significant differences did not identify themselves on these variables, but it is interesting to see where the levels of use vary. The undocumented category in this table represents situations in which the practitioner did not record the usage of these products. No data describing influence of drugs of abuse were summarized.

Table 2-5   Social drug use (tobacco, alcohol, caffeine)

Variable	Patients < 65 yrs old	Patients ≥ 65 yrs old	Total
Tobacco use			
None	1651 (53.9%)	884 (42.7%)	2535 (49.4%)
<1 pack per day	266 (8.7%)	65 (3.1%)	331 (6.4%)
>1 pack per day	115 (3.7%)	34 (1.6%)	149 (2.9%)
History of tobacco dependency	175 (5.7%)	299 (14.4%)	474 (9.2%)
Undocumented	857 (28.0%)	790 (38.1%)	1647 (32.1%)
Alcohol use			
No use	1222 (39.9%)	787 (38.0%)	2009 (39.1%)
<2 drinks/week	574 (18.7%)	329 (15.9%)	903 (17.6%)
2–6 drinks/week	204 (6.7%)	41 (2.0%)	245 (4.8%)
>6 drinks/week	89 (2.9%)	16 (1.0%)	105 (2.0%)
History of alcohol dependency	27 (0.9%)	28 (1.4%)	55 (1.1%)
Undocumented	948 (30.9%)	871 (42.0%)	1819 (35.4%)
Caffeine use			
None	503 (16.4%)	295 (14.2%)	798 (15.5%)
1–2 cans-cups/day	831 (27.1%)	493 (23.8%)	1324 (25.8%)
>2 cans-cups/day	719 (23.5%)	359 (17.3%)	1078 (21.0%)
History of caffeine dependency	52 (1.7%)	29 (1.4%)	81 (1.6%)
Undocumented	953 (31.1%)	889 (42.9%)	1842 (35.9%)

Types of Common Medical Conditions

In a generalist practice, practitioners frequently see the same types of problems over and over again. Clinical experience is based upon learning how to antici-pate and manage similar problems on a repeated basis. Therefore, it is helpful to know the most frequent medical conditions evaluated in practice, especially when the practitioner is new to practice. These data will help the practitioner to anticipate what he/she is likely to encounter on a daily basis, and at the very least, this list can become a learning agenda for students and new practitioners.

Table 2-6 lists the ten most common medical conditions. Six of the ten most frequently encountered medical conditions are similar in the two groups, while four important conditions differ. In the younger group, depression, asthma, allergic rhinitis, and treating menopausal symptoms occur in 11–13% of patients. In the older group, patients with ischemic heart disease, cardiac dysrhythmias, hypothyroidism, and/or insomnia are frequently encountered.

Table 2-6   Ten most common medical conditions

Patients < 65 yrs old ($n = 3064$)		Patients ≥ 65 yrs old ($n = 2072$)	
Medical condition	No. of patients (%)	Medical condition	No. of patients (%)
Hypertension	1151 (37.8%)	Hypertension	1190 (57.4%)
Hyperlipidemia	572 (18.7%)	Hyperlipidemia	721 (34.8%)
Diabetes	543 (17.7%)	Diabetes	616 (29.7%)
Peptic ulcer disease	428 (14.0%)	Arthritis	595 (28.7%)
Allergic rhinitis	409 (12.9%)	Osteoporosis	535 (25.8%)
Osteoporosis	380 (12.4%)	Peptic ulcer disease	458 (22.1%)
Menopausal symptoms	362 (11.8%)	Hypothyroidism	311 (15.0%)
Arthritis	361 (11.8%)	Cardiac dysrhythmias	276 (13.3%)
Asthma	354 (11.6%)	Ischemic heart disease	258 (12.4%)
Depression	344 (11.2%)	Insomnia	250 (12.1%)

Although the differences in the types of medical conditions seen in the two age groups appear quite minor, it is instructive to observe the high level of comorbidities suggested by the higher levels of incidence in patients in the older group. This is especially important because many practitioners have chosen to focus on the care of certain diseases, either ignoring or minimizing the impact that comorbidities can have on these *managed* disease states (diabetes, asthma, or hyperlipidemia). It should be encouraging to the student that the 10 most frequent medical conditions managed with drug therapy in patients less than 65 years old represented 52% of all of the conditions seen, and the 10 most frequent medical conditions managed with drug therapy in patients 65 years old or older represented 50% of all of the conditions seen.

A learning agenda designed to maximize student exposure to patients requiring pharmacotherapy for these most common conditions will greatly enhance student competence and confidence. This approach is also beneficial in that there are now numerous drug products available to treat or prevent virtually all of the most frequently encountered conditions. For example, for patients with hypertension, we have hundreds of individual drug products, several classes of agents (diuretics, beta-blockers, ACE inhibitors, aldosterone antagonists, and calcium channel blockers), and even numerous combination products demonstrated to be efficacious at reducing blood pressure. New national guidelines make it clear that a more aggressive approach to the identification, management, and control of hypertensive patients will be necessary.[4]

Similarly, for patients with major depression, practitioners have over two dozen efficacious products approved for treatment. Therefore, a learning agenda constructed around seeing patients with common medical conditions will also serve to provide the student with a broad exposure to important forms of pharmacotherapy.

For the benefit of the students of pharmaceutical care practice, Table 2-7 displays the 25 most frequently encountered medical conditions in all patients (the two age groups combined) throughout their entire course of care, in decreasing order of frequency. This list represents 70.5% of all the medical conditions cared for in the sample as a whole (27,148 medical conditions).

Table 2-7   Twenty-five most common medical conditions

Most common medical conditions	No. of patients (%)	Percent of conditions
Hypertension	2839 (55.3%)	10.6
Hyperlipidemia	1698 (33.1%)	6.4
Diabetes	1420 (27.6%)	5.2
Arthritis	1270 (24.7%)	4.7
Osteoporosis	1239 (24.1%)	4.6
Peptic ulcer disease	1175 (22.9%)	4.3
Allergic rhinitis	989 (19.3%)	3.0
Depression	825 (16.1%)	2.9
Menopausal symptoms	780 (15.2%)	2.8
Hypothyroidism	649 (12.6%)	2.4
Migraine/headache	613 (11.9%)	2.3
Insomnia	594 (11.6%)	2.2
Asthma	591 (11.5%)	2.2
Pain (general)	522 (10.2%)	1.9
Anxiety	513 (10.0%)	1.9
Cardiac dysrhythmias	444 (8.6%)	1.6
Ischemic heart disease	437 (8.5%)	1.6
Myocardial infarction	400 (7.8%)	1.5
Angina pectoris	369 (7.2%)	1.4
Constipation	362 (7.1%)	1.4
Stroke/CVA prevention	354 (6.9%)	1.3
Back pain	332 (6.5%)	1.2
Congestive heart failure	330 (6.4%)	1.2
Obesity	274 (5.3%)	1.0
COPD/emphysema	230 (4.5%)	0.9

Table 2-8   Most frequent drug use in all patients

Drug products	No. of patients (%)
Oral antidiabetics	1155 (22.5)
Diuretics	1090 (21.2)
Salicylates	1061 (20.7)
ACE inhibitors	1021 (19.9)
HMG CoA reductase inhibitors (statins)	975 (19.0)
Nonsteroidal anti-inflammatory agents (NSAIDs)	956 (18.6)
Beta-blockers	929 (18.1)
Multiple vitamin preparations	928 (18.1)
Calcium blockers	896 (17.4)
Calcium supplements	797 (15.5)
Antiasthmatic-beta adrenergics	740 (14.4)
Estrogen & progestins	719 (14.0)
Anti-infectives	624 (12.1)
Vitamin E	591 (11.5)
Narcotic analgesics	549 (10.7)
Thyroid hormones	524 (10.2)
Nitrates	524 (10.2)
Insulins	496 (9.7)
Cough & cold products	444 (8.6)
Selective serotonin reuptake inhibitors (SSRIs)	432 (8.4)
Proton pump inhibitors	424 (8.3)
Antihistamines	408 (7.9)
Ophthalmic preparations	361 (7.0)
Warfarin	352 (6.9)
Laxatives	338 (6.6)
Benzodiazepines	337 (6.6)
Antacids	333 (6.5)
H2 antagonists	322 (6.3)
Antiasthmatic-steroid inhalants	318 (6.2)
Vitamin C	318 (6.2)
Potassium supplements	314 (6.1)
Dermatologic preparations	311 (6.1)
Nasal steroids	298 (5.8)
Corticosteroids	278 (5.4)
Cardiac glycosides	274 (5.3)
Anticonvulsants	273 (5.3)
Cyclooxygenase-2 inhibitors (COX-2)	257 (5.0)
Hypnotics	231 (4.5)
Tricyclic antidepressants	223 (4.3)
Alternative medicines	184 (3.6)
Oral contraceptives	85 (1.7)

The data presented in this chapter describes documented experiences in ambulatory patients. Although pharmaceutical care provided to hospitalized patients is less well documented, national figures published by the Agency for Healthcare Research and Quality (AHRQ) demonstrate similar patterns of common diseases among hospitalized individuals.[5]

In 1997, nearly 60% of all hospitalized patients were female. Excluding the delivery of healthy newborns and trauma admissions, 5 of the top 10 conditions for which people were admitted to the hospital through the emergency department were related to cardiovascular problems including congestive heart failure, myocardial infarction, chest pain, ischemic heart disease, and cardiac dysrhythmias. Patients with depression, asthma, and chronic obstructive lung disease were also among the most frequently hospitalized patients in the United States. Hypertension is the most common comorbidity in hospitalized patients, which is a coexisting condition that is not the main reason for the hospital stay, but can make hospital stays more expensive and complicated. Also similar to ambulatory patient data was the observation that about a third of patients have two or more comorbidities. These national inpatient figures are similar to those outpatient data from pharmaceutical care practices, suggesting that common medical conditions that are not properly managed or effectively prevented in ambulatory patients can lead to emergency department visits and hospitalizations.[5]

As described earlier, we often have multiple drug products or classes from which to choose therapy for an individual patient. Table 2-8 represents practice-based use of medications by class.

Table 2-8 displays the most frequently encountered drug therapies in all patients (the two groups combined) throughout the entire course of care, in decreasing order of frequency. This list represents 75% of all of the drug therapies taken by the patients. Table 2-9 displays the types of drug products by rank order of frequency of use for the two patient groups. The drug products most frequently used by patients in the younger group were nonsteroidal anti-inflammatory agents (NSAIDs) and angiotensin-converting enzyme inhibitors (ACE). In the older patient group, the two most frequently used products were diuretics and salicylates.

DRUG THERAPY PROBLEMS IDENTIFIED AND RESOLVED

The unique and valuable contribution of the pharmaceutical care practitioner is to identify patients' drug therapy problems. It is obvious that problems cannot be resolved unless they are identified, and perhaps even more importantly, they cannot be prevented unless they are anticipated. Therefore, one

Table 2-9 Frequency of drug use by category

Drug products	Rank order for younger patients ($n = 3064$)	Rank order for older patients ($n = 2072$)
Oral antidiabetics	3	3
Diuretics	10	1
Salicylates	12	2
ACE inhibitors	2	8
HMG CoA reductase inhibitors (statins)	7	4
Nonsteroidal anti-inflammatory (NSAIDs)	1	10
Beta-blockers	8	7
Multiple vitamin preparations	9	6
Calcium blockers	11	5
Calcium supplements	13	9
Antiasthmatic-beta adrenergics	4	19
Estrogen & progestins	5	16
Anti-infectives	6	27
Vitamin E	19	12
Narcotic analgesics	14	22
Thyroid hormones	23	13
Nitrates	31	11
Insulins	17	23
Cough & cold products	15	32
Selective serotonin reuptake inhibitors (SSRIs)	18	29
Proton pump inhibitors	21	24
Antihistamines	16	36
Ophthalmic preparations	40	14
Warfarin	38	15
Laxatives	33	18
Benzodiazepines	28	25
Antacids	32	21
Histamine-2 antagonists	30	26
Antiasthmatic-steroid inhalants	20	34
Vitamin C	29	28
Potassium supplements	35	20
Dermatologic preparations	24	37
Nasal steroids	22	39
Corticosteroids	26	33
Cardiac glycosides	41	17
Anticonvulsants	25	35
Cyclooxygenase-2 inhibitors (COX-2)	34	30
Hypnotics	36	31
Tricyclic antidepressants	27	40
Alternative medicines	37	38
Oral contraceptives	39	41

of the most significant contributions of this practice can be measured in the number and type of drug therapy problems identified in these patients.

Pharmaceutical care practitioners identified and resolved drug therapy problems in 42% of these patients during their first assessment. One in five patients had multiple drug therapy problems.

One-third of the patients in the younger group (34.3%) experienced one or more drug therapy problems at the initial visit to the pharmaceutical care practitioner. This number represents patients who had a severe enough problem that action was taken at the time of the encounter. It should also be mentioned that this number does not include those drug therapy problems identified and resolved at later encounters throughout the care of the patient, only on the initial visit.

Over half of the patients in the older group (53.6%) experienced one or more drug therapy problems at the time of the initial assessment. Table 2-10 displays the frequency distribution for the two groups. The patients in the younger group experienced from 0 to 12 drug therapy problems while the older group experienced from 0 to 8 drug therapy problems.

During the development of this practice, few clinicians anticipated that the frequency of drug therapy problems would be so significant in the ambulatory population. It should not come as a surprise, however, because the literature reports a staggering amount of drug-related morbidity and mortality as well

Table 2-10 Frequency distribution of drug therapy problems in patients

No. of drug therapy problems	Patients < 65 yrs old No. of patients (%) (n = 3064)	Patients ≥ 65 yrs old No. of patients (%) (n = 2072)
1	607 (19.8%)	550 (26.5%)
2	247 (8.1%)	305 (14.7%)
3	118 (3.8%)	138 (6.7%)
4	44 (1.4%)	60 (2.9%)
5	16 (0.5%)	30 (1.4%)
6	11 (0.4%)	21 (1.0%)
7	3 (0.1%)	4 (0.2%)
8	3 (0.1%)	3 (0.1%)
9	1 (0.0%)	0 (0.0%)
10	1 (0.0%)	0 (0.0%)
11	0 (0.0%)	0 (0.0%)
12	1 (0.0%)	0 (0.0%)
Total	1052 (34.3%)	1111 (53.6%)

as an economic burden that now exceeds $177 billion annually in the United States.[6,7] It is often difficult to translate such large numbers into a daily workload. However, the numbers have been consistent since the beginning of this practice. Nearly one-half of all patients entering a community or clinic pharmacy will have a drug therapy problem. The impact of this practice on patient care is significant.

Types of Drug Therapy Problems

There were a total of 3995 drug therapy problems identified and resolved in these 5136 (total sample) patients during their first pharmaceutical care encounter. These drug therapy problems involved 4849 individual medications as some drug therapy problems involve multiple medications. The drug therapy problems can be classified according to the seven categories displayed in Table 2-11.

The most important observation about these data is that the distribution is virtually identical in the two age groups. Although there were more drug therapy problems identified in the older group as compared to the younger group, the types of problems identified were about the same. These figures have been consistent over the 10 years this practice has been in place.

Figure 2-4 displays the frequency and categories of drug therapy problems experienced by the two groups of patients.

The frequency distribution of drug therapy problems often surprises new practitioners. Most practitioners expect compliance problems to be the most common. Toxic doses (doses too high) and adverse drug reactions are

Table 2-11   Distribution of drug therapy problems by category

Drug therapy problem category	Patients < 65 yrs old No. of drug therapy problems (% of total)	Patients≥ 65 yrs old No. of drug therapy problems (% of total)
Unnecessary drug therapy	133 (7.2%)	143 (6.7%)
Additional drug therapy needed	586 (31.6%)	644 (30.1%)
Ineffective drug	121 (7.6%)	104 (4.9%)
Dosage too low	390 (21.0%)	497 (23.2%)
Adverse drug reaction	284 (14.3%)	269 (12.6%)
Dosage too high	74 (4.0%)	102 (4.8%)
Noncompliance[a]	265 (14.3%)	383 (17.9%)
Subtotals	1853 (100.0%)	2142 (100.0%)

[a]Patient is considered noncompliant only when the drug therapy is determined to be clinically indicated, effective, and safe, yet the patient is not taking medication as intended.

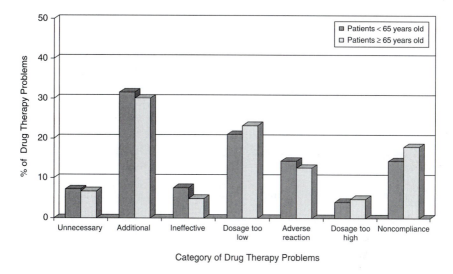

Figure 2-4   Drug therapy problems by category.

also expected to contribute significantly to drug therapy problems, however this is not the case in pharmaceutical care practice. Patients are considered to be noncompliant only after their drug therapy has been determined to be appropriately indicated, effective, and safe for the specific patient. Because a patient's drug therapy is first evaluated for appropriateness and then effectiveness before adverse reactions are considered a possibility, many problems are eliminated before an adverse reaction is considered. Noncompliance represented only 14 and 18% of the drug therapy problems in the two patient groups.

Pharmaceutical care practitioners constantly assess drug therapy for effectiveness, so drug therapy problems in which the dosage is too low can quickly be identified and corrected. It is important to note that patients receive inadequate (ineffective) dosage regimens two or three times more frequently than they receive too much drug. These data validate many of the problems, struggles, and concerns experienced by patients in the current health care system. Modern pharmacotherapy has advanced to the point where for most common indications, there are not only several product choices at the practitioner's disposal, but a dosage regimen can be individually designed to ensure that the goals of therapy are achieved and the patient's therapy is effective.

These practice-based findings describe the scope of problems created in our health care system with today's drug use process. Without pharmaceutical care, many patients do not receive the drug products they require to combat common illnesses, dosages are frequently inadequate to provide relief, and instructions are vague or confusing resulting in poor clinical results. Pharmaceutical care practice addresses each of these common problems in an organized, personalized approach, designed to improve each patient's medication experience. Identifying and resolving drug therapy problems improves the effectiveness and safety of drug therapy.

Causes, Frequency, and Distribution of Drug Therapy Problems

The ability to identify the cause of a drug therapy problem makes resolving it straightforward. Stating the cause of the problem defines the intervention that the practitioner must make. There is a tremendous amount of knowledge to be gained from evaluating the most common causes of the drug therapy problems.

Tables 2-12 to 2-18 describe the distribution of causes of drug therapy problems identified for each of the seven categories of drug therapy problems. This information often reflects the intervention made by practitioners to resolve the problem.

> **Example** In the first category, unnecessary drug therapy, when no valid medical indication for the drug therapy occurred, the medication was discontinued. When two drug products were being used for a condition when only one product was indicated, one of the products was discontinued. Taking action to resolve the drug therapy problem is quite straightforward, but the assessment that led to the decision that a drug therapy problem existed is dependent on the knowledge and skills of a qualified pharmaceutical care practitioner.

In almost half of the cases in this category, no medical indication could be found for the drug therapy being taken (see Table 2-12). Frequently, patients are not aware of the reason (or indication) they are taking the drug in the first place and therefore sometimes continue to take the medication much longer than necessary. Without proper instructions, patients may not understand when to discontinue a certain medication or if it is safe to stop taking it. This leads to wasted money and time, as well as causing unnecessary confusion in the patient's life.

The need for additional pharmacotherapy as treatment or prevention (see Table 2-13) is substantial among patients seen by the pharmaceutical care practitioner. Prevention is often forgotten or lost in a health care system geared to respond to diseases, illnesses, and acute disorders. Among the older patients, over 40% of the additional medications required were for preventive purposes. These included initiation of daily aspirin to prevent myocardial infarction or

Table 2-12 Type of drug therapy problem—Unnecessary
drug therapy

Cause of the problem	Patients < 65 yrs old[a]	Patients ≥ 65 yrs old[b]
No valid medical indication for the drug therapy at this time	64 (48.1%)	78 (54.6%)
Multiple drug therapies are being used for a condition that requires single drug therapy	49 (36.8%)	53 (37.1%)
Medical condition is more appropriately treated with nondrug therapy	13 (9.8%)	6 (4.2%)
Drug therapy is being taken to treat an avoidable adverse reaction associated with another medication	4 (3.0%)	5 (3.5%)
Drug abuse, alcohol use, or smoking is causing the medical problem	3 (2.3%)	1 (0.7%)

[a]Number of drug therapy problems (%) $n = 133$.
[b]Number of drug therapy problems (%) $n = 143$.

Table 2-13 Type of drug therapy problem—Needs additional
drug therapy

Cause of the problem	Patients < 65 yrs old[a]	Patients ≥ 65 yrs old[b]
Medical condition requires the initiation of drug therapy	235 (40.1%)	225 (34.9%)
Preventive drug therapy is required to reduce the risk of developing a new condition	228 (38.9%)	274 (42.6%)
Medical condition requires additional drug therapy to attain synergistic or additive effects	123 (21.0%)	145 (22.5%)

[a]Number of drug therapy problems (%) $n = 586$.
[b]Number of drug therapy problems (%) $n = 644$.

Table 2-14 Type of drug therapy problem—Ineffective drug therapy

Cause	Patients < 65 yrs old[a]	Patients ≥ 65 yrs old[b]
Drug product is not the most effective product for the indication being treated	79 (65.3%)	64 (61.5%)
Medical condition is refractory to the drug product	24 (19.8%)	17 (16.4%)
Dosage form of the drug product is inappropriate	10 (8.3%)	21 (20.3%)
Drug is not effective for the medical problem	8 (6.6%)	2 (1.9%)

[a]Number of drug therapy problems (%) $n = 121$.
[b]Number of drug therapy problems (%) $n = 104$.

stroke, calcium supplements to minimize the risk of osteoporosis, and immunizations to prevent pneumonia or the flu.

Ineffective drug therapy requires changing the product (see Table 2-14). These problems most commonly included situations in which the patient was taking a drug that was not the most efficacious, or the patient simply was not responding. However, no drug product works 100% of the time. You will always find patients who do not benefit from products known to be highly efficacious.

The second most frequent type of drug therapy problem is due to inadequate dosing (see Table 2-15). Most of the medications we have available today can be effective in a large majority of patients, but only if the patient receives an adequate dosage regimen. These data support the observation that too often pharmacotherapy is initiated using a low or conservative dosage regimen in order to *see what will happen*. However, due to the lack of vigilant monitoring, follow-up, and evaluation of pharmacotherapy throughout the health care system, the dosage is seldom increased to provide effective results. Most frequently the correct drug product was selected, but the dose or the dosing interval was inadequate for the patient to benefit. Pharmaceutical care practitioners increase drug dosages in order to provide effective therapy far more often than they decrease dosages.

Adverse drug reactions occur frequently (see Table 2-16). Many are not preventable because they are not related to the dose of the drug the patient is taking.[8,9] Establishing the connection between the adverse response and a specific drug product allows for its rapid resolution. Most adverse drug reactions require discontinuation of the drug product involved.

Table 2-15 Type of drug therapy problem—Dosage too low

Cause	Patients < 65 yrs old[a]	Patients ≥ 65 yrs old[b]
Dose is too low to produce the desired response	231 (59.2%)	298 (60.0%)
Dosage interval is too infrequent to produce the desired response	133 (34.1%)	173 (34.8%)
Drug interaction reduces the amount of active drug available	19 (4.9%)	21 (4.2%)
Duration of drug therapy is too short to produce the desired response	7 (1.8%)	5 (1.0%)

[a]Number of drug therapy problems (%) $n = 390$.
[b]Number of drug therapy problems (%) $n = 497$.

Table 2-16 Type of drug therapy problem—Adverse drug reaction

Cause	Patients < 65 yrs old[a]	Patients ≥ 65 yrs old[b]
Drug product causes an undesirable reaction that is not dose-related	184 (64.8%)	139 (51.7%)
Safer drug product is required due to risk factors	39 (13.7%)	28 (10.4%)
Drug interaction causes an undesirable reaction that is not dose-related	31 (10.9%)	39 (14.5%)
Dosage regimen was administered or changed too rapidly	21 (7.4%)	35 (13.0%)
Drug product causes an allergic reaction	9 (3.2%)	6 (2.2%)

[a]Number of drug therapy problems (%) $n = 284$.
[b]Number of drug therapy problems (%) $n = 269$.

Table 2-17   Type of drug therapy problem—Dosage too high

Cause	Patients < 65 yrs old[a]	Patients ≥ 65 yrs old[b]
Dose is too high	48 (64.9%)	62 (60.8%)
Dosing frequency is too short	19 (25.7%)	24 (23.5%)
Duration of drug therapy is too long	4 (5.4%)	12 (11.8%)
Drug interaction occurs resulting in a toxic reaction to the drug product	3 (4.0%)	4 (3.9%)
Dose of the drug was administered too rapidly	1 (1.4%)	0 (0.0%)

[a]Number of drug therapy problems (%) $n = 74$.
[b]Number of drug therapy problems (%) $n = 102$.

Excessive dosages most frequently involved high doses or dosing frequencies that were too short (see Table 2-17). It is interesting to note that high dosages were identified in both age groups at approximately the same frequency. Again, dose and interval must both be assessed and corrected to ensure that the patient's pharmacotherapy is safe.

Noncompliance can be considered an issue of behavior; therefore, resolving noncompliance problems requires a change in behavior, sometimes on the patient's part and sometimes on the part of the practitioner (see Table 2-18). It is noteworthy that approximately 30–40% of noncompliance is due to behavioral aspects on the patient's part (prefers not to take and/or forgets to take medications). These data mean that noncompliance due directly to patient behavior was identified in only about 5–7% of patients. On the other hand, 60–70% of noncompliance problems require changes on the part of the health care practitioner or the system in order for the patient to be able to take the medication as intended (patient does not understand instructions, product is too expensive, patient cannot swallow or self-administer).

Patients have made it clear that health care practitioners do not do an adequate job of explaining medication instructions. The most frequent cause of noncompliance was that the patient did not understand how to use the drug product. Also, practitioners frequently encountered situations in which the patient simply preferred not to participate in the pharmacotherapy that was recommended or prescribed. These data indicate that forgetfulness is less commonly the cause of noncompliance than many clinicians want to believe. Our younger patients forgot as frequently as the older patients. All noncompliance has a root cause, and only by determining why the patient is not compliant, can an effective solution be implemented.

Table 2-18   Type of drug therapy problem—Noncompliance

Cause	Patients < 65 yrs old[a]	Patients ≥ 65 yrs old[b]
Patient did not understand instructions	128 (48.3%)	149 (38.9%)
Patient prefers not to take the medication	72 (27.2%)	81 (21.2%)
Patient forgets to take medication	35 (13.2%)	31 (8.1%)
Drug product is too expensive for the patient	25 (9.4%)	110 (28.7%)
Patient cannot swallow or self-administer the drug product appropriately	3 (1.1%)	9 (2.3%)
Drug product is not available for the patient	2 (0.8%)	3 (0.8%)

[a]Number of drug therapy problems (%) $n = 265$.
[b]Number of drug therapy problems (%) $n = 383$.

Common Medical Conditions and Common Drug Therapy Problems

Table 2-19 displays the medical conditions most frequently associated with drug therapy problems for the two patient groups. This list can help the new practitioner be sensitive to common medical conditions and associated drug therapy problems.

The practice-based results described in Table 2-19 demonstrate that patients over 65 years of age often have considerable difficulty in obtaining effective and safe pharmacotherapy for arthritis (rheumatoid or osteo arthritis). This occurs despite the constant development of new, efficacious antiarthritic drug products and disease modifying antirheumatic agents including the cyclooxygenase-2 inhibitors, rofecoxib, (Vioxx), celecoxib, (Celebrex), interleukin-1 receptor antagonists, anakinra, (Kineret), and the tumor necrosis factor receptor blocking agent, etanercept, (Enbrel).

Arthritis is the leading cause of disability among Americans over the age of 15. Seven million Americans experience arthritis-related limitations on every day activities like walking, dressing, and bathing. The medical costs for treating arthritis and lost wages that result from this disease total more than $82 billion annually.[10] It is clear that pharmaceutical care practice has the potential to directly benefit many who suffer from damaging chronic disorders.

Table 2.19 Most common drug therapy problems and associated medical conditions

Patients < 65 yrs old		Patients ≥ 65 yrs old	
Diabetes	Needs additional drug therapy	Arthritis	Needs additional drug therapy
Depression	Needs additional drug therapy	Arthritis	Dosage too low
Asthma	Needs additional drug therapy	Hypertension	Needs additional drug therapy
Asthma	Dosage too low	Anxiety	Needs additional drug therapy
Menopausal symptoms	Needs additional drug therapy	Hyperlipidemia	Needs additional drug therapy
Hypertension	Needs additional drug therapy	Hypertension	Dosage too low
Allergic rhinitis	Needs additional drug therapy	Arthritis	Adverse drug reaction
Diabetes	Dosage too low	Arthritis	Noncompliance
Hyperlipidemia	Needs additional drug therapy	Ischemic heart disease	Needs additional drug therapy
Allergic rhinitis	Dosage too low	Diabetes	Dosage too low

The five medical conditions most frequently associated with each category of drug therapy problem are displayed in Table 2-20. This table suggests problems with pharmacotherapy for certain medical conditions that can be anticipated and dealt with before serious drug therapy problems develop. The order of the medical conditions reflects the frequency of drug therapy problems (with the most frequent listed first). Although there is not a noticeable difference between the two groups because the same medical conditions are common in both groups, there are individual differences in each of the problem categories.

Note that older patients suffering from arthritis commonly experience drug therapy problems of all types. Arthritis (osteo or rheumatoid arthritis) is the most frequent medical illness associated with five of the seven categories of drug therapy problems. Similarly, in the younger group, patients with depression are among those who most frequently experience drug therapy problems in five of the seven categories. This is despite the availability of numerous antidepressive agents demonstrated to be effective and safe for use in general practice.

Again, for the benefit of the new practitioner, Table 2-21 displays those medical conditions associated with drug therapy problems (in decreasing frequency). Note that this table combines the two groups of patients and is quite similar to Table 2-7 that lists the 25 most common medical conditions in these patients. These practice-based results demonstrate that drug therapy problems occur in patients with virtually any and all medical conditions. This is most likely due to the overall lack of a rational approach to drug therapy in general and not due to any particular disease or drug characteristics.

The 25 medical conditions most frequently involved in drug therapy problems represented 75.4% of all of the medical conditions in patients who had one or more drug therapy problem of any type ($n = 5136$ patients).

It is perhaps obvious that drug categories most commonly involved in drug therapy problems are consistent with the medical conditions associated with drug therapy problems. Because of the large range of therapeutic alternatives available to today's practitioners, it is instructive to review those medications that were frequently involved in drug therapy problems before selecting products for individual patients. Table 2-22 displays these data in decreasing order of frequency.

It is instructive to note that four of the five drug categories most frequently associated with the drug therapy problem category *needs additional drug therapy* were the same for both age groups (salicylates, calcium supplements, analgesics, and antacids). These categories represent inexpensive products, which are generally available without a prescription and are very efficacious at preventing or treating serious illnesses. It is common for pharmaceutical care practitioners to identify unmet drug-related needs and provide effective preventative or palliative pharmacotherapy.

Table 2-20 Five most common medical conditions involved in each type of drug therapy problem

Drug therapy problem	Patients < 65 yrs old	Patients ≥ 65 yrs old
Unnecessary drug therapy	Allergic rhinitis Hypertension Back pain Asthma Menopausal symptoms	Hypertension Constipation Anxiety Arthritis Hypertension
Needs additional drug therapy	Asthma Depression Menopausal symptoms Hypertension Allergic rhinitis	Arthritis Hypertension Anxiety Ischemic heart disease Hyperlipidemia
Ineffective drug	Hypertension Depression Hyperlipidemia Asthma Anxiety	Hypertension Hyperlipidemia Anxiety Peptic ulcer disease Arthritis
Dosage too low	Asthma Diabetes Allergic rhinitis Hypertension Menopausal symptoms	Arthritis Hypertension Diabetes Hyperlipidemia Constipation
Adverse drug reaction	Depression Hypertension Hyperlipidemia Allergic rhinitis Asthma	Arthritis Hyperlipidemia Hypertension Menopausal symptoms Anxiety
Dosage too high	Asthma Depression Menopausal symptoms Anxiety Hypertension	Arthritis Diabetes Angina pectoris Congestive heart failure Constipation
Noncompliance	Asthma Diabetes Depression Hypertension Anxiety	Arthritis Hyperlipidemia Hypertension Diabetes Allergic rhinitis

Table 2-21 Twenty-five most common medical conditions involved in drug therapy problems ($n = 5136$)

Medical condition	No. of patients with drug therapy problems (%)
Hypertension	606 (11.8)
Diabetes	538 (10.5)
Osteoporosis	531 (10.3)
Hyperlipidemia	323 (6.3)
Arthritis	271 (5.3)
Asthma	180 (3.5)
Peptic ulcer disease	165 (3.2)
Allergic rhinitis	133 (2.6)
Depression	113 (2.2)
Myocardial infarction	105 (2.0)
Menopausal symptoms	97 (1.9)
Cardiac dysrhythmias	89 (1.7)
COPD/emphysema	81 (1.6)
Ischemic heart disease	76 (1.5)
Constipation	72 (1.4)
Hypothyroidism	71 (1.4)
Migraine/headache	68 (1.3)
Insomnia	67 (1.3)
Pain-generalized	63 (1.2)
Angina pectoris	61 (1.2)
Tobacco use	59 (1.2)
Back pain	54 (1.1)
Stroke/CVA prevention	44 (0.9)
Congestive heart failure	42 (0.8)
Anxiety	38 (0.7)

It is also interesting to note that older patients often receive too high of a dose of warfarin, while the younger patients are often underdosed. These findings are similar to other clinical trials in which about half of the patients receiving warfarin are inadequately protected from thromboembolism.[11]

Table 2-23 displays the number of drug therapy problems associated with the different classes of drugs for the entire patient sample. These 25 classes of drugs were involved in two-thirds of all drug therapy problems identified. The most frequent therapies involved in drug therapy problems are not the most expensive, or the most complex, but the most common. It is noteworthy that the first three categories of products are not prescription products, but instead common over-the-counter medications.

Table 2-22 Five most common drug categories involved in each type of drug therapy problem

Drug therapy problem	Patients < 65 yrs old	Patients ≥ 65 yrs old
Unnecessary drug therapy	Beta-blockers NSAIDs B-complex vitamins Steroid inhalants Anti-inflammatory agents	H2-antagonists Nitrates Benzodiazepines Salicylates Proton pump inhibitors
Needs additional drug therapy	Salicylates Calcium supplements Smoking deterrents Antacids Analgesics	Salicylates Calcium supplements Nonnarcotic analgesics Multiple vitamins Antacids
Ineffective drug	Narcotic analgesics NSAIDs Nonsedating antihistamines Calcium blockers ACE inhibitors	Salicylates Nonnarcotic analgesics NSAIDs HMG CoA reductase inhibitors (statins) Narcotic analgesics
Dosage too low	Sulfonylureas Insulin Biguanides ACE inhibitors Warfarin	Calcium supplements Sulfonylureas ACE inhibitors HMG CoA reductase inhibitors (statins) Calcium blockers
Adverse drug reaction	NSAIDs ACE inhibitors SSRI (selective serotonin reuptake inhibitors) Salicylates Beta-blockers	NSAIDs Salicylates Beta-blockers Calcium blockers HMG CoA reductase inhibitors (statins)
Dosage too high	Sulfonylureas Beta adrenergic inhalants Thyroid hormone Tricyclic antidepressants Salicylates	Salicylates Warfarin HMG CoA reductase inhibitors (statins) Cardiac glycosides Analgesics
Noncompliance	Steroid inhalants HMG CoA reductase inhibitors (statins) Beta-adrenergic inhalants Calcium blockers SSRI (selective serotonin reuptake inhibitors)	HMG CoA reductase inhibitors (statins) Beta-adrenergic inhalants Calcium blockers ACE inhibitors Beta-blockers

Table 2-23   Twenty-five classes of drugs most commonly involved in drug therapy problems of all types ($n = 5136$)

Drug class	No. of drug therapy problems (%)	Cumulative % of total drug therapy problems
Calcium supplements	422 (10.6%)	10.6
Salicylates	292 (7.3%)	17.9
Nonsteroidal anti-inflammatory agents (NSAIDs)	167 (4.2%)	22.1
HMG CoA reductase inhibitors (statins)	156 (3.9%)	26.0
Sympathomimetics	136 (3.4%)	29.4
Angiotensin converting enzyme (ACE) inhibitors	127 (3.2%)	32.6
Calcium blockers	112 (2.8%)	35.4
Nonnarcotic analgesics	107 (2.7%)	38.1
Beta-blockers	103 (2.6%)	40.7
Warfarin	102 (2.6%)	43.3
Steroid inhalants	99 (2.5%)	45.8
Sulfonylureas	96 (2.4%)	48.2
Narcotic analgesics	91 (2.3%)	50.5
Biguanides	88 (2.2%)	52.7
Insulin	79 (2.0%)	54.7
Nitrates	72 (1.8%)	56.5
Antacids	69 (1.7%)	58.2
Alternative medicines	65 (1.6%)	59.8
Selective serotonin reuptake inhibitors [SSRIs]	63 (1.6%)	61.4
Thyroid hormones	60 (1.5%)	62.9
Laxatives	55 (1.4%)	64.3
Proton pump inhibitors	52 (1.3%)	65.6
Cough/cold combinations	38 (1.0%)	66.6
Smoking deterrents	33 (0.8%)	67.4
Antihistamines-nonsedating	32 (0.8%)	68.2

LEVEL OF PATIENT COMPLEXITY

The level of patient complexity is determined by evaluating the patient's number of medical conditions, the patient's number of medications, and the patient's number of drug therapy problems (refer to Chapter 4).[1,12,13] The Assurance Pharmaceutical Care software used to create this database automatically calculates this level from the documentation of the practice. The level of patient complexity will determine the amount of resources, time, and effort involved in caring for the patient's drug-related needs. The variable of complexity also determines the level of reimbursement for the practitioner. Patient complexity represents a standard approach to estimating resources required to provide care to patients. Some patients present with additional challenges including difficulties with language, hearing, or vision that can make providing care more difficult. However, in general the determination of patient complexity serves as the basis for workload and reimbursement.

Figure 2-5 displays the two groups of patients. The level of complexity is higher for the older group. Although this is as expected, the fact that there are twice as many patients in Levels 3, 4, and 5 for the older group as for the younger group speaks to the effort and resources required to care for the elderly. This should be noted when establishing a new pharmaceutical care practice. The amount of time scheduled for an encounter and the amount of time required for documentation and follow-up will be greater for this group of patients as compared to the younger group.

Figure 2-5 represents a typical distribution of patients in a generalist's practice with the majority of patients' drug-related needs represented by the Level 1 and Level 2 criteria and 12–25% of patients' needs at Levels 3 through 5. Patient complexity dictates workload in clinical practice; therefore, it is important to understand the needs of all of the patients within your practice. It is important to become efficient at providing pharmaceutical care for patients with less complex needs (Levels 1 and 2) in order to have the

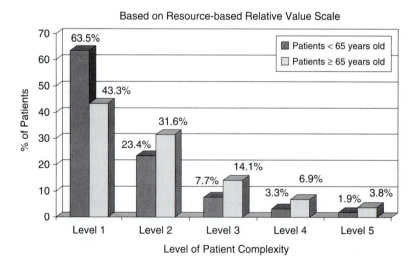

Figure 2-5 Patient complexity.

resources and time to provide appropriate care for your patients with more complex drug-related needs. Note that the older patient group generally has more complex needs than the younger group. This *shift to the right* means that more resources will be required to provide pharmaceutical care for the older group than for the younger group of patients.

INTERVENTIONS MADE IN CARE PLAN DEVELOPMENT

Once drug therapy problems were identified, care plans were developed for each patient. An evaluation of the data illustrates how practitioners intervened to resolve drug therapy problems and achieve the goals of therapy for each medical condition. Table 2-24 presents these data. Pharmacists are often surprised that so many drug therapy problems are resolved directly with the patients themselves. A common misperception is that the practitioner must contact the physician or the health plan directly to resolve most of the drug therapy problems. This is not the case in a practice that provides direct patient care. The majority of the work occurred between the patient and the practitioner providing the care.

Pharmaceutical care is a patient-centered practice. In this sample, 77.6% of the interventions made on behalf of the younger patients were directed toward the patient. Even more of the interventions made on behalf of the older group (81.7%) were made directly with these patients. Only 21.4% of the interventions made for the younger group required physician intervention, while 18.1% of them required direct physician intervention in the older group. In these cases, the original prescriber was personally consulted in order to change the drug product or dosage regimen. In many cases, the patient was informed of the suggested changes in drug therapy and took those recommendations to his/her physician at the next medical visit, at which time the patient and the physician agreed to the changes.

We have found this to be a much more efficient use of physician and patient time. By supplying the patient with a written record of all of his/her medications, indications, instructions, and recommendations for improvement, the patient and the physician are provided the complete set of information required to make appropriate drug therapy decisions at the next physician visit. The use of collaborative practice agreements can also facilitate the resolution of many drug therapy problems.

A quick review of these interventions demonstrates that students studying to become pharmaceutical care practitioners must learn how to initiate

Table 2-24 Interventions made to resolve drug therapy problems

	Patients < 65 years old No. of interventions (%)	Patients ≥ 65 years old No. of interventions (%)
Required patient intervention only		
Initiate new drug therapy	358	451
Change drug product	58	81
Change dosage regimen	293	352
Discontinue drug therapy	129	138
Initiate laboratory test monitoring	126	204
Education beyond OBRA	330	430
Provided medication reminder device	43	54
Removed patient barrier	126	131
Other	209	59
Total	1672 (77.6%)	1905 (81.7%)
Required physician intervention		
Initiate new drug therapy	146	130
Change drug product	88	45
Change dosage regimen	107	93
Discontinue drug therapy	56	72
Initiate laboratory monitoring	33	54
Other	30	26
Total	460 (21.3%)	420 (18.1%)
Required protocol/carrier intervention		
Initiate new drug therapy	4	0
Change drug product	6	1
Change dosage regimen	4	0
Discontinue drug therapy	1	4
Other	8	1
Total	23 (1.1%)	6 (0.2%)
Total no. of interventions	**2155**	**2326**

new drug therapies, change products, individualize dosage regimens, use laboratory tests to evaluate therapy, and discontinue drug therapy safely.

It is noteworthy that the situation in pharmaceutical care is different than that in dispensing pharmacy as only 1 and 0.2%, respectively, of the interventions in the two groups involved the insurance carrier or protocol manager in order to resolve the problem. The category of *other* in this table refers to interventions that were so patient-specific that they could not be categorized into one of the other intervention categories.

PATIENT OUTCOMES

Pharmaceutical care can have a very positive impact on patients' clinical outcomes. This clinical impact is most comprehensively represented by the patient's status at the follow-up evaluation. This evaluation compares the patient's status at the initial assessment with what is occurring at follow-up. This evaluation compares actual patient outcomes against the parameters that reflect the goals of therapy for each patient's pharmacotherapy for each medical condition. If a practitioner can impact the status of a patient at follow-up, then that practitioner has positively impacted a patient's life. Data in this section describe the size and nature of the impact the pharmaceutical care practitioner can have.

There were 2720 patients who were less than 65 years old, who had at least one follow-up visit evaluating the status of the same medical condition(s). The follow-up evaluations of patients with multiple medical conditions are coordinated, if possible, so the outcomes of all of the patient's drug therapies can be evaluated during the same visit. This represented 9169 total medical conditions in which outcomes of pharmacotherapy were evaluated in these 2720 patients. These patients became the sample for this portion of the analysis.

There were 1772 patients who were 65 years old or older, who had at least one follow-up visit evaluating the status of the same medical condition(s). This represented 9582 total medical conditions evaluated. These patients became the sample for this portion of the analysis.

Table 2-25 displays the status of patients at the most recent evaluation following pharmaceutical care services. To be meaningful, it is necessary to present the definitions of each of the clinical outcome status terms because the meaning of each is specific.

Consolidating these data into positive and negative categories explains the impact pharmaceutical care can have on patient outcomes. In both groups, practitioners produced positive outcomes in 90% of the patients' medical conditions at follow-up. This figure is impressive in any context, but in the context of pharmaceutical care it is very noteworthy. These results have been produced in patients experiencing drug therapy problems and in patients whose drug therapy has been changed, initiated, and/or discontinued. These patients have had practitioners intervene in their drug therapy, and positive results were realized (Table 2-26).

The identification and resolution of drug therapy problems coupled with the establishment and achievement of measurable goals of therapy were critical in producing these positive clinical results.

When these data are further analyzed, the full impact of the practice itself can be seen. Table 2-27 compares the patient's status at the first

Table 2-25 Patient outcome status at the most recent follow-up evaluation

Patient status	Patients < 65 yrs old (n = 2720)		Patients ≥ 65 yrs old (n = 1772)		Definition criteria
	No. of conditions	%	No. of conditions	%	
Resolved	847	9.2	411	4.3	Goals achieved, therapy completed
Stable	5639	61.5	6453	67.4	Goals achieved, therapy continued
Improved	995	10.8	946	9.9	Adequate progress being made, continue same therapy
Partially improved	815	8.9	874	9.1	Progress being made, adjustments in therapy required
Unimproved	514	5.6	510	5.3	No progress yet, but continue same therapy
Worsened	235	2.6	223	2.3	Decline in health status, adjust therapy
Failure	113	1.2	98	1.0	Goals not achieved, discontinue current therapy, replace with new therapy
Expired	11	0.1	67	0.7	Patient died

Table 2-26 Comparison of outcome status at follow-up evaluation

Status	Patients < 65 yrs old (n = 2720)		Patients ≥ 65 yrs old (n = 1772)	
	No. of conditions	%	No. of conditions	%
Positive outcome[a] (resolved, stable, improved, partially improved)	8296	90.5	8684	90.6
Negative outcome[b] (unimproved, worsened, failure, expired)	873	9.5	898	9.4

[a]Positive outcomes defined as goals of therapy being achieved.
[b]Negative outcome defined as goals of therapy not met.

encounter with the status of that same patient at follow-up. We see that 84% of the medical conditions requiring drug therapy, which were not already stable at the time of the first pharmaceutical care encounter, improved (69%) or remained the same (15%) through the provision of pharmaceutical care.

The positive impact of pharmaceutical care practice on patients is remarkable. Although the clinical impact on the patient is considered to be the most important, pharmaceutical care also impacts health care costs.

Table 2-27 Comparison of goals met at follow-up evaluation

Outcomes	Patients < 65 yrs old (n = 2720)		Patients ≥ 65 yrs old (n = 1772)	
	Goals of therapy at first encounter	Goals of therapy at most recent encounter	Goals of therapy at first encounter	Goals of therapy at most recent encounter
Goals met	6161 (67.2%)	8296 (90.5%)	7434 (77.6%)	8684 (90.6%)
Goals not met	888 (9.7%)	873 (9.5%)	1005 (10.5%)	898 (9.4%)
Initial therapy	2120 (23.1%)	0 (0.0%)	1143 (11.9%)	0 (0.0%)

Validation of Care Provided by Pharmaceutical Care Practitioners

A significant portion of care provided to patients evaluated in this sample was provided by practitioners in the Fairview Clinic System in Minneapolis-St. Paul, Minnesota. Recently, a study was undertaken to determine the quality of the therapeutic determinations made by practitioners in the course of providing pharmaceutical care.[14] A 12-member panel of physicians and pharmaceutical care practitioners reviewed randomly selected blinded patient records (documented in the Assurance system described earlier in the chapter) and used an implicit review process to evaluate the clinical credibility of therapeutic determinations made and documented by pharmaceutical care practitioners.

In 2524 patients receiving pharmaceutical care, a total of 5780 drug therapy problems was resolved. A total of 4779 evaluations of clinical decisions was made in the evaluation. Goals achieved increased from 74% at the initial visit to 89% at the patients' latest encounter.

The panel was asked to validate the decisions documented by the pharmaceutical care practitioner in the areas of indication for drug therapy, identification of drug therapy problems, interventions to resolve drug therapy problems, clinical status of the patient's medical condition being treated with drug therapy, and the economic impact of the pharmaceutical care service provided to the patient.

Panelists indicated agreement with the practitioner's evaluations in 94.2% of cases, whereas a neutral opinion was made in 3.6% of the cases and disagreement occurred in 2.2% of the cases. Intraclass correlation coefficients ranged from 0.73 to 0.85. The authors concluded that the decisions made by pharmaceutical care practitioners were valid or clinically credible based on the evaluations and comments of peer review panels.[14] With the clinical results of the practitioner's care validated, the economic impact was evaluated.

THE ECONOMIC IMPACT OF THE PRACTICE

The impact of pharmaceutical care on drug product costs was analyzed separately from the impact on health care costs because they represent different decisions. Table 2-28 demonstrates that practitioner decisions both increase drug costs and decrease drug costs depending on the patient's needs. Drug costs are generally increased when medication is added to a patient's regimen in order to prevent or treat medical problems that are not being treated appropriately. As previously noted, this occurred frequently ($n = 2355$). The drug costs for a patient were often decreased ($n = 1317$)

Table 2-28   Impact of pharmaceutical care on medication costs

Medication interventions	Patients < 65 yrs old	Patients ≥ 65 yrs old	Total
Interventions	$n = 1098$	$n = 1257$	$n = 2355$
Total increase in medication costs for a 90-day period	$58,559	$64,075	$122,634
Average increase in medication costs per intervention	$53.33	$50.97	$52.07
Interventions	$n = 509$	$n = 808$	$n = 1317$
Total decrease in medication costs for a 90-day period	$45,309	$100,410	$145,719
Average decrease in medication costs per intervention	$89.02	$124.27	$110.64

when medication use was decreased or discontinued due to toxicities, adverse reactions, or unnecessary drug therapy.

Pharmaceutical care can minimize drug costs. The data in Table 2-28 suggest that practitioners initiate therapy with less expensive products and discontinue more expensive drug therapies. When new drug therapies were initiated or dosages or compliance were increased, the average medication costs went up by $52 over a 3 month period. When medication use was decreased by discontinuing drugs or reducing dosages, the average savings was $110 over a 3 month period. The ninety day time period was used to ensure a conservative estimate of savings. The net change was to decrease the patient's drug costs by approximately $58 per occurrence.

These data demonstrate that the cost of the drug product is rarely the primary issue.

Health Care Savings

Even more significant than drug costs are the costs associated with medical care in general. When a practitioner can save a clinic visit, an employee work day, or an emergency room visit, the practitioner has saved the patient and the health care system a substantial amount of money. All health care savings documented by the pharmaceutical care practitioners were reviewed and audited by an independent analyst. This method of estimating health care cost savings has been found to be valid when assessed by a peer review process.[14]

The documented health care savings for these two patient groups were indeed substantial. These figures are displayed in Table 2-29. Over $1.2 million in nondrug health care expenses were avoided through the provision of pharmaceutical care. These results were calculated using the U.S. National Average Expenses for 2001.

A substantial portion of nondrug savings results from eliminating the need for unnecessary clinic visits due to inappropriate or inadequate drug therapy results. With the pharmaceutical care practitioner resolving drug therapy problems and thus making the patient's pharmacotherapy more effective and safe, physician office visits primarily to respond to medication-related issues were avoided.

Substantial savings were also realized by avoiding a total of 31 hospitalizations and 148 emergency department visits due to drug-related morbidity. Each time the practitioner determined that either a hospital admission or an emergency department visit was avoided, additional documentation of agreement by the patient and or the patient's primary physician was required. This additional level of requiring a second source to verify savings was not burdensome as these two types of savings occurred in approximately 7 of every 1000 pharmaceutical care encounters.

These validated savings represent an average of $297 per patient receiving pharmaceutical care. In the younger group the average savings was $258, while in the older patients, an average of $355 in health care expenses was avoided.

These data are based on published national averages and are quite conservative.[16–22] They only include savings that might be realized as a direct consequence of the pharmaceutical care encounter. They do not account for any longer term savings that occurred as a result of implementing preventive drug therapies such as aspirin to prevent myocardial infarction and stroke, calcium supplement to prevent osteoporosis and fractures, or immunizations to prevent the flu or pneumonia.

The resource-based relative value scale described in Chapter 14 was used to determine the cost of providing pharmaceutical care.[1,12,13] The charge for each encounter was determined based on the complexity of the patient's drug-related needs and averaged $29.42 per encounter (refer to Fig. 2-5). Taking into account all 26,238 patient encounters, including those at which no savings occurred, the savings to cost ratio was 2:1. These data support the observation that pharmaceutical care not only improves patient health,

Table 2-29 Health care savings from pharmaceutical care services

Health care savings[*]	Patient < 65 yrs old 3064 patients 18,363 encounters		Patients ≥ 65 yrs old 2072 patients 7,875 encounters		Totals $ Savings
	No. of events	$ Savings	No. of events	$ Savings	
Clinic outpatient visit avoided ($265/visit)[16]	908	$240,620	1089	$288,585	$529,205
Specialty office visit avoided ($304/visit)[17]	69	$20,976	101	$30,704	$51,680
Employee work days saved ($237/day)[18]	102	$24,174	10	$2,370	$26,544
Laboratory service avoided ($24/test)[19]	118	$2,832	223	$5,352	$8,184
Urgent care visit avoided ($82/visit)[17]	29	$2,378	22	$1,804	$4,182
Home health care visit avoided ($271/visit)[20]	7	$1,897	9	$2,439	$4,336
Long-term care admission avoided ($56,000/1 year)[17,21,22]	4	$224,000	2	$112,000	$336,000
Emergency department visit avoided ($452/visit)[17,20]	70	$31,640	78	$35,256	$66,896
Hospital admission avoided ($16,091/admission)[22]	15	$241,365	16	$257,456	$498,821
Totals		$789,882		$735,966	**$1,525,848**

[*]Health care savings are represented by U.S. national averages for 2001.

Table 2-30 Referrals to identify problems early and prevent illness

Referral	Patients < 65 yrs old No. of events	Patients ≥ 65 yrs old No. of events	Total No. of events
Clinic office visit	31	66	97
Specialty office visit	5	8	13
Laboratory preventive monitoring	50	104	154
Emergency department referral	3	3	6
Hospital referral	0	3	3

but it also saves health care resources. For every dollar invested in the provision of pharmaceutical care to ambulatory patients, $2.00 can be saved by reducing the need for other health care services. Pharmaceutical care that ensures the appropriate and rational use of modern, effective pharmacotherapies is one of the most cost-effective health care services available to patients.[15]

One of the responsibilities of the pharmaceutical care practitioner is to refer the patient to another practitioner if he/she is in need of other expertise. This saves the patient from suffering and experiencing future problems and can also save the health care system a tremendous number of medical services (costs) in the future. Table 2-30 describes the number of times referrals were made in each of the two groups. Pharmaceutical care practitioners made timely referrals to medical colleagues in clinics, emergency departments, or hospitals 119 times. These referrals were always made to identify a medical problem early in order to prevent serious morbidity from occurring.

SUMMARY

Pharmaceutical care can benefit many patients. The impact of this practice has been well documented and includes clinical improvement, health care savings, and sometimes both. Positive outcomes were documented in over 90% of cases and $250–$350 in health care savings can be realized in patients receiving pharmaceutical care. In today's health care system, more and more complex pharmacotherapy is used to help patients treat and prevent illness. The need for pharmaceutical care is increasing. More than at any other time in history, there is an opportunity for practitioners who are willing to accept a new set of responsibilities to have a dramatically positive impact on the lives of patients. Chapter 3 describes these new practitioner responsibilities.

EXERCISES

2-1 The data from practice suggest that no single variable (age, number of medical conditions, or number of drug therapies) predicts whether the patient will experience a drug therapy problem. What reasons would you give to explain this?

2-2 Describe how the complexity level of a patient's care impacts the workload and resources required to provide pharmaceutical care.

2-3 Using the philosophy of pharmaceutical care practice, explain why the majority of interventions to resolve drug therapy problems are made directly between the patient and the pharmaceutical care practitioner.

2-4 Which points would you make in a presentation to a health care administrator who wants to know the clinical and economic impact of pharmaceutical care?

REFERENCES

1. Cipolle, R., Strand, L.M., Morley, P.C. *Pharmaceutical Care Practice*. New York: McGraw Hill; 1998.
2. Hensrud, D.D., Engle, D.D., Scheitel, S.M. Underreporting the use of dietary supplements and nonprescription medications among patients undergoing a periodic health examination. *Mayo Clinic Proc.* 1999; 74(5):443–447.
3. Klepser, T.B., Doucette, W.R., Horton, M.R., Buys, L.M., Ernst, M.E., Ford, J.K., Hoehns, J.D., Kautzman, H.A., Logemann, C.D., Swegle, J.M., Ritho, M., Klepser, M.E. Assessment of patients' perceptions and beliefs regarding herbal therapies. *Pharmacotherapy* 2000; 20(1):83–87.
4. National High Blood Pressure Education Programs. The Seventh Report of the Joint National Committee of High Blood Pressure. *Hypertension* 2003 Dec; 42(6):1206–52.
5. Elixhauser, A., Yu, K., Steiner, C., Bierman, A.S. *Hospitalization in the United States, 1997: HCUP Fact Book No. 1.* www.ahrq.gov/data/hcup/factbk1/hcupfbk1.pdf accessed on 2/18/03, Agency for Healthcare Research and Quality: Rockville, MD; 2000.
6. Johnson, J.A., Bootman, J.L. Drug-related morbidity and mortality. *Am J Health Syst Pharm* 1997; 54(5):554–558.
7. Ernst, F.R., Grizzle, A.J. Drug-related morbidity and mortality: updating the cost-of-illness model. *J Am Pharm Assoc* 2001; 41(2):192–199.
8. Otero, M.J., Dominguez-Gil, A., Bajo, A.A., Maderuelo, J.A. Characteristics associated with ability to prevent adverse drug reactions in hospitalized patients—a comment. *Pharmacotherapy* 1999; 19(10):1185–1187.
9. Stergachis, A., Hazlet, T.K. Chapter 8: Pharmacoepidemiology, in: Dipiro, J.T., et al. (eds), *Pharmacotherapy—A Pathophysiologic Approach*. New York: McGraw-Hill; 2002, p. 94.
10. A Closer Look at Arthritis. www.npcnow.org/issues_productlist/pdf/ arthritis%20final.pdf, National Pharmaceutical Council & The Arthritis Foundation.
11. Bungard, T.J., Ackman, M.L., Geotham, H., Tsuyuki, R.T. Adequacy of Anticoagulation in Patients with Atrial Fibrillation Coming to a Hospital. *Pharmacotherapy* 2000; 20(9):1060–1065.

12. AMA, *American Medical Association. Medicare Physician Payment Reform: The Physicians' Guide*, vol. 1. Chicago: American Medical Association; 1992.

13. AMA, *American Medical Association: Medicare RBRVS: The Physicians' Guide 2000*: Chapter 4: The Physician Work Component; Gallagher, P.E. (ed), Chicago: American Medical Association: 2000, p. 26–37.

14. Isetts, B.J., Brown, L.B., Schondelmeyer, S.W., Lenarz, L.A. Quality assessment of a collaborative approach for decreasing drug-related morbidity and achieving therapeutic goals. *Arch Intern Med* 2003; 163(15):1813–1820.

15. ACCP, American College of Clinical Pharmacy: A vision of pharmacy's future roles, responsibilities, and manpower needs in the United States. *Pharmacotherapy* 2000; 20(8):991–1020.

16. *Statistics 1998–2002:* www.cms.hhs.gov/statistics/health-indicators/t1.asp, Centers for Medicare & Medicaid Services.

17. HCCA, *2002 Physicians Fee and Coding Guide.* Augusta, GA: Health Care Consultants of America, Inc.; 2001.

18. *2000 to 2001 Supplementary Surveys Change Profile United States*, U.S. Census Bureau, Demographic Surveys Division, Continuous Measurement Office.

19. www.cms.hhs.gov/providers/pufdownload/clfdown.asp. CMS. Accessed May 20, 2003.

20. American Diabetes Association—Tables for Economic Costs of Diabetes in the US in 2002. *Diabetes Care* 2003; 26(3):917–932.

21. www.research.aarp.org/health/fs10r_nursing.htm, AARP. Accessed May 2003.

22. www.research.aarp.org/health/fs86_cna.htm, AARP. Accessed May 2003.

THREE

THE PRACTITIONER'S RESPONSIBILITIES

Key Concepts

1. *The pharmaceutical care practitioner's responsibility is to determine that all of the patient's drug-related needs are met at all times. This means that (a) all of a patient's drug therapy is used appropriately for each medical condition; (b) the patient's drug therapy is the most effective available; (c) the patient's drug therapy is the safest possible; and (d) the patient is able and willing to take the medication as intended.*

2 *The pharmaceutical care practitioner's responsibilities include the identification, resolution, and prevention of drug therapy problems.*

3 *The pharmaceutical care practitioner's responsibilities are to ensure that the goals of therapy are met for each of the patient's medical conditions and desired outcomes are achieved.*

4 *These responsibilities are fulfilled by caring for each patient as an individual in a way that benefits the patient, minimizes harm, and is honest, fair, and ethical.*

5 *The pharmaceutical care practitioner fulfills these clinical responsibilities by meeting the standards for professional and ethical behavior prescribed within the philosophy of pharmaceutical care practice.*

6 *The standards for professional behavior include providing pharmaceutical care at a specified standard of care, being ethical in all decision-making, displaying collegiality, collaborating, maintaining competency, applying research findings where appropriate, and being sensitive to limited resources.*

7 *It is the pharmaceutical care practitioner's responsibility to hold colleagues accountable to the same standards of professional performance. The success of the practice will depend upon it.*

8 *Do the very best you can for every patient. In all cases, do no harm. Tell the patient the truth. Be fair. Be loyal. Recognize that the patient is the ultimate decision maker. Always protect your patient's privacy.*

Becoming a patient care provider is not complicated, but it requires the development of a number of dimensions of both character and behavior. In this chapter, we will discuss the responsibilities of the pharmaceutical care practitioner that will shape both. We will begin with the most visible of responsibilities in practice: identifying and meeting a patient's drug-related needs. Then we will discuss the responsibilities involved in caring for a patient. The ethical responsibilities of the practitioner are discussed in the second section of this chapter. The principles and the behaviors consistent with these responsibilities are presented. Finally, the standards for professional behavior are discussed.

PRACTICE RESPONSIBILITIES

The pharmaceutical care practitioner provides direct patient care. This means that the first responsibility is to the patient. When individuals choose to become pharmaceutical care practitioners, they make a commitment to meet the patient's drug-related needs whenever and wherever they might arise. Although such practitioners will work with a number of other health care providers, managers, and administrators, they will be accountable to patients first and colleagues second. Placing patients' needs before personal needs and all other obligations is central to pharmaceutical care practice.

Providing direct patient care means taking responsibility for a patient's drug-related needs—one patient at a time. It is important to provide comprehensive care of the same quality to all patients. Although the interventions may differ based upon the specific needs of each patient, the practitioner will always perform the same set of core functions.

All of the following responsibilities must be met for each patient, and they are considered nonnegotiable with respect to providing pharmaceutical care.

Understand who the patient is and what he/she wants from the practitioner   Practitioners make all clinical decisions in the context of a specific patient. Many patient parameters influence decisions regarding drug therapy. It is important to become familiar with, and knowledgeable about, the whole patient and to create a pharmacologically relevant description of this individual.

This can be accomplished when clinicians understand the patient's medication experience. The medication experience includes the patient's description of his/her beliefs, preferences, concerns, and behaviors concerning drug therapy, as well as the medication history, current medication record, social drug history, allergies, and alerts.

Assess each patient's medical conditions and associated drug therapies for appropriate indication, effectiveness, safety, and the patient's compliance   It is essential to assess the patient's medical conditions and drug therapies to determine if each of the medications is appropriately indicated for the medical condition or illness, if it is the most effective product available for that indication, if the dosage regimen will be effective or if it will produce toxicity, if the patient is experiencing any adverse effects from the medication, and the degree to which the patient has been compliant. This assessment ensures that all the patient's medical conditions that can benefit from drug therapy are being managed with medication and determines if the patient's medication is being taken in a manner that results in the desired outcomes.

This means that a number of clinical questions about a patient's pharmacotherapy must be asked:

- Is the medication necessary?
- Is it the best product?
- What is the correct dose?
- How frequently and for what duration should the patient take it?
- Will it cause side effects?
- Does it interact with other medications?
- Does the patient understand how to use the product?
- Is the patient able and willing to use the drug product?

The answers to these questions will guide practitioners in making decisions in a logical manner using the systematic, rational decision-making process of the Pharmacotherapy Workup. A consistent and rational approach is necessary because many decisions will have important consequences for the patient. This process is thorough and logical so when positive outcomes occur, clinicians can understand why these transpired, and learn from the experience. Similarly, when the patient experiences a negative outcome, it is essential to take corrective action, and learn from this experience. Drug therapy can be effective but not safe or safe but not effective. A standard, rational approach determines the most effective pharmacotherapy and the safest pharmacotherapy for this patient.

Identify drug therapy problems because they interfere with achieving the goals of therapy   Drug therapy problems can occur anywhere in the medication use process, from product selection to treatment outcome. Pharmaceutical care practitioners will identify these problems because no other practitioner systematically and comprehensively evaluates the patient's medications for drug therapy problems. This contribution is unique and significant because drug therapy problems that prevent patients from experiencing the full benefit of effective and safe drug therapy occur in many patients who require pharmacotherapy. Drug therapy problems are costly to the patient in terms of pain and suffering. Treatment failures are also costly in terms of hospitalizations, additional clinic visits, and lost days at work or school.

Develop a plan that establishes the desired goals of therapy for each of the patient's medical conditions   All forms of pharmacotherapy are intended to achieve specific positive effects. These goals of therapy guide the selection of drug products and determine the acceptable risk in selecting each dosage regimen. Establishing achievable goals of therapy requires an understanding of the patient's preferences because goals represent a negotiation between practitioner and patient. Goals of therapy establish the criteria upon which the outcomes of all pharmacotherapy are evaluated, both positive and negative.

Make appropriate interventions to resolve drug therapy problems, achieve the goals of therapy, and prevent drug therapy problems from occurring   Resolving drug therapy problems benefits the patient directly. Practitioners intervene to resolve drug therapy problems by taking actions such as changing the drug product, increasing the dosage regimen, decreasing the dosage, discontinuing drug therapies, or providing additional medications to prevent illness. Another benefit derived from the pharmaceutical care practitioner is preventing drug therapy problems. When a specific patient is at an unacceptably high risk of developing a side effect, toxicity, or experiencing a treatment failure, the practitioner identifies these individual risks and takes action to prevent the problems from occurring. From the patient's perspective, this responsibility can be one of the most important.

Pharmaceutical care practitioners intervene whenever possible to positively influence the patient's medication experience. Educating patients, perhaps referring patients to other helpful practitioners, providing advice and support, obtaining necessary services or technologies, and helping the patient to obtain affordable medication may all be necessary to optimize patient outcomes from drug therapies.

Follow-up with the patient to evaluate the results of pharmacotherapies, recommendations, and other interventions   The responsibility to follow-up with the patient is absolute. In fact, if there is no follow-up, the patient may interpret this to mean that no one cares about him/her. If there is no follow-up, you will not know if the drug therapy was effective or if it caused harm. It is unacceptable to make recommendations and intervene with drug therapies in a patient's life without determining the outcome of actions. It is vital to determine the patient's progress toward achieving the goals of therapy, assess the effectiveness of medications, and assess whether any safety issues have developed. This is where clinicians are held accountable for their actions. They learn from decisions and patient experiences. The follow-up evaluation works to strengthen the therapeutic relationship.

Continue to manage your patient's drug therapy until the goals of therapy are achieved   Once responsibility is taken for a patient's medications, it is necessary to follow-up until a successful outcome has been achieved. It shows a lack of professional responsibility to assume that someone else will accept the responsibility or that patients will *manage* on their own. Continuous, excellent care is necessary for patients to benefit optimally from their medications.

The professional responsibilities described above prescribes the activities performed on a daily basis when pharmaceutical care is provided. It will be important to learn the knowledge and skills necessary to fulfill these responsibilities in an efficient and effective manner. However, knowledge and skills are not enough to guarantee success in practice. A philosophy of practice is required to explain how these responsibilities should be conducted.

THE PRACTITIONER'S PHILOSOPHY OF PRACTICE

All of the values described in this chapter constitute the foundation of the practitioner's philosophy of practice. The practitioner must internalize the philosophy of practice before he or she cares for patients.

Definition   A philosophy of practice is a set of values that guides the behavior of a professional. It helps the practitioner determine what is important, how to set priorities, and how to make clinical decisions and judgments. The philosophy of practice prescribes how a practitioner should practice on a daily basis. It is a set of rules the practitioner must follow to meet the standards of practice.

All practitioners within a profession adhere to the same philosophy of practice thus creating uniform behavior and standards. Without a common set of values, each practitioner would be free to use a different approach and establish different standards of care, and therefore could not be held accountable to patients or colleagues. This randomness of commitment, actions, and services would be harmful and confusing to patients and others within the health care system.

Note   The philosophy of pharmaceutical care practice requires the acceptance of the social obligation to minimize drug-related morbidity and mortality. Practitioners accomplish this by meeting the expectations of the caring paradigm: assessing the patient's drug-related needs, bringing the necessary resources to meet those needs, and following up to determine that the needs have been met.

THE RESPONSIBILITY TO CARE

From the discussion of the practice in Chapter 1 and the responsibilities just described, it is clear that *the concept of care is foundational to pharmaceutical care practice*. Within the context of health, care derives from two different—but complementary—concerns:

1. The technical dimensions of taking care of patients.
2. Caring for or about a particular patient, thereby demonstrating a concern for and commitment to the well-being of another person, usually a stranger.[1]

The first of these has already been quite extensively explained. While it is essential that competent practitioners focus on the therapeutic agent in question, there is much more to the provision of pharmaceutical care.

The second concern identifies the patient as the *center of attention*. Authentic caring as a practice involves an understanding of the patient's needs, goals, and concerns. Care is *the moral integrity* of any professional's practice.[1,2]

Understanding the patient as an individual and taking the time to *know* the patient's medication experience, which is explained in detail in Chapter 5, allows the clinician to achieve an "understanding of the 'whole patient' in his life situation."[3] This important point cannot be over emphasized.

In order to balance the technical dimensions of taking care of patients, the practice of pharmaceutical care was designed to be patient-centered. For many decades medicine and nursing have fought to maintain the patient-centeredness of their practices, so it is important that pharmaceutical care begins with a strong understanding of and commitment to patient-centered practice.

Patient-centered Approach

Patient-centeredness places the patient at the *center of attention*, at all times, in all situations, regardless of the practitioner's demands, time constraints, or personality characteristics. Patient-centeredness prescribes the behavior of the practitioner toward the patient during the patient care process.

When thinking and acting in a caring manner with the patient at the center of the practice, practitioners will:[4]

- place the patients' needs, wants, and preferences before their own;
- serve as advocates and do what is best for the patient, regardless of what it requires on their part;
- treat patients as individuals—be sensitive to cultures and belief systems, without being patronizing or condescending;

- respect patients' time and priorities by committing full attention to them;
- remain conscious of patients' value system, and be prepared to identify and resolve ethical dilemmas in an honest and straightforward manner.

When these behaviors become internalized and reflect a commonly held standard to which practitioners adhere on a daily basis, a patient-centered approach to practice will develop.

The patient-centered approach considers the patient as a whole individual whose health care needs generally, and drug-related needs specifically, are the primary concern of the practitioner.[4,5] The patient is seen as an individual with rights, knowledge, and experience, all of which are necessary for the practitioner to fulfill his or her responsibilities.[5] This approach requires that the practitioner treat the patient as a partner in care planning and always as the ultimate decision maker, because the patient experiences the ultimate consequences of pharmacotherapy. Most importantly, this approach prevents the patient from being seen as a repository for drugs to be assessed and evaluated. It also prevents the individual from being defined as a conglomerate of organ systems and drug reactions. Such objectification is unacceptable to the pharmaceutical care practitioner.

A patient-centered approach means that all of the patient's concerns, expectations, and understanding of his or her illness—and associated pharmacotherapy—become the practitioner's responsibility. In addition, the patient-centered approach insists that the patient's needs, not the practitioner's preferences, *drive* the practice of pharmaceutical care. In a pragmatic sense, this means that the practitioner will start with the patient's needs and provide care until all of these needs are met. This means that the practitioner will do whatever is necessary to meet the drug-related needs of the patient.

The patient-centered approach prescribes behaviors as we just described, but it does more than that. It prescribes the values that must drive the practitioner in his/her interaction with the patient. Decisions will be made that affect another individual using knowledge and experience not possessed by that person. These decisions can lead to dramatic consequences, which are often positive, but are sometimes negative. Essential to the practice of pharmaceutical care is a set of values that can guide the appropriate decisions in situations where there is uncertainty, where there are multiple acceptable answers, where there may be ethical dilemmas, and where it can be difficult to know what to do. Let us consider the role that values play in patient care.

THE VALUES INVOLVED IN CARING FOR PATIENTS

Pharmaceutical care practice is inherently value-laden. Values, or that which we consider worthy, are central to all interventions in the lives of others. As Guttman observes:

> Values are embedded in all facets of the intervention process and both influence and serve as justification for the choice of the intervention goals and objectives.[6]

For the pharmaceutical care practitioner, this fact is of vital importance. Clinical intervention is much more than the accurate, competent application of technical knowledge to the resolution of health problems. It is also the value-laden context in which the clinician struggles with the process of decision-making, judgment, and justification for choices made.

The first step to dealing with these situations successfully on a daily and patient-specific basis, is to separate your personal values from the professional values that are required to provide care to others. This is difficult for new, young practitioners because in order to separate one set of values from another, one must be conscious of what one's personal values are. To become conscious of these values, it is necessary to engage in critical thinking in an area usually referred to as *values clarification.*

Values clarification is an essential step in the development of a pharmaceutical care practitioner as it leads to greater self-awareness. Practitioners who engage in a reflective process to become more conscious of what they value or consider worthy, do the following:

- Understand one's beliefs and behaviors, which includes knowing what one does and does not support, and communicating this to others.
- Choose one's beliefs and behaviors by evaluating values received from others, which includes examining alternatives and their consequences, then deciding what are one's own.
- Act on these beliefs with a consistent pattern that reinforces actions supportive of the values.[6–8]

A personal set of values will include political views, religious beliefs, social norms, personal preferences, and influence from personal experiences. Practitioners must become consciously aware of these personal values so that they know when they create conflict in the practice setting.

Note Problems can develop in practice when practitioners confuse personal values with professional values and when they impose personal values onto the patient.

Personal values must be kept separate from professional values, because personal values are private while professional values are public and prescribed by the practicing community.

From Values to Ethics

The leap from values to ethics is in reality a short one. Values help to shape what is individually conceived as right and wrong, and this drives the decisions and interventions made in practice. Ethics is a system of understanding what motivates and determines our behavior, based upon individual conceptions of right and wrong.[9] Moreover, ethics helps us to address the question "What should I do in this situation?" Ethics offers a formal process for applying moral dimensions to our actions.[9]

A strong case can be made for including ethical reflection within the context of pharmaceutical care practice. Indeed, we argue that such a focus is essential to practice and is closely tied to care. Accepting responsibility for the outcomes of another person's drug therapies is not a complex commitment, but it is a serious commitment.

Husted and Husted[2,10] put forward the following decision-making principles as *natural* in all interactions:

- Every patient has a right to be treated according to his/her unique character.
- Every patient has a right to decide and act on his/her own values to fulfill individual life plans.
- Every patient has a right to expect complete objective information and the emotional support necessary to act effectively on that information.
- Every patient has the right, alone or through a health care professional, to the control of his/her time and effort.
- Every patient has a right to expect whatever benefit is possible in the health care setting and to expect no avoidable harm.
- Every patient has a right to expect that agreements established with the health care professionals will be kept.[10]

Such principles as these provide ethical justification for a certain standard of care. Hence, they are useful for practitioners to *push against* while exploring their personal values and ethical positions. Can you readily and unreservedly accept these principles? How do they affect your professional obligations, responsibilities, and duties to patients? What will you do when you cannot accept any one of these? These questions, and others, are important to ask at all stages of values/ethics exploration.

Ethics in Practice

The practice of pharmaceutical care will create situations that have the potential to involve ethical dilemmas. Two individuals (patient and practitioner) perhaps from different cultures, with different values and levels of knowledge are meeting to address life-changing issues of disease and treatment. This is occurring in a society that is increasingly dependent on technology and that has limited financial resources coupled with an increased demand for services. Any one of these situations can lead to an ethical dilemma.

Every practitioner must be prepared to recognize, and even prevent, situations with moral and ethical implications. This requires the practitioner be prepared with (1) insight of his/her own values, cultural norms, moral development, and ethical principles; (2) time, focused attention, and sensitivity to recognize subtle clues that may indicate a situation is laden with ethical components; and (3) the knowledge and aptitude for making logical, fair, and consistent decisions.

Basic professional behavior can go a long way in helping to avoid ethical dilemmas. Each of these important behaviors is based on an ethical principle and is described in Table 3-1 below. Pharmaceutical care practitioners will learn these behaviors and make them a consistent part of every day practice.

It is useful to briefly discuss each of these and place them in the context of pharmaceutical care.

Beneficence   The ethical practitioner will want to do what is best for the patient. While perhaps exceptionally well-informed on pharmacological matters, we have seen that in itself, this does not mean that the practitioner knows best. Clearly, when the centrality of the patient and his/her preferences

Table 3-1   Basic professional behaviors expected in practice

Professional behavior	Ethical principle
Do the very best you can for every patient	Beneficence
In all cases, do no harm	Nonmaleficence
Tell the patient the truth	Veracity
Be fair	Justice
Be loyal	Fidelity
Allow the patient to be the ultimate decision maker	Autonomy/paternalism
Always protect your patient's privacy	Confidentiality

are considered, deciding what is best under any circumstance involves more than professional opinion and alternatives. For example, deciding the burdens and benefits of therapeutic protocols cannot be carried out without the involvement of the patient. Patients will decide what risks to take, what benefits they desire, and what burdens they are willing and able to endure.

While the *expert* may be capable of calculating the technical dimensions of risk and uncertainty based on empirical evidence, once this is communicated to the patient, he/she must decide the course of action. Beneficence—doing what is best for the patient—is therefore negotiated between two parties rather than imposed even if what is best for the patient seems to be *clinically obvious*.

> **Rule** A simple rule of thumb is to consider all available information, engage in free noncoercive discussion with the patient, facilitate decisions that derive from this individual, and serve his/her best interests.

Nonmaleficence All health care practitioners are familiar with the Hippocratic principle of *primum non nocere, or above all, do no harm.* This can be seen as linked to the principle of beneficence. However, while we may all agree that any principles opposed to inflicting harm must be accepted, it is reasonable to suggest that wherever there is risk, there is the potential to harm.[11]

At no time should the pharmaceutical care practitioner aggressively force a treatment on a patient. No matter what justification is offered, whether in the name of pharmaceutical science, clinical evidence, or practitioner preference, the clinician who performs without due regard for the patient's considerations acts maleficently. In this sense, the end does not justify the means.

Veracity It sounds simple to insist that practitioners tell the truth at all times. Keep in mind that there are many questions that must be explored. Should we tell the truth at all times? Is it ever ethical not to tell the patient the truth? Can telling the truth harm people? If so, under what circumstances? Can we lie when we consider it in the best interest of our patients? Does lying sometimes protect people? Why not deceive a patient if it promotes his/her health and recovery? Does this particular patient want bad news? Will a bleak prognosis harm the patient? Why not withhold certain information? Is nondisclosure a form of lying? Do we need to tell the patient everything? Don't we confuse patients with all this information?

These are but a few of the questions that emerge in any discussion related to truth-telling. There are no formulaic answers unless one adopts the position that the truth will be told at all costs regardless of the consequences. While we endorse the ethical principle of veracity, and believe honesty to be a highly regarded part of character, we also recognize that in practical terms, grounded in the realities of human suffering, individual practitioners are fallible creatures, and often lack the emotional strength necessary to tell the complete truth if they are convinced that it will harm the patient. Emotional strength, conscience, and often clinical judgment can present barriers to truth-telling.

Those providing care devote considerable time reflecting upon the nature and practice of truth-telling and its place in the therapeutic relationship. Can there be trust based on deception and lies? Does it matter how small the lie, how insignificant the deception? What if it worked, and the patient recovered? Those who provide care, respect patients, and recognize the importance of trust in the therapeutic relationship must ask themselves how they can transmit peace of mind to those who willingly place themselves in the hands of strangers.

Does it really come down to a personal choice? Not exactly. Truth-telling may be a skill that can be learned with practice. Providing patients with bad news is difficult and sometimes heartbreaking. It may seem easier to equivocate, be vague, or even mumble. Rest assured, in the end, *the truth will win out*. Individuals in trouble, often weak, vulnerable, and impoverished in spirit, seem to find the truth.

In the end, the principle of veracity can only serve the best interests of the patient. Sensitivity and thoughtful communication skills on the part of the pharmaceutical care practitioner can be learned and *polished* with experience.[12-14] Once initial formative trust is established and a therapeutic relationship is developed, honesty should be unconditional and reciprocal. In order to accomplish this it is useful to make honesty a part of therapeutic discourse. Outline the expectation of truth, emphasize its importance, and nurture its development. Only when truth is a central piece of a relationship can a care plan be created with any hope of success.

Justice Justice is an ethical principle "that relates to fair, equitable, and appropriate treatment in the light of what is due or owed to persons. The principle of justice recognizes that giving to some may deny receipt to others."[7] Frequently, patient circumstances raise serious considerations of fairness and justice. Not all patients can afford essential drugs. Is it appropriate to accept what are generally described as *the morals of the marketplace*? Clearly, practitioners, who are predominantly employees, cannot *give away the store*. What are their responsibilities to the poor who need assistance? What of the uninformed patient who does not understand insurance options and limitations? Is it ethical to refuse to serve uninsured patients? This has become a serious issue when practitioners claim that insurance does not *pay enough* to cover expenses.

Once again there is no easy fix for issues arising from questions of justice. At the outset the problem is systemic in that the distribution of goods and services in a market-driven economy is always going to be inequitable, uneven, and—for many, of questionable fairness. Presently in the United States, we do not have a national health system, and there is no common acceptance of the idea that health care is a fundamental social right. Given the prevailing realities of our social norms and values, pharmaceutical care practitioners must resolve problems within the context of what *is*, not what *ought to be*. Most practitioners are aware of such matters and will endorse a pragmatic approach to each case as it presents itself.

In effect, it is reasonable to expect the ethical pharmaceutical care practitioner to make every effort to treat all patients equally and assist those who are legitimately disadvantaged by locating information and programs that will meet their needs. This is not to suggest that all pharmaceutical care practitioners should become social workers, but rather to know the health care system in general and policies in particular and use this information to solve a patient's problems of access to care and pharmaceuticals.

Practitioners will be expected to adhere to the principle of equality in so much as they care for patients as equals regardless of ethnicity, class, gender, or sexual preference. Discrimination of any kind is unacceptable, unethical, and intolerable.

Fidelity   This is an ethical principle that relates "to the concept of faithfulness and the practice of keeping promises."[7] Pharmaceutical care practitioners are granted authority to practice by a society that regulates competition through licensure and thereby protects the self-interests of the profession. In a real sense, such a social contract provides privileges to an elite group, and in doing so demands accountability. Burkhardt and Nathaniel, while specifically referring to nurses, put the case well:

> The process of licensure is one that ensures no other group can practice within the domain of (pharmaceutical care) as defined by society and the profession. Thus, to accept licensure and become legitimate members of the profession mandates that (pharmaceutical care practitioners) uphold the responsibilities inherent in the contract with society.[7]

While we have inserted *pharmaceutical care practitioner* where they had written *nurse*, the same conditions apply. Pharmaceutical care practitioners are expected to "be faithful to the society that grants the right to practice."[7] Moreover, they are expected to:

> Keep the promise of upholding the profession's code of ethics, to practice within the established scope of practice and definition of (pharmaceutical care), to remain competent in practice, to abide by the policies of employing institutions, and to keep promises to individual patients.[7]

To be a pharmaceutical care practitioner is to make and keep promises to patients. Of course, it can readily be seen that fidelity is related to trust as an essential part of any meaningful therapeutic relationship.

Promises can be hard to keep in patient care, particularly when they are based on hope or reassurance. The often heard *I promise—you will be all right*, meant to reassure, and perhaps motivate the patient, all too often cannot deliver the promised outcome. In short, there can be no absolute promises, or immutable duty to keep them.[7] The ethical pharmaceutical care practitioner should keep in mind "that in every case, harmful consequences of the promised action should be weighed against the benefits of keeping the promise."[7]

Autonomy　No one is entirely self-governing. For the purpose of ethics discourse, however, the concept of autonomy refers to a patient having the freedom to make choices for him or herself. In this sense, it implies that an individual is free from coercion or threat and can make informed decisions as a free agent. This does not mean that other individuals play no role in influencing the choices people make, rather, it means that individual choices are respected and subsequent interventions are predicated on respect. This is particularly true when the patient's choices conflict with those of the practitioner. Respect for patients is mandatory. Without it there can be no trust, no therapeutic relationship, and no care.

Of course everything has limits. In the case of autonomy, while respect should be ever present, there are serious considerations to be taken into account when formulating a care plan. Does the patient have a clear understanding of all important facts and values? How do I know if the patient is cognitively competent and can make informed, autonomous decisions? Is the confused patient acting autonomously? These questions may sound rhetorical, but they are frequently asked, and uncertainty is common. Some patients—children and the mentally incompetent, for example—are not thought capable of making autonomous decisions.

Respect for the patient's autonomy is essential in pharmaceutical care practice. Trust, and the necessary therapeutic relationship—the *covenant*[15]— cannot become a shared reality unless, and until, respect is established.

Failure to take this foundational principle seriously makes a mockery of any claim to have provided care, and most certainly offers very little assistance that is meaningful to those seeking help.

Paternalism is not the answer   Setting aside the child or otherwise dependent patient, there are very few occasions when paternalism should be acted upon. Paternalism refers to "the practice of overriding or ignoring preferences of patients to benefit them or enhance their welfare."[16] Moreover, paternalism represents the judgment that beneficence takes priority over autonomy.[16]

Pharmaceutical care is committed to *informed* patient preference. As stated earlier, the pharmaceutical care practitioner and the patient form a therapeutic alliance where the patient is given to understand the pharmaceutical care practitioner's responsibilities and duties and, most importantly, understands his/her personal responsibilities in relation to those of the practitioner. In effect, both the practitioner and patient must have a clear understanding of the rules, roles, and responsibilities central to the therapeutic relationship. Without such an understanding there can be no meaningful relationship that produces positive outcomes.

The authoritative and univocal allocation of pharmaceutical fact[17] and value does not result in productive communication. It is equally doubtful that such an approach will result in too much informed consent or compliance. Therefore, it can be argued that it is both ethically and therapeutically more appropriate to engage in dialogue and develop meaningful two-way communication that maximizes cooperation and meaningful understanding of all facets of the pharmaceutical care experience.

Respect for autonomy is not simply an ethical imperative but it also receives a legal mandate in some instances. For example, the Patient Self-Determination Act of 1990[18] mandates that in all institutions receiving Medicare or Medicaid funding patients must receive written information explicitly stating

- their right to accept or refuse treatment;
- their rights under existing state laws regarding advance directives;
- any policies the institution has regarding the withholding of life-sustaining treatment.

The logical consequence of respect for autonomy and person can only be understood as respect for patient preference. Ethically, it should be the individual's desires, aspirations, and priorities that form the nucleus of pharmaceutical care. Such a view of patient-centered care sets an agenda where the pharmaceutical care practitioner acts as advocate for the patient's well-being.

Pharmaceutical care practice is not possible without due regard to the full implications of patient autonomy and informed consent. Indeed, upon reflection, it is noteworthy that pharmacotherapy is the most common form of treatment found on a daily basis, yet very little attention is focused on consent. While surgery, a much less common invasion on mind and body, requires written consent based on substantive information, pharmacotherapy relies on a less rigorous process of an entirely verbal nature. Some would argue that written consent for every prescription written and filled is not practical or desirable. Traditional patient education practices too often manifest as warnings, technical procedures, and verbal renderings of *package inserts*. While no one doubts the usefulness of accurate information, a pharmaceutical care practitioner monologue too often ensues.

Patient-centered care requires an ethical and clinical commitment to a therapeutic relationship in which accurate, therapeutically optimal drug therapy and drug information is discussed. Options are examined, and the patient communicates a strong sense of understanding. The practitioner has acted ethically and in a clinically appropriate manner when both parties have reached a common understanding of purpose and goals, and a care plan has been jointly negotiated and agreed upon.

Confidentiality   The trust that is built between practitioner and patient is compromised without the assurance of confidentiality. The duty to protect patient confidentiality emerges from a relationship based upon trust.

As a clinician with clearly defined pharmaceutical care responsibilities, you have a duty, within the context of the therapeutic relationship to protect a patient's personal information from public view. This is a well-known fact of clinical life. The expectation of confidentiality is essential to further the free exchange of information between patient and practitioner and should not be taken lightly. Patients must feel that anything they say, the nature of their disease or illness, the medications they take, or any other matter they regard as *private* will be respected.

If the pharmaceutical care practitioner displays a respectful attitude and protects privacy at all times even a nondrug-related transaction can contribute to a relationship that embodies trust and eventually has some therapeutic value. It is simple—at all times, confidentiality is the rule.

These practice responsibilities, the patient-centered approach to pharmaceutical care, and the ethical principles involved in patient care all lead to a set of standards for professional performance. Although these standards are quite self-evident, their statement in an explicit and complete manner is necessary to finish the subject of practitioner responsibilities.

THE STANDARDS FOR PROFESSIONAL BEHAVIOR

Note Caring for others is a privilege that is reserved for those individuals who are uniquely well prepared and who adhere to standards for professional behavior.

All health care professionals are expected to learn and execute a set of behaviors that set them apart because they are working with patients to make decisions that can have significant consequences. The behavior and the standards expected are described as the Standards for Professional Behavior. These were developed for pharmaceutical care practice by adapting those developed for other patient care providers.[4]

These standards refer to the behaviors expected of practitioners who belong to an identifiable group of professionals. Each practitioner is not only expected to adhere to the standards him or herself but to hold his or her colleagues accountable for similar behavior. Even though practitioners are seldom evaluated in any formal or consistent manner, all practitioners *know* whether a colleague is able to maintain these standards in practice on a daily basis.

New practitioners need to internalize the meaning of each standard and become comfortable with the level of expectation associated with the successful application of each standard in practice. Table 3-2 summarizes the seven professional behaviors expected of all pharmaceutical care practitioners. These standards were adapted from nursing, medicine, dentistry, and veterinary models of standards for professional behavior.[19]

One of the cornerstones of a profession is that it is self-regulating. Colleagues hold other colleagues accountable for the quality of the work that is performed. This starts with self-evaluation. It is important to be reflective in practice so that each practitioner comes to know the quality of his/her work. This helps each practitioner improve in practice and contributes to maintaining high standards of professional performance.

The standards of professional performance applied to the practice of pharmaceutical care are described below. The criteria to measure adherence to each standard are also described.

Standard I: Quality of Care

The practitioner evaluates his/her own practice in relation to professional practice standards and relevant statutes and regulations.

Table 3-2 Standards of professional performance for pharmaceutical care practitioners[19]

Category	Standard
Quality of care	The practitioner evaluates his/her own practice in relation to professional practice standards and relevant statutes and regulations.
Ethics	The practitioner's decisions and actions on behalf of patients are determined in an ethical manner.
Collegiality	The pharmaceutical care practitioner contributes to the professional development of peers, colleagues, students, and others.
Collaboration	The practitioner collaborates with the patient, family and/or care-givers, and health care providers in providing patient care.
Education	The practitioner acquires and maintains current knowledge in pharmacology, pharmacotherapy, and pharmaceutical care practice.
Research	The practitioner routinely uses research findings in practice and contributes to research findings when appropriate.
Resource allocation	The practitioner considers factors related to effectiveness, safety, and cost in planning and delivering patient care.

Measurement criteria

1. The pharmaceutical care practitioner uses evidence from the literature to evaluate his/her performance in practice.
2. The pharmaceutical care practitioner seeks peer review on a continual and frequent basis.
3. The pharmaceutical care practitioner utilizes data generated from his/her practice to critically evaluate performance.

A significant amount of discussion has already focused on ethical behavior in practice. Its presence here only helps to emphasize the relative importance of this behavior. Second to providing high quality care is providing care in an ethical manner.

Standard II: Ethics

The practitioner's decisions and actions on behalf of patients are determined in an ethical manner.

Measurement criteria

1. The practitioner maintains patient confidentiality.
2. The practitioner acts as a patient advocate.
3. The practitioner delivers care in a nonjudgmental and nondiscriminatory manner that is sensitive to patient diversity.
4. The practitioner delivers care in a manner that preserves/protects patient autonomy, dignity, and rights.
5. The practitioner seeks available resources to help formulate ethical decisions.

It is common knowledge among experienced practitioners that it is impossible to become a great practitioner without the support and assistance of colleagues. This is especially true as a patient care provider. It is impossible to know everything, experience everything and make the *right* decision in all cases. Therefore, the need to be collegial becomes absolutely necessary. In the end it serves the patient's best interest, but it also serves the practitioner's purpose as well.

Standard III: Collegiality

The pharmaceutical care practitioner contributes to the professional development of peers, colleagues, and others.

Measurement criteria

1. The practitioner offers professional assistance to other practitioners whenever asked.
2. The practitioner promotes relationships with patients, physicians, nurses, and other health care providers.

Patient care, perhaps more than any other activity imaginable, is collaborative. The patient is complex. Patient care is complex. The health care system is complex. Collaboration makes all of this manageable, even enjoyable. The practice of pharmaceutical care has been developed to make collaboration relatively easy and productive. Take advantage of this and become comfortable with all patient care practitioners, for the patient's benefit.

Standard IV: Collaboration

The practitioner collaborates with the patient, significant others, and health care providers in providing patient care.

Measurement criteria

1. The patient is seen as the ultimate decision maker, and the practitioner collaborates accordingly.
2. The practitioner collaborates with the patient's health care providers whenever it is in the best interest of the patient.

The professional behavior described as education is closely associated with the first standard of providing care. It is virtually impossible today to remain competent without a rigorous schedule of continuing education and collegial interaction. You owe it to your patient, yourself, and your colleagues to invest both time and energy in remaining current with your knowledge and competent in your skills. The volume and rate of knowledge expansion makes this a necessity today.

Standard V: Education

The practitioner acquires and maintains current knowledge in pharmacology, pharmacotherapy, and pharmaceutical care practice.

Measurement criteria

1. The practitioner uses the skills of reflectivity to identify areas where knowledge needs to be supplemented.
2. The practitioner continually updates knowledge with journal subscriptions, current texts, practitioner interactions, and continuing education programs.

The expectation that research will serve as the basis for decision making in practice is expressed as evidence-based practice. This is a requirement when a practitioner makes decisions that will impact another person. Because our knowledge of drug therapy, human physiology, and pathology is incomplete, clinicians make decisions in areas of uncertainty on a daily basis. The appropriate method for dealing with this is to use our knowledge well, understand the limits of the knowledge, and be able to recognize when science is inconclusive on a topic.

Standard VI: Research

The practitioner routinely uses research findings in practice and contributes to research findings when appropriate.

Measurement criteria

1. The practitioner uses research results as the basis for practice.
2. The pharmaceutical care practitioner systematically reviews the literature to identify knowledge, skills, techniques, and products that are helpful in practice and implements them in a timely manner.
3. The practitioner approaches his/her practice with a perspective to conduct applied research in practice when appropriate.

All health care resources are limited whether it be time, personnel, knowledge, or access to the latest technology. Decisions made by practitioners need to recognize this, but always put the patient's best interest first.

Standard VII: Resource Allocation

The practitioner considers factors related to effectiveness, safety, and cost in planning and delivering patient care.

Measurement criteria

1. The pharmaceutical care practitioner is sensitive to the financial needs and resource limitations of the patient, the health care providers, and the institutions with which he/she interacts.
2. Decisions are made by the pharmaceutical care practitioner to conserve resources and maximize the value of those resources consumed in practice.

Becoming a patient care practitioner is about being prepared to meet, and exceed when necessary, professional practice standards on behalf of the patient. These activities become part of the clinician's personality, and executing them becomes a way of life. Pharmaceutical care practitioners will come to expect this behavior of themselves and colleagues. The following represent healthy practice behaviors for pharmaceutical care practitioners.

1. Insist on knowing or learning the facts before acting or speaking (*evidence-based practice*).
2. Always follow through—find the answer and find it soon—*never let unknowns last.*
3. Set an example both personally and professionally. People respect you, and they will emulate you—*act like it.*
4. Be a colleague who can be trusted.

5. Hold yourself and your colleagues to the standards of practice.
6. Attend to appearance and be conscious of the impact it has on others.
7. Practice ethically.

SUMMARY

Every patient places his/her welfare in the practitioner's hands each time an agreement to provide care is made. The patient gives up a significant amount of freedom when seeking help or advice about medications. The circumstances of patient care make it necessary that practitioners demonstrate to the public, to society and to all patients, that they will promise to think and act in a professional manner. Patients need to know the values, priorities, and ethics that will be used when a professional makes decisions about his/her care.

EXERCISES

3-1 List three characteristics that differentiate a practitioner's philosophy of practice from an individual's personal philosophy of life.

3-2 What is meant when someone says, "As a professional it is imperative that you act ethically?"

3-3 Two practitioners are being observed as they practice. One is behaving in a patient-centered manner and the other is not. Describe at least three behaviors that could be observed that can differentiate the two practitioners.

3-4 Review your life and work experiences and describe situations where the following principles were involved:
  (*a*) Truth-telling
  (*b*) Confidentiality
  (*c*) Fairness
  (*d*) Autonomy

REFERENCES

1. Reich, W.T. Historical dimensions of an ethic of care in health care. *Encyclopedia of Bioethics*. New York: Macmillan; 1995.
2. Husted, G.L., Husted, J.H. *Ethical Decision-Making in Nursing and Health Care*, 3rd ed. New York: Springer; 2001.

3. Weed, L.L. *Medical Records, Medical Education, and Patient Care*. Chapter 2: The Database, Case Western Reserve, Cleveland, OH: University Press; 1971, p. 18.

4. Wilkinson, J.M. *Nursing Process: A Critical Thinking Approach*, 2nd ed. Menlo Park, CA: Addison-Wesley Nursing; 1992, pp. 16–17.

5. Stewart, M., Brown, J.B., Weston, W.W., McWhinney, I.R., McWilliam, C.L., Freeman, T.R. *Patient-Centered Medicine: Transforming the Clinical Method*. Thousand Oaks, CA: Sage Publications; 1995, pp. 37–41.

6. Guttman, N. *Public Health Communication Interventions*. Thousand Oaks, CA: Sage Publications; 2000, p. 1.

7. Bukhardt, M.A., Nathaniel, A.K. *Ethics and Issues in Contemporary Nursing*, 2nd ed. New York: Delmar; 2002, pp. 57–59.

8. Simon, S.B., Howe, L.W., Kirschbaum, H., *Values Clarification: A Handbook of Practical Strategies for Teachers and Students*. New York: Hart; 1995.

9. Towsley-Cook, D.M., Young, T.A. *Ethical and Legal Issues for Imaging Professionals*. St. Louis, MO: Mosby; 1999, p. 3.

10. Husted, G.L., Husted, J.H. *Ethical Decision Making in Nursing and Health Care*, 3rd ed. New York: Springer; 2001, p. 8.

11. Hebert, P.C. *Doing Right: A Practical Guide to Ethics for Medical Trainees and Physicians*. Toronto: Oxford University Press; 1996, pp. 13–20.

12. Tindall, W.N., Beardsley, R.S., Kimberlin, C.L. *Communication Skills in Pharmacy Practice: A Practical Guide for Students and Practitioners*, 3rd ed. Malvern, Pennsylvania: Lea & Febiger; 1994.

13. Lipkin, M.J., Putman, S.M., Lazare, A. The *Medical Interview: Clinical Care, Education, and Research*. New York: Springer; 1995, p. 10.

14. Cole, S.A., Bird, J. *The Medical Interview: The Three-Function Approach*. St. Louis, MO: Mosby; 2000, pp. 127–128.

15. Hepler, C.D., Strand, L.M. Opportunities and responsibilities in pharmaceutical care. *Am J Pharm* 1990; 53 (Winter Suppl.): 75–155.

16. Jonsen, A.R., Siegler, M., Winslade, W.J. *Clinical Ethics: A Practical Approach to Ethical Decisions in Clinical Medicine*, 5th ed. New York: McGraw-Hill; 2002, p. 50.

17. Parrish II, R.H. *Defining Drugs: How Government Became the Arbiter of Pharmaceutical Fact*. New Brunswick: Transaction Publishers; 2003.

18. Ulrich, L.P. *The Patient Self-Determination Act: Meeting the Challenges in Patient Care*. Washington, DC: Georgetown University Press; 1999.

19. ANA, *American Nurses Association. Standards of Clinical Nursing Practice*. Kansas City, MO: ANA; 1991.

FOUR

THE PATIENT'S ROLE

Key Concepts

1 *The therapeutic relationship is a partnership developed with the patient for the specific purpose of providing care to optimize the medication experience.*

2 *The quality of care that the practitioner can provide depends greatly on the quality of the therapeutic relationship developed with the patient.*

3 *A strong therapeutic relationship facilitates the retrieval of the necessary information from the patient so that clinical decisions can be made.*

4 *The relationship established with each patient will be unique. Both practitioner and patient bring values, experiences, and*

*expectations to the therapeutic relationship. Be aware of and
sensitive to what both bring because many times they differ.*

5 *Developing successful therapeutic relationships involves skills
that can be learned and improved daily.*

6 *Treating the patient in a confidential manner is the greatest
respect afforded to him/her.*

THE THERAPEUTIC RELATIONSHIP DEFINED

The relationship that develops between the patient and the practitioner is a
very important component of pharmaceutical care. Both the quality of the
care provided and the success of the treatments implemented depend to a
great extent on the quality of this unique relationship which is termed *the
therapeutic relationship.*

Definition The therapeutic relationship is a partnership or alliance
between the practitioner and the patient formed for the purpose of optimizing the patient's medication experience.[1]

The therapeutic relationship requires recognition of certain responsibilities on the part of the patient and the practitioner. It is based on trust,
respect, authenticity, empathy, and commitment.

We use the term *therapeutic* because this distinguishes it from other
relationships including familial, friendly, customer, or professional. The
therapeutic relationship has the specific purpose of facilitating the
exchange of information and expertise so that patients can achieve the best
possible results from drug therapies. The first function of the face-to-face
interaction with the patient is to build and maintain an effective therapeutic
relationship.

An effective relationship takes the form of a partnership with the patient.
This partnership serves as the foundation for the entire assessment process
as well as future follow-up evaluations. There will always be a relationship
between practitioner and patient, and it is your responsibility to maintain
the quality of that relationship. A good therapeutic relationship means that
you can provide good care to your patient, whereas an excellent therapeutic relationship allows you to provide excellent care. Therefore, it should
come as no surprise that a badly maintained therapeutic relationship often
results in unsatisfied patients and even litigation. The therapeutic relationship can make this much of a difference.

The nature of the information that is shared by your patient can be quite technical, often personal, occasionally embarrassing, and frequently difficult to describe. Therefore, the therapeutic relationship must be supported by trust, honesty, cooperation, sensitivity, empathy, and confidentiality. It will take time to develop a relationship with these qualities, but the continuous nature of pharmaceutical care practice facilitates the establishment and growth of a positive therapeutic relationship. Achieving a positive therapeutic relationship is an active rather than passive process. It is an act of caring for and about a person. It focuses on the whole person and not simply a biological specimen, organ system, disease state, or drug product in any reductionist sense.

BUILDING THE THERAPEUTIC RELATIONSHIP

Therapeutic relationships will vary because each patient is different, and each practitioner is different. However, there are certain characteristics and behaviors that facilitate building the therapeutic relationship with your patient. There are characteristics about yourself and behaviors toward your patient that make a noticeable difference in the quality of relationship that can be built. These are listed in Table 4-1.

Table 4-1 Characteristics and behaviors associated with the therapeutic relationship

Characteristics about yourself	Behaviors you manifest toward your patient
Honesty/authenticity/open communication	Putting the patient's needs first
Empathy/sensitivity	Offering reassurance Seeing the patient as a person
Patience and understanding	Mutual respect/trust
Competence	Cooperation/collaboration
Assuming responsibility for interventions	Caring
Being held accountable for the decisions and recommendations made	Building confidence Supporting the patient Offering advocacy Paying attention to the patient's physical and emotional comfort

This list includes characteristics and behaviors that are central to the philosophy and practice of pharmaceutical care. The therapeutic relationship links a practitioner's philosophy of practice to the real world of the patient. In this way, the therapeutic relationship provides an ethic of practice.

THE IMPACT OF THE THERAPEUTIC RELATIONSHIP

The time and effort invested in developing a strong therapeutic relationship will serve you well in practice. This relationship will make it easier to elicit necessary information from the patient, positively influence the patient's decisions, and learn from the patient.

The Patient as the Primary Source of Information

In all patient care practices the patient is the primary source of information. The patient either knows everything the practitioner needs to learn about the case or has primary access to the necessary information. Often we think of the medical chart, laboratory values, or the physician as the primary source of information, but all of these sources are secondary to the patient him/herself. The medical chart is often a translation of patient information. Laboratory values can be helpful, and whenever we need them, we can obtain them from the patient or request that the patient obtain them from the physician's office. Often we can generate the data firsthand in practice by gathering it ourselves (i.e., blood pressure, glucose, cholesterol), or by ordering the test directly from the laboratory.

The stronger your therapeutic relationship is with the patient, the more likely you can gather all of the personal medication use and history information necessary to make sound clinical decisions. One of the most important results of a positive therapeutic relationship between a patient and a practitioner is the shared decision-making applied to goals of therapy. Goals of therapy establish the direction, the intensity, the risks, and even the duration of drug therapies to be employed. Negotiation and agreement between patient and practitioner must be accomplished for positive outcomes to be possible. Through the therapeutic relationship, patients must be willing to participate in establishing achievable goals of therapy.

It would be a mistake to underestimate the value of the patient's input into the assessment of drug-related needs and the identification and resolution of drug therapy problems. Over 75% of all drug therapy problems identified and resolved in pharmaceutical care practice are resolved directly with the patient. This is similar to other primary care providers in which the vast majority of issues are resolved between patient and practitioner. The quality of the therapeutic relationship will greatly impact your ability to accomplish these objectives.

The Patient as Decision Maker

The patient is the ultimate decision maker in his/her health care. This is especially true for drug therapy decisions. Prescribers decide only what medication and dosage regimen to suggest, and the patient makes all the other decisions. Patients decide what medications—both prescription and non-prescription—they will actually take and what they will not. Patients also decide how much to take, how frequently to take it, and how long they will continue to take it. Because only the medication that the patient decides to take has an impact on the patient's condition, the patient's decision-making process is very important to understand.

The practitioner has to positively influence the patient's decisions to create a positive medication experience. This requires a good therapeutic relationship. If you ever have difficulty influencing your patient's decisions about drug therapy, reevaluate your relationship with the patient. It usually holds at least part of the explanation.

The relationship between a patient and a health care professional should always be therapeutic in its most literal sense. We are always striving to help the patient achieve the most positive therapeutic results possible. However, drug therapy can be dangerous or frightening. It can be confusing. It can be distressing to some patients. These emotions are implicit in the pharmaceutical care process, and therefore, a significant portion of what the practitioner contributes to the patient is made possible only through a close, respectful, mutually rewarding therapeutic relationship. In situations of uncertainty, it will help to recall direction provided by Cipolle: "Treat each patient as you would treat your own grandmother."[2]

The Patient as Teacher

Practitioners will learn more from their patients than they learn from most textbooks. Books, professors, and experts can teach you a significant amount, but only your patient can teach you what you need to know about him/herself and the impact drug therapy has. Never assume your patient has the same values and views about his/her drug therapy as you do. Learn what the patient's views are and use his/her information to develop better goals and assure positive outcomes. Patients have a wealth of information about their diseases and drug therapy. This is especially true for patients with chronic diseases. Not only have they lived the experience firsthand, but they can often describe how drug therapy actually impacts their daily lives.

Patients frequently have multiple medical problems and are using several medications. Each patient presents a new combination or mixture of diseases, illnesses, personal characteristics, and drug therapies. This is an experience we can retrieve only from the patient. You will benefit tremendously if you allow your patients to teach you about their diseases and their drug therapy. It is an efficient and effective way to learn. In contrast to material learned from a textbook, practitioners retain all that they learn from their patients. The asset that allows you to learn optimally from your patients is a strong therapeutic relationship.

THE PATIENTS' RIGHTS AND RESPONSIBILITIES

What the Patient Can Expect

Although your patient may not have previously experienced pharmaceutical care, he/she will have received care from other health care practitioners and will have learned to expect certain behaviors from a clinician. These expectations often remain unspoken; however, you can be certain that your patients will look for the following behaviors from you each time care is provided. These expectations and your ability to meet them will have a significant impact on the quality of the therapeutic relationship you will develop with your patient.

Patients expect you to care about what they want   Experienced practitioners acknowledge what the patient wants and addresses these wants directly. Patients may not be able to express what this is in the most sophisticated clinical terms, and they may not have the same understanding as you regarding what would be therapeutically best, but they know what they want. When patients feel they are getting what they want, they are usually satisfied.

Patients only care how much you know, when they know how much you care. There will be times when what your patient wants conflicts with what you consider to be in the patient's best interest. Successful resolution of these dilemmas requires that you put the patient first. What you think your patient needs is applied in the context of what your patient wants, what your patient expects, and what your patient is willing to do.

Patients will expect you to put their needs first, before your own Patients expect their drug-related needs to dictate what you do and when you do it. Patients' needs establish your priorities and direct your clinical activities. When you fully recognize that your patient's needs are the focus of what you do, you will understand what it means to have a patient-centered practice. This is the cornerstone of pharmaceutical care practice.

Patients expect compassion and understanding of them as individuals All patients are different. Each has unique beliefs, experiences, emotions, and understandings of health and the use of medications. Patient care practitioners hold the patient's personal beliefs and customs in high regard. You will have to be informed about patients' beliefs and customs from many different cultural backgrounds because the decisions you will make must be sensitive to them and reflect your patient's wishes. Taking time to understand the individual patient's medication experience will demonstrate your interest in the patient.

The patient expects you to possess the technical knowledge and the clinical experience and confidence it takes to apply that knowledge to their individual case Compassion is only part of what the patient expects. You must be competent in your work. The patient will expect a similar experience and level of service from all pharmaceutical care practitioners. Patients should be able to expect practitioners to have and to meet specific practice standards that are consistently and comprehensively applied to all patients. Patients will expect pharmaceutical care practitioners to be competent at what they do, to create a written record of the care that is provided, and to follow-up to verify that the desired goals of therapy have been achieved. When you see a patient for the second time, he/she will expect you to remember what was said and done the last time—or at least to have a written record of it.

Patients expect to receive the appropriate medication for their medical problems, and they expect the medication to work Because you have the knowledge and skills to meet this expectation, patients have a right to expect you to do whatever is necessary to ensure that they achieve the results they want from their medication. They expect you to provide this without taking unnecessary risks in the process. This does not seem difficult, but the data suggest that in today's health care system, we are having a difficult time meeting this expectation.[3]

If the drug therapy is not effective, the patient expects you to find one that will be. If the drug product needs to be changed, they expect you to change it. If the dose needs to be altered, they expect you to alter it so it is effective, yet safe. There are several medications that are efficacious for most medical conditions or illnesses. Find one that works for the patient.

Patients will expect you to be realistic and honest about what they can expect from their medications   All patients are unique, so some will want to know everything about their medications: how they work and what they do, both positively and negatively. Virtually all patients want to have some level of understanding about the goals of therapy so that they will know if their drug therapy is working. Some patients will want you to make all the decisions without explaining much at all about their drug therapy other than how to take it. You will have to determine the level at which your patient wants to understand details about drug therapy.

When you put a drug product (a chemical entity) about which we know a great deal into a patient (a complex biological system), the outcome cannot be predicted with full certainty. The more experience you have, the better you will be at predicting the outcome. There is so much that is still under investigation concerning drug therapy. In most situations there is no *right* answer. We are always making our best clinical judgment at the time. The patient has a right to know how certain you are about the potential positive and negative outcomes of drug therapy. You selected the drug therapy based upon effectiveness and safety, so be certain to explain how often this product works. If the data indicate that the drug is effective in 75% of cases, then your patient can expect it to work in three out of four cases.

Patients will expect you to be their advocate for all their drug-related needs   This will require that a special relationship develop between you and your patient, similar to the relationship patients have with other patient care providers. This relationship will demand that you respect every patient and his/her values, views, preferences, and wishes when making decisions about medications. What the patient wants and needs become your major concerns in practice. Your patients should be able to expect that you will provide the very best drug therapy possible. They should expect that you will provide the most effective drug therapy available in every circumstance. They will also expect you to keep their safety as a high priority. As a clinician, your advocacy for effectiveness and safety takes precedence over other considerations such as convenience and cost.

Patients will expect you to be accountable for the decisions you make and the advice you give   Whatever happens to the patient as a result of pharmacotherapy, positive or negative, you must take responsibility. The out-comes of drug therapies are your responsibility. Encourage the patient to contact you when questions arise or problems develop. Although you will work closely with the patient and his/her prescribing practitioners, always take responsibility for the outcomes resulting from drug therapy. The patient needs to know that you will be there for him/her regardless of the outcome. The patients needs to know that you will find solutions to his/her problems.

Patients will expect you to know when to refer them to someone with different expertise   Don't try to be a dietician, an exercise physiologist, or a psychiatrist. It is important that you know the scope and breadth of your responsibilities (pharmacotherapy) and that you know where the boundaries of your expertise lie. Modern pharmacotherapies can improve the lives and overall health of many people. Focus your attention on maximizing the benefits of all drug therapies. Consultation and referrals serve a vital role in today's health care system. When referring a patient to another health care practitioner it is important to be clear about the purpose of the referral, provide all of the relevant drug therapy documentation you have describ-ing your patient's needs, and help your patient understand what questions to ask or what service to seek.[4]

The Patient's Responsibilities

With rights come responsibilities. It is important to be cognizant of your patients' expectations and aware of their responsibilities. Meeting the patient's drug-related needs requires the patient's participation and coop-eration. Simply stated, you can expect your patients to

1. provide you with accurate and complete information;
2. participate in the establishment of goals of therapy;
3. contribute to the care plan as agreed upon (act on the education and instructions they received, collect important outcome parameters, keep appointments);
4. maintain a diary of medication use, signs, and symptoms, and test results if needed to evaluate effectiveness, safety, and compliance;
5. notify you of changes and/or problems with their drug therapy so you can act on them before they become harmful;
6. ask questions whenever they arise.

   In Chapter 6, you will be introduced to a number of specific techniques that will help you to develop a therapeutic relationship with your patients;

however, there are a number of general behaviors that will always impact the impression you have on your patients:

1. Attend to your appearance and be conscious of the impact it has on the patient.
2. Be conscious of the impact the appearance of your surroundings has on the patient.
3. The vocabulary and language that you use to greet the patient will set the tone of the meeting.
4. Listen and give attention to the patient, he/she will be expecting it.

Issues of Confidentiality

Maintaining a patient's privacy is the greatest test of the respect a practitioner gives a patient. Practitioners can claim to be fair and loyal, they can argue they are patient-centered, they can attest to a positive therapeutic relationship, and yet if the patient's privacy is not protected, then they have failed on all of these accounts.

Patient confidentiality has always been a concern in health care. However, since April 14, 2003, it is of even greater concern. New patient privacy standards were developed as a result of the Health Insurance Portability and Accountability Act (HIPAA).[5] The U.S. Federal Government intervened to establish a new standard for patient confidentiality with the HIPAA requirements. These guidelines require a higher expectation and a more diligent adherence to the precept of *always protect your patient's privacy*.

HIPAA regulations are designed to protect the privacy and security of individual health information. Patients have the right to request a copy of their medication information. They also have the right to amend any information that is incorrect or incomplete. Patients also have the right to request that practitioners communicate about health matters in a specific way, for example, only by mail or e-mail, or at a certain location such as only at work or only at home.

SUMMARY

Every time a patient and a practitioner meet or communicate it is done in the context of their therapeutic relationship. A positive therapeutic relationship helps the patient to believe and trust in the drug therapies and advice provided and it helps the practitioner to feel confident that positive results can be achieved.

EXERCISES

4-1   Discuss four factors that can impact the quality of a therapeutic relationship positively and four factors that might impact it negatively.

4-2   Discuss the variables that could impact the length of time it might take to develop a strong therapeutic relationship with a patient. How long do you anticipate it will take?

4-3   Discuss how a therapeutic relationship is different from a friendship or a customer relationship and why it needs to be different.

4-4   Describe the potential impact on clinical outcomes if your patient
   (a) actively participates in establishing goals of therapy;
   (b) agrees to follow the care plan instructions;
   (c) records medication use and keeps a diary of evidence of improvement in his/her condition;
   (d) informs you of any changes in medication use.

REFERENCES

1. Cipolle, R., Strand, L.M., Morley, P.C. *Pharmaceutical Care Practice*. New York: McGraw Hill; 1998.
2. Cipolle, R. Drugs don't have doses...people have doses. *Drug Intell Clin Pharm* 1986; 20: 881–882.
3. Kohn, L.T., Corrigan, J.M., Donaldson, M.S. (eds). *To Err is Human: Building a Safer Health System*. Washington, D.C.: National Academy Press; 1999.
4. Billings, J.A., Stoeckle, J.D. *The Clinical Encounter: A Guide to the Medical Interview and Case Presentation*. St. Louis, MO: Medical Publishers of Mosby-Year Book, Inc.; 1989, pp. 270–272.
5. Available at: www.ahc.umn.edu/ahc_content/about/privacy/index2.cfm, University of Minnesota. Accessed April 15, 2003.

CHAPTER FIVE

THE PATIENT'S MEDICATION EXPERIENCE

Key Concepts

1. *The medication experience is the sum of all the events in a patient's life that involve medication use.*

2. *The patient's medication experience is the context in which all good drug therapy decisions are made.*

3. *The patient's medication experience will have a significant influence on the decisions patients make about taking medication.*

4. *The three dimensions of the medication experience are the patient's description of the medication experience, the medication history, and the current medication record.*

5. *The patient's medication experience includes the patient's description of his/her expectations, wants, concerns, understanding, preferences, attitudes, beliefs, cultural, ethical, and religious influences on medication taking behavior.*

6. *The patient's medication experience includes the history of immunizations, social drug use, medication allergies, adverse*

drug reactions, health alerts/health aids/special needs, relevant past medication use, and current medication use.

7 *The patient's current medication record will include all medical conditions and associated indications for drug therapies, the drug products being used, the dosage regimens the patient is actually taking, the duration of therapy, and the patient's response to each of the therapies.*

THE PATIENT'S MEDICATION EXPERIENCE DEFINED

We have already discussed the importance of the therapeutic relationship in providing pharmaceutical care. This relationship will determine how successful you can be at the human dimension of caring for patients. A second important variable in your success, a variable that will affect your ability to make good therapeutic decisions, is how well you understand your patient's medication experience.

The medication experience is a new concept in health care. Practitioners have always completed medication histories and created medication records that list drug therapies taken in the past or currently being taken, but no other patient care practitioner has systematically determined how the patient *feels* about taking his/her medications, and how the patient actually takes his/her medications. This level of inquiry requires time and attention to the details involved in rational drug therapy. The physician has learned to understand the patient's views of his/her disease as a description of illness, so too must the pharmaceutical care practitioner understand the patient's perception of his/her medication as the medication experience.[1]

The patient medication experience reveals how patients make personal decisions about medications. It includes the evidence of medications that were effective and those that failed in the past, and it tells you what drug therapy is currently prescribed and how the patient is actually taking it. There is no more important information about your patient than the medication experience. Because it describes his or her attitudes and beliefs about medications, it has a very powerful influence on the outcomes of drug therapy. In fact, a practitioner cannot make sound clinical decisions without a good understanding of the patient's medication experience.

Definition The *patient's medication experience* is the sum of all the events a patient has in his/her lifetime that involve drug therapy. This is the patient's personal experience with medications. This lived experience shapes the patient's attitudes, beliefs, and preferences about drug therapy. It is these characteristics that principally determine a patient's medication taking behavior.

The patient's medication experience consists of three related entities:

1. The patient's description of the experience he/she has had with medications;
2. A comprehensive medication history, including immunizations, allergies, adverse drug reactions, and social drug use patterns;
3. A complete record of the patient's current medications and associated medical conditions.

The patient's medication experience is the patient's personal approach to the use of medicines—why the patient believes or feels a certain way about drug therapy. Some patients have little or no well-formed medication experience, others who have taken numerous medications may have developed distinct beliefs or preferences. It is shaped by patients' traditions, religion, culture, and what they have heard and learned from others. All of these factors will influence whether patients take a medication or not, how they will use the medication, whether they believe it will be effective, and whether they believe the medication will be harmful. The patient's medication experience influences the confidence he/she has in your abilities to help, whether you are an experienced clinician or if this is your first encounter.

Example   Some patients will express a high level of frustration with past drug therapies that have failed to produce any benefit. This negative experience can influence that patient's expectations of your recommended drug therapy unless you recognize and directly address the patient's negative impressions. Also, patients may prefer not to use medications while at work or at school. Incorporating this common patient preference into your pharmacotherapy decisions can greatly enhance compliance and outcomes.

The patient's medication experience can be strongly influenced by others including friends and family members. This is especially true of young patients and individuals who have little or no personal experience with medications. It is not only helpful to become familiar with your patient's understanding and beliefs concerning medications, but also learn how those beliefs are influenced by others.

Your primary responsibility as a pharmaceutical care practitioner is to improve each patient's medication experience—to make it better than it was before you provided care. The medication experience is the context in which you will do all of this work, and it is the portion of the patient's life you will influence most.

Each patient has a unique medication experience. Some patients will have a very short, concise medication experience either because they are young, they have taken very few medications, or they have never been ill. Others, especially the elderly with multiple medical conditions, will have an extensive medication experience and require a significant amount of time to communicate it to you. Sometimes, these specific beliefs or preferences concern only a limited scope of pharmacotherapy, such as a patient with a chronic back ailment who has endured numerous therapeutic attempts with nonsteroidal anti-inflammatory drugs (NSAIDs) and now feels these medications will not be effective to manage his/her back pain.

It will not be useful to make assumptions about your patient's medication experience or to generalize from one patient's experience to another. Taking the time to understand each patient's individual medication experience is a valuable investment in your time. Not putting forth the effort to understand a patient's medication experience will impede your decision-making ability and reduce the likelihood of your patient experiencing positive outcomes.

> **Example**   Some patients have strong religious beliefs that inhibit them from taking oral contraceptives to prevent pregnancy. Others may rely on traditional or folk medicines to maintain health and only seek conventional pharmacotherapy for acute illnesses.

Practitioners learn to make decisions in all of these unique patient contexts. It is the reason each patient must be treated as an individual.

UNDERSTANDING THE PATIENT'S MEDICATION EXPERIENCE

There are three dimensions to the patient's medication experience, and all three are important in pharmaceutical care practice: the patient's description of the medication experience, the medication history, and the current medication record.

The Patient's Description of the Medication Experience

Early in the assessment process, practitioners encourage patients to describe their medication experience.

The first dimension of the patient's medication experience is constructed with the following information:

- What is the patient's general attitude toward taking medication?
- What does the patient want/expect from his/her drug therapy?
- Describe any concerns the patient has about his/her drug therapy.
- To what extent does the patient understand his/her medications?
- Are there cultural, religious, or ethical issues that influence the patient's willingness to take medications?
- Describe the patient's medication taking behavior.

Patient's general attitude toward taking medications   The patient's medication experience represents the sum total of the impact of events in the patient's life that have formed the patient's impressions, beliefs, concerns, understanding, and preferences about the use of medications to manage certain health problems.

Over time and with experience, patients develop attitudes toward and beliefs about drug therapy generally and specifically. Negative attitudes and beliefs that patients may develop include "Drugs don't work, they only cause more problems," or "I don't take medications." Overly positive attitudes include "There must be a drug I can take to solve this problem."

> **Example**   Individuals who use herbs may have a less positive perception of the safety of prescription therapies and a more favorable attitude regarding the impact of herbs on their health.[2]

These attitudes and beliefs work to establish specific preferences that each patient has about taking medications. These preferences will directly impact whether or not a patient will take medication and how the patient will take the mediation. Therefore, it is important to understand this portion of the patient's medication experience. It is likely that you will need to influence the patient's attitudes and beliefs about drug therapy. It is necessary to know what your patient believes before you attempt to change those beliefs or attitudes.

Patient's wants and expectations   Establishing what your patient wants is the most productive place to begin an assessment. This is for two common sense reasons. In order to provide a service that a patient feels is valuable, it must be perceived to be doing what he/she wants it to do. The best way to determine what another person wants is to ask. The other, and more pragmatic reason to begin an assessment by determining what your patient wants, is that virtually all patients already know this.

Every patient who walks into a clinic, an office, or a pharmacy is there for a purpose. Some people may have difficulty describing what they want in terms that the practitioner can fully understand. Some may be hesitant to share their goals with someone with whom they have not yet established a strong therapeutic relationship. Some may feel as though what they want is not very important to the practitioner. Some patients may feel that the practitioner is too busy with other issues to deal with their personal issues.

You may experience all of these situations in your practice, but understand that all patients you care for have a good idea of what they really want. The better you are at discovering what that is, the better you will serve your patients. If you provide services that people want, you will engender their loyalty. If you can determine what your patients want and reassure them that you intend to help them achieve a positive experience from their medications, then patients will have full confidence that you have their best interest in mind. This establishes the basis for the trust that is needed to build a strong therapeutic relationship. It also assures your patient that you intend to be comprehensive in your care. A caveat: remember that sometimes what a patient wants is not necessarily what he/she needs. Needs and wants must be discussed and resolved. Discuss these distinctly different issues with the patient (refer to Chapter 10 for a process to resolve ethical dilemmas).

> **Example** In the situation when the patient describes that he/she wants to "not have to take so many pills every day," the practitioner will need to make every effort to minimize the number or frequency of doses the patient is required to take every day. During the assessment, the practitioner may determine that other, clinically important drug therapy problems need to be resolved, however it is still important to address the patient's original stated request to reduce daily doses.

There will be plenty of opportunity to interpret what the patient wants relative to your professional decision of what is needed, later in the assessment. However, if you fail to determine what your patient wants from his/her medications, you have no reference point.

Patient concerns Patients frequently express what they want in terms of concerns they have about the medication itself or how it must be taken.[3] Patient concerns are frequently the reason they want to see a pharmaceutical care practitioner. Common concerns include risks of taking a certain medication, side effects experienced, and confusion over how to take a medication or why it is being taken. Concerns can be more expansive if the patient is afraid to take medications in general because of previous problems experienced. It is important to know all of a patient's concerns because they can have a dramatic impact on the patient's medication taking behavior. Patients who feel that their concerns are not being attended to by the practitioner often do not take medications as intended. Concerns related to medications are a major cause of noncompliance.

Past experiences with medications have a significant impact on the patient's willingness to take them in the future, so take the time required to understand the patient's concerns.

> **Example** The patient may be afraid to take an antibiotic because a friend or another family member once had a bad experience with a drug which was also used to treat an infection. Even if the two anti-infectives are completely different, such as amoxicillin and erythromycin, and even if the infections were different, such as pneumonia and urinary tract infection, you must recognize and address this patient concern to have a successful outcome.

Patients' understanding of drug therapy Each patient's medication experience leads to a unique understanding of his/her drug therapies. The patient may present with a thorough and comprehensive understanding of all his/her drug therapies or may understand very little about the medications. Other patients will know more than you do about both their disease and their drug therapy. Your patient's level of understanding will determine the extent to which you will need to educate and explain the effectiveness and safety instructions. Experienced practitioners are certain to elicit the patient's level of understanding before embarking on a time-consuming patient drug information and education campaign.

Achieving the patient's goals of therapy depends on the patient having a clear understanding of why each medication is being taken, the name of each medication (in a way the patient understands), the dosage and dosing schedule for each medication, the clinical and laboratory measures that will be used to determine a successful outcome, and the clinical and laboratory measures that can be used to detect if any safety/risk issues occur. The pharmaceutical care practitioner needs to elicit enough information from the patient to determine how well he/she understands medications.

Cultural, ethical, and religious issues The impact that society has on shaping individual attitudes and beliefs has been widely documented and broadly accepted.[4-7] Therefore, it is important to understand the social context of each patient. Within that social context lie religious beliefs, traditions, and social expectations that can all impact a patient's attitudes and beliefs about the efficacy of the medication, its appropriateness, and the proper way to administer it. Again, this information is relevant because it shapes the patient's medication taking behavior or compliance. Practitioners frequently need to influence this behavior to optimize the patient's response to medications.

The practitioner must accommodate religious practices, traditional beliefs, and cultural norms that may be very different from his/her own. All of these belief systems may directly influence a patient's willingness to comply with the recommended drug therapy. Unfamiliarity with issues or differences in views commonly introduces ethical dilemmas into practice.

> **Example** Many Native Americans value a process of group decision-making by the family that may need to be balanced with the concept of personal autonomy.[8]

Ethical dilemmas do not have to be negative experiences. They can serve as discussion topics between the practitioner and the patient. It is important to emphasize that the patient is always the final decision maker, and he/she must give consent to the practitioner's influence on whether and how to take a drug product. A systematic process for resolving ethical dilemmas when they arise is discussed in Chapter 10.

Patient's medication taking behavior All of the previous components of a patient's medication experience—a patient's expectations, concerns, understanding, beliefs, attitudes, preferences, culture, and religion can influence what is described as the patient's medication taking behavior.

> **Note** A patient's medication taking behavior describes the decisions a patient makes and acts upon related to the use of drug products and dosage regimens.

These behaviors include whether a patient chooses to obtain and take the medication, how the patient takes the medication, whether the patient chooses to refill a prescription, or if the patient chooses to be compliant. These behaviors frequently need to be positively reinforced to obtain the desired results from therapy. Some patients may not believe that the drug therapy the clinician recommended will work. Therefore, the patient may not even have the prescription filled or purchase the product. The practitioner needs this information to make good decisions.

Some portions of your patient's description of his/her medication experience may be confusing or missing. Complicated brand and generic names, complex dosing schedules, and multiple instructions can all contribute to a patient having incomplete information or recall about the medication and how it was taken. It may require both time and patience to elicit this information.

Pharmaceutical care practitioners will use the patient's description of the medication experience as the context or meaning for the medication history. The medication experience explains how past medications impacted the patient and therefore, how the patient currently makes decisions about drug therapy. Without understanding the medication experience first, a medication history is simply a list of drug products purchased in the past.

The Medication History

A comprehensive medication history is conducted for very specific reasons. The record of medications used in the past to treat or prevent medical conditions or illnesses provides information that is essential when making current therapy decisions. Effectiveness of therapies used in the past can direct future drug selections. Safety issues from the patient's history serve as warnings to avoid reexposing the patient to harm. Medications, primarily vaccines used to immunize the patient against communicable diseases, are the mainstay of preventive drug histories.

Following is a list of the components of a comprehensive medication history. Not all of this information will be available or useful in every case.

The second dimension of the patient's medication experience contains a comprehensive medication history and includes:

- an immunization record;
- a history and quantification of social drug use;
- medication allergies and characteristics of the allergic response;
- a description of any adverse reactions to medications;
- health alerts and/or special needs of the patient;
- a historical account of relevant medication use (success/failures).

Keep in mind, you are trying to identify drug-related needs (for example, the patient requires an immunization), identify a drug therapy problem (patient is allergic to penicillin,) or gather information that will help you select medications that will be effective in the future (hydrochlorothiazide did not work in the past). Medication histories focus on the discovery of information that is most likely to be relevant to improving your patient's future medication experience. Collect only that information you will use to make decisions for and with your patients.

Immunizations The immunization record includes the documentation of childhood and/or adult vaccinations received and a plan to meet current guidelines. Pharmaceutical care practitioners should be aware that guidelines for vaccinations change quite frequently so it is important to keep an up-to-date protocol. This record can become very useful for the patient because there are few health care professionals or institutions who maintain a current record of all of the patient's vaccinations, and yet it is frequently required for travel, school enrollment, participation in athletics, or emergency care. Maintaining accurate immunization records for patients and their family members is a valuable service.

History of social drug use   Social drug use in the context of pharmaceutical care includes tobacco, caffeine, alcohol, and drugs of abuse. It should be made clear to the patient that this information is important because all of these compounds can alter the absorption, distribution, metabolism, and elimination of many other prescription and nonprescription products, in addition to causing a number of health problems themselves. Care must be taken not to be judgmental about the behavior of patients, nor to introduce any personal beliefs or prejudices with regard to the use of these substances. Practitioners will assess the impact of the social drug use on the selection, dosing, and safety of the patient's pharmacotherapies.

Medication allergies   Medication allergies can be confusing to patient and practitioner alike. Frequently patients have been told they had an allergic reaction, or they suspect an allergic reaction themselves, when he/she actually experienced an adverse reaction to a drug product.

> **Definition**   Allergic drug reaction: Unfavorable physiological response to an allergen (the drug) to which the patient develops an immune response (antibodies) and through the release of chemical mediators (immunoglobulins, complement, cytokines) experiences symptoms including urticaria, eczema, dyspnea, bronchospasm, diarrhea, rhinitis, laryngospasm, and anaphylaxis. Subsequent exposure can result in more serious symptoms and consequences.[9] The reaction often resolves after the drug is discontinued, but may require emergency treatment.
>
> Adverse drug reaction: A harmful, undesirable, or unintended effect of a drug administered at dosages normally used in patients for prophylaxis, diagnosis, or therapy. Type A adverse drug reactions are most commonly extensions of the known but undesirable pharmacology of the drug. Type B reactions are idiosyncratic and unrelated to the pharmacology or dosage and are therefore unpredictable.[9,10]

Care should be taken to be specific when gathering drug allergy information from the patient. Be sure to include the nature of the allergic response, the product that caused the reaction, and the timing of the reaction. Patients should not be exposed to a product that has produced a true allergic reaction, so a portion of your responsibility is to separate true allergic responses from adverse drug reactions. This may be difficult with the limited history and/or memory the patient has of the event. In all cases, the reaction should be noted with documentation to describe the circumstance. This information will directly impact your choice of drug products to be used in a patient.

Adverse drug reactions   Adverse reactions to past medications can manifest themselves in a number of ways: gastrointestinal problems (nausea, vomiting), dermatological problems (rashes, hives), central nervous system changes (drowsiness, irritability), and many others. Again, it is important to be specific about the product and the dosage regimen that resulted in the adverse outcome. The timing of the problem in relation to taking the medication, the severity, the duration, and the resolution of the problem should all be noted.

Alerts and special needs   Most patients have specific issues or preferences that will help them to be more comfortable, more functional, or simply happier when taking medications. The patient may have impaired hearing or sight loss, may have problems walking up stairs, or require oxygen therapy. The patient may use a cane, a wheelchair, or crutches. The patient may not speak English. Any alerts, special needs, or health aids used by the patient to assist in medication administration or to optimize the outcomes of drug therapies should be noted as part of the medication history so that accommodation can be made. This is an opportunity to individualize your care.

History of relevant medication use   Patients often can provide tremendously useful information about previous medication use. What has been effective, what has failed? It is likely that this will be the case again. What the patient will not take—for whatever reason—and what does the patient feel good about taking due to previous experience? This information can save a significant amount of time and energy, but more importantly, it can save the patient suffering and inconvenience. Take time to elicit this information and listen closely. Be sure to include the original reason the patient was taking the medication, the product, the dosage regimen, the start and stop dates, and the response the patient experienced. In general, practitioners use 6 months as a guide to determine how far back to investigate medication histories in patients with extensive past treatments.

Some patients may have difficulty providing specific drug names, dosages, and dates due to memory loss or complexity of the information. This is frequently the case when the patient speaks a different language and/or has acquired the medication in a different country.

The patient will provide you with significant help if you let him/her. The medication history is an important context in which to evaluate the medications currently being taken. It is worth repeating here that a medication history is never completed as an end in itself, but provides information for decision-making during the assessment and care planning process.

The Current Medication Record

The third component of the patient's medication experience is the current medication record.

> **Note**   The current medication record includes all of the patient's current medical conditions or illnesses and how well they are being managed with drug therapy. The current medication record includes the indication, drug product, dosage regimen, duration of therapy, and clinical results to date.

Patients frequently interpret a question about current medications to mean only those medications written as prescriptions by a physician. Time and care should be taken to assess all the products a patient is currently taking for therapeutic purposes (regardless of source and category of product). All of the products being taken can impact other products as well as the medical condition of the patient.

There is a specific way to organize the information describing your patient's current drug therapies. Practitioners establish the connections between the clinical indication, the specific drug product, the dosage regimen actually taken by the patient, the length of therapy, and the response the patient has experienced from each drug regimen. All of these data are necessary to make clinical decisions. The relationship between indication, drug product and dosage, and response is among the most important clinical information the pharmaceutical care practitioner contributes to care.

Indication   Indication is the clinical reason the patient is taking the medication.

Patients take medications for a variety of reasons. Treating a disease that has been diagnosed by a physician is only one of several categories of indications for drug therapies. Drugs are often used before a formal diagnosis can be established. Medications are frequently used to prevent a medical condition or illness from developing. Many forms of pharmacotherapy are used to simply alleviate uncomfortable signs or symptoms.

The current medication record serves as the basis for practitioners to make clinical judgments as to the appropriateness of the indication for each medication the patient is currently taking. Patients have many personal reasons for taking supplements, alternative products, and nonprescription medications. Symptoms, prevention, and medical problems can all be indications for medications. When you record your patient's current medication record, drug therapies are grouped by indication.

Drug product   The drug product should be noted by generic and brand names (if applicable). The color or appearance of products vary—especially in generic products—and this can be very confusing to the patient, so you may need to include the manufacturer of generic products.

Dosage regimen   The dosage regimen is made up of several components. Each of these can influence the outcomes, and practitioners must be exact and complete when describing the dosage regimen the patient is actually taking. The dosage regimen includes the dose (usually in milligrams (mg)) of the medication, the frequency of administration (usually times per day), and the duration of treatment (for 2 weeks). It will be difficult to evaluate the appropriateness of the medication regimen if any of this information is missing.

The *dose* most often represents the amount of active ingredient that the patient takes or applies each time he or she self-administers the drug product. The dose could also be administered by a nurse or some other health care provider. However, in general, the dose is the amount of drug the patient takes (or is given) each time. The *strength* is how much active drug is contained in the dosage form (tablet or capsule, liquid). For injectable medications, strength is usually described in terms of *concentration* of active drug per volume of liquid.

> **Example**   An aspirin tablet containing 325 mg of acetylsalicylic acid provides a dose of 325 mg of aspirin. The strength of the tablet is said to be 325 mg. If the patient takes two of these tablets, the dose taken was 650 mg. In the United States, aspirin tablets commonly have a strength of 81 or 325 mg. Example: 1 milliequivalent (mEq) of potassium chloride (KCl) per milliliters (mL) of 5% dextrose in water would be expressed as a concentration of 1 mEq/ml.

The term *dosage* is used to describe the total amount of drug the patient takes over a given amount of time.

Example   If your patient takes two aspirin tablets containing 325 mg each, and takes the same dose four times each day, then the dosage would be described as 650 mg four times a day (or a daily dosage of 2600 mg).

The *dosing interval* describes the time between consecutive doses.

Example   Every 12 hours or every 6 hours. In some cases, dosing intervals can be measured in days, weeks, or months.

The *duration of therapy* describes the total time (most often expressed in days, weeks, or months) the patient has been taking the same medication.

Example   Many antibiotic drug regimens instruct the patient to complete a full 10-day course of therapy to ensure effectiveness. This would be described as a duration of therapy of 10 days.

When describing the patient's dosage regimen of a medication currently being taken, all of the components (product, dose, dosing interval, and duration) are important in order to make valid clinical decisions about how to optimize your patient's medication experience.

It is also important to emphasize that the dosage regimen recorded here must be the one the patient is actually taking. If this is not the one prescribed by the physician then that difference is noted. Be aware of both, but your clinical decisions are always based on what the patient is actually taking.

Start date   The start date of medications is especially important if you are assessing the possibility of an allergic reaction or the onset of an adverse reaction to a medication. It is also important in assessing whether a certain drug therapy has had enough time to produce the desired response. Treatment failures are a significant drug therapy problem, and time to response is an important item of information in assessing treatment failures.

Response   The patient's response to a medication should be evaluated relative to the desired goal of therapy for the specific medical problem. Pharmaceutical care practitioners use a standard set of definitions for terms to describe the patient's response to drug therapy (refer to Chapter 9). The terms *stable, improved, partially improved, worsened, resolved*, and *failed* all have specific meaning when used to describe the patient's response to current medications. Standard terminology will allow a colleague (or even yourself over time) to understand exactly what is occurring in a patient. The description of the patient's response needs to include both positive and negative responses, if applicable. For example, how well is this drug therapy working for your patient at the time you are gathering the current medication record?

This is a good time to emphasize that no information should be elicited from a patient unless you are going to use it. Each item of information you collect needs a purpose and a specific reason to apply it to make better decisions for the patient. Chapter 6 describes the relevant patient information required to make an assessment of the patient's drug-related needs.

SUMMARY

Every time a patient uses a medication or decides not to take a drug, he/she has a medication experience. This personal experience serves as the basis for making medication-related decisions in the future. Therefore, the more you understand about your patient's past and present medication experience the more likely positive outcomes will be realized.

Your patient's expression of preferences, needs, expectations, and concerns will form the basis for the majority of what will occur in the assessment, care plan, and evaluation. It is important to remember that these early patient impressions are most important because they reflect how your patient sees the situation. Your clinical decisions, impression, advice, and knowledge must all be related to your patient's view of his/her medication experience, what has worked in the past and what drug therapies he/she is currently taking. The patient's medication experience is the context in which the practitioner does all of his/her work. It is important to understand it and to be able to use it to benefit the patient.

EXERCISES

5-1 Write at least one paragraph describing your own personal medication experience. After you are finished, read it aloud and reflect on the meaning of the words you have chosen to describe the experience. What did you describe: feelings, expectations, concerns, experiences, beliefs?

5-2 Select two acquaintances you know to be taking at least two different medications. Ask each one (separately) to describe his/her medication experience to you. Reflect on the meaning of the words each one chose to describe the experience. What did they describe: feelings, expectations, concerns, experiences, beliefs? How were the two similar? How were their experiences different?

5-3 Give a specific example of how each of the following can influence drug taking behavior:

(a) Cultural and traditional practices

(b) Religious beliefs

(c) Different primary language

5-4 Define and differentiate the following pairs of concepts:

(a) Drug allergy and adverse drug reaction

(b) Dose and dosage regimen

REFERENCES

1. Radley, A. *Making Sense of Illness: The Social Psychology of Health and Disease.* Chapter 1: Explaining Health and Illness: An Introduction. London: Sage Publications; 1999.
2. Klepser, T.B., Doucette, W.R., Horton, M.R., Buys, L.M., Ernst, M.E., Ford, J.K., Hoehns, J.D., Kautzman, H.A., Logemann, C.D., Swegle, J.M., Ritho, M., Klepser, M.E. Assessment of patients' perceptions and beliefs regarding herbal therapies. *Pharmacotherapy* 2000; 20(1): 83–87.
3. Smith, R.C. *The Patient's Story: Integrated Patient-Doctor Interviewing.* Chapter 3: Patient Centered Process, Boston, MA: Little, Brown and Company; 1996, p. 25–53.
4. Brown, P. *Perspectives in Medical Sociology*, 2nd ed. Chapter 2: Social Class, Health, and Illness, Dutton, D.B. Prospect Heights, IL: Waveland Press, Inc.; 1989, p. 23–46.
5. Conrad, P., Kern, R. *The Sociology of Health and Illness*: *Critical Perspectives*, 2nd ed. Chapter 2: Social Class, Susceptibility, and Sickness; Syme S.L. and Berkman, L.F., New York: St. Martin's Press; 1986.
6. Morley, P.C., Wallis, R. *Culture and Curing: Anthropological Perspectives on Traditional Medical Beliefs and Practices.* Chapter 1: Culture and the Cognitive World of Traditional Medical Beliefs: Some Preliminary Considerations. Morley, PC, p. 1–18, London: Peter Owen; 1979.
7. Mechanics, D. *Medical Sociology*, 2nd ed. Chapter 1: Man, Health, and the Environment. New York: Free Press; 1978.
8. Coulehan, J.L., Block, M.R. *The Medical Interview: Mastering Skills for Clinical Practice*, 4th ed. Chapter 10: Cultural Competence in the Interview, p. 155–169. Philadelphia, PA: F.A. Davis Company; 2001, p. 156.
9. Stergachis, A., Hazlet, T.K., Chapter 8: Pharmacoepidemiology. *Pharmacotherapy—A Pathophysiologic Approach.* New York: McGraw-Hill; 2002, p. 94.
10. Seeger, J.D., Xiaodong, S., Schumock, G.T. Characteristics associated with ability to prevent adverse drug reactions in hospitalized patients. *Pharmacotherapy* 1998; 18(6): 1284–1289.

THE ASSESSMENT

Key Concepts

1. *The purpose of the assessment is to determine if the patient's drug-related needs are being met and if any drug therapy problems are present.*

2. *Know your patient by understanding his/her medication experience before making any decisions about his/her drug therapy.*

3. *Elicit only relevant information necessary to make drug therapy decisions.*

4. *Always assess the patient's drug-related needs in the same systematic order. First determine if the indication is appropriate for the drug therapy. Second, evaluate the effectiveness of the drug regimen for the indication. Third, determine the level of safety of the drug regimen. Only after determining that the drug therapy selected or being used by the patient is appropriately indicated, effective, and safe, should you evaluate the patient's compliance with the medication.*

5. *Documentation includes the clinician's assessment of how well the patient's drug-related needs are being met and a description of the drug therapy problems present.*

PURPOSE, ACTIVITIES, AND RESPONSIBILITIES

The purpose of the assessment is to determine if a patient's drug-related needs are being met. In order to accomplish this, the practitioner gathers, analyzes, researches, and interprets information about the patient, the patient's medical conditions, and the patient's drug therapies. Individuals can have drug-related needs whether they are taking medications or not.

This chapter describes how all of these activities combine to create an assessment of the patient's drug-related needs. A consistent format will be used to describe the standards of care and the corresponding measurement criteria that apply to the assessment step of the patient care process.

The assessment step in the patient care process is the most important of the three. It requires work on the part of the clinician and cooperation on the part of the patient. There are standard sets of issues and questions the practitioner must constantly think about and analyze throughout the assessment. The assessment interview is the means through which the practitioner encourages the patient's participation in the patient care process. The assessment interview influences all other components of the patient care process. It influences communication, data accuracy, clinical decision-making, ethical judgements, patient compliance, patient satisfaction, practitioner satisfaction, and clinical outcomes.

There are essential clinical skills that each practitioner must develop in order to conduct a productive assessment. These include inquiry, listening, and observational skills. You must be committed to learning and to teaching yourself the skills you will use to assess the drug-related needs of your patients.

To be successful, you must understand and master the basic skills as well as the pharmacotherapy knowledge required to conduct a comprehensive assessment of your patient's drug-related needs because over a 40-year career, a clinician will conduct over 160,000 patient assessments.[1]

> **Note** All of your subsequent activities, clinical decisions, care planning, interventions, and evaluation are dependent upon your ability to fully assess your patient's drug-related needs and identify drug therapy problems.

The thoroughness and organization of the assessment play a major role in determining how effective you will be as a practitioner and whether your patients will receive the maximum benefit from your work.

There is structure to the assessment so that the practitioner can be logical, systematic, and comprehensive in the work that must be accomplished. The activities and responsibilities of the assessment are shown in Table 6-1.

Table 6-1 Activities and responsibilities in the assessment

Activities	Responsibilities
Meet the patient	Establish the therapeutic relationship
Elicit relevant information from the patient	Determine who your patient is as an individual by learning about the reason for the encounter, the patient's demographics, medication experience, and other clinical information
Make rational drug therapy decisions using the Pharmacotherapy Workup	Determine whether drug-related needs are being met (indication, effectiveness, safety, compliance)
	Identify drug therapy problems

During each assessment interview the three responsibilities of developing the therapeutic relationship, assessing drug-related needs, and identifying drug therapy problems are simultaneously at work, and each function influences the other two. Practitioners in training need to expend considerable effort to develop the knowledge and skills required for each of these essential tasks; however, you can work on developing one skill at a time so as not to become overwhelmed with the task at hand.

During every assessment, the pharmaceutical care practitioner must collect information and make clinical decisions concerning the relevance of the patient's demographics, medication experience, immunization history, allergies and adverse reactions, medication history, and current medical conditions and drug therapies. This is accomplished through clinical assessment and inquiry skills and the use of the Pharmacotherapy Workup.

The assessment and inquiry functions are accomplished by the use of two sets of questions. One is a structured set of questions the practitioner must learn to ask him/herself about the patient, diseases, and drug therapies and their interrelatedness. The other set is the questions the practitioner can address directly to the patient to elicit the information necessary to properly assess all of the patient's drug-related needs. It is important to learn how to effectively collect information directly from your patient. A few basic skills can help in this most important clinical endeavor. The mark of an effective practitioner is one who can combine the skills of asking appropriate assessment questions and analyzing the patient, disease, and drug data in a logical, structured manner.

The Pharmacotherapy Workup directs you through a logical decision-making process that allows you to evaluate the appropriateness, effectiveness, and safety of each of the patient's medications and determine the ability and willingness of the patient to be compliant with the drug therapy.

Standard of Care 1: Collection of Patient-specific Information

Standards of care have been developed for the major activities in practice: the assessment, care plan, and follow-up evaluation. These standards apply to the care that the practitioner provides for individual patients. These standards are applicable to all practice sites, diseases, patients, and drug therapy categories because they represent the generalist practitioner's responsibilities to provide pharmaceutical care.

The standards of care are presented throughout Chapters 6, 8, and 9 so the practitioner knows the performance expected when providing pharmaceutical care. The complete set of standards for the practice of pharmaceutical care can be found in the Appendix. The first standard of care for the assessment (there are three in all) is given below.

STANDARD 1: THE PRACTITIONER COLLECTS RELEVANT PATIENT-SPECIFIC INFORMATION TO USE IN DECISION-MAKING CONCERNING ALL DRUG THERAPIES.

Measurement criteria

1. Pertinent data are collected using appropriate interview techniques.
2. Data collection involves the patient, family and care-givers, and health care providers when appropriate.
3. The medication experience is elicited by the practitioner and incorporated as the context for decision-making.
4. The data are used to develop a pharmacologically relevant description of the patient and the patient's drug-related needs.
5. The relevance and significance of the data collected are determined by the patient's present conditions, illnesses, wants, and needs.
6. The medication history is complete and accurate.
7. The current medication record is complete and accurate.
8. The data collection process is systematic and ongoing.
9. Only data that are required and used by the practitioner are elicited from the patient.
10. Relevant data are documented in a retrievable form.
11. All data collection and documentation is conducted in a manner that ensures patient confidentiality.

MEETING THE PATIENT

The first responsibility involved in the patient-practitioner interaction is to establish an effective therapeutic relationship so the practitioner can collect, analyze, and use relevant patient-specific information to understand who the patient is and what he/she wants. Meeting and greeting your patient is a very important step in establishing this relationship.

You must meet and greet a person you may have never met before, describe all of his or her drug-related needs, identify drug therapy problems, design a plan to resolve those problems as well as achieve therapeutic goals, and make certain that your patient experiences the maximum effectiveness from every medication. To accomplish all of this, it is important to start in a positive direction with each patient. The therapeutic relationship begins the moment you first meet your patient. Make greeting him or her a positive experience for both of you.

Introducing Yourself

How you introduce yourself sends a very distinct message. If you are a student, make certain your patient understands that you have a preceptor, mentor, or staff member who is fully responsible for the care being provided and is available if needed.

Decide how you want to be addressed. Your patients most often address you in the same manner in which you introduce yourself. Consider whether you want your patients to use your given name, surname, and/or applicable prefixes. Your patients will usually follow your lead. As an example, you might introduce yourself as *Sally, Sally Brown, Ms. Sally Brown, Dr. Sally Brown,* or *Dr. Brown.* Keep in mind that written materials you provide to your patients might also have your name on them, and it will be helpful if you are consistent. Furthermore, your colleagues and other staff in the patient care areas will also address you in the presence of your patients, and it will be less confusing if everyone calls you by the same name and/or title.

Addressing your patient in a proper manner is essential to begin a positive, respectful relationship. Addressing adult patients as Mr., Ms., or Mrs. is most often appropriate. Children usually prefer to be addressed by their first names. Correct pronunciation of your patient's name is important to him/her. If you are unsure of how to correctly say or pronounce it, ask how he/she would like to be addressed and how he/she pronounces his/her name.

During the assessment interview the patient's perception of your professional expertise is based on many factors including your dress and demeanor, quality and relevance of your comments, your ability to elicit relevant information, your ability to provide meaningful information, feedback, and explanations, as well as your attitude of confidence. If you are well prepared to meet and help your patient, you will find your patients are forthcoming, open, and appreciative of your work.

The Physical Environment

The assessment interview can be personal and involve the exchange of sensitive information. The physical environment you choose to practice in reflects you and the choices that you make as a practitioner. A semi-private or private space must be provided for you to conduct an assessment of your patient's drug-related needs. Unlike a physical examination, the assessment of a patient's drug-related needs rarely requires a fully private area. An environment in which the patient feels comfortable and assured that others cannot hear the conversation is often sufficient. However, some patients will need to speak with you in private about some drug-related issues, and therefore it is advisable to have a fully private space available for those occasions.

Keep the area where you meet with patients clean and organized. It is their space, not yours. Only have materials available that you intend to use to help patients such as informational brochures, patient records, access to the internet, or samples of products or drug administration devices for demonstration. If you have large supplies of these items, only keep a minimal supply in the patient care area. Keep in mind that most of these items are new to your patients and can be distracting during the assessment interview.

A comprehensive assessment requires focused work on the part of the practitioner. First, you will need to focus on your patient and his or her needs. This means that how you feel personally, how your day is going, what is on your mind, what you were just doing, and what you will be doing later must all be set aside. Your patient has come to see you. You need to give each patient your full and undivided attention. This person trusts that you will do your very best to help. The patient believes you can and do care about his/her well-being. He or she will believe that you have the skills and knowledge to help. He or she needs to feel comfortable and know that at this moment you are committed to helping with whatever drug-related issue he/she may have.

Taking Notes

You will often need to take notes during the assessment. At times you may want to record the patient's words verbatim as he/she describes the medication experience. Documentation is an essential standard of practice that you must meet. It is important that your patient feels comfortable with this. Take the time to explain how essential it is for your records to reflect what is truly happening with the patient and his/her medications.

Assure your patient that all records you make are considered confidential. You can only make good decisions and provide good advice with good data. Well-meaning decisions based upon bad or missing information can become bad decisions. When you use a computer to document care, be careful not to focus your attention on the machine at the expense of your patient. Once you have computerized your pharmaceutical care records, you will find that only very minimal note taking is required.

ELICITING INFORMATION FROM THE PATIENT

During the assessment, a significant amount of information is needed from the patient. It is important to be clear about what information is relevant to the patient's case so that only the information you will use is gathered, otherwise time and resources are wasted. The information that is necessary for the assessment is represented in Table 6-2.

All of this information is necessary in all patient encounters; however, each patient is different and will require a different level of detail in each of these data categories.

Getting Started

No two patients have exactly the same medication experience. Student practitioners need to embrace these individual differences and not become frustrated that every patient, and every drug regimen, does not respond in the same manner.

The first two challenges for the student practitioner are to learn what information is necessary to help each patient and how to effectively gather the necessary patient-specific information. The *what* includes information that describes the personal characteristics of the patient that influence the use and outcomes of drug therapies. The *how* involves becoming skilled in eliciting patient-specific information by employing open-ended questions that help the patient to tell his/her story and then delving into relevant areas in search of sufficient detail to make the necessary clinical decisions.

Table 6-2   Patient information required for the assessment

Demographic information	Patient's medication experience	Clinical information
Age Weight, height Gender Pregnancy status Living arrangements Occupation	Patient's attitude toward taking medication and description of wants, concerns, understanding, beliefs, and behaviors	Reason for the encounter
	Medication history Immunization history Allergies and adverse drug reactions Social drug use Special needs	Relevant medical history
	Current medication record Medical conditions—all related drug therapies (indication—product-dosage-outcome)	Review of systems

Elicitation techniques that encourage the patient to state his or her full range of concerns and questions and that help the patient stay actively involved in the assessment process, lead to a more valid assessment of needs and problems, more comprehensive data, greater patient satisfaction, better patient compliance, and more positive clinical outcomes.

Introductions such as the following can be useful to inform your patient of what to expect:

- I would like to talk with you today in order to gather some information about your medications and determine how we can best meet your needs.
- Today we will review all of your drug therapies, so we can make certain that you get the results you want from all of your medications.

Keep in mind that your primary goal is to determine what your patient wants and needs from you. You will find it helpful to present open-ended questions during most of the assessment interview. Open-ended questions ask what, when, why, where, who, and how. They allow the patient to fully respond and facilitate complete descriptions of needs, wants, concerns, and experiences.[1-3]

The first information you will need from your patient is the reason for the present encounter. The following questions may help to initiate this discussion:

- What can I do for you today?
- How can I help you today?

If you have provided care for this patient in the past, you can open the assessment with:

- I am glad you came to see me today. Tell me how you have been feeling since the last time we talked.
- Tell me how well your new medications have been working for you.

Reason for the Encounter

The patient's primary reason(s) for the encounter anchors and directs the practitioner's assessment process. The primary reason for the encounter can be variable and may be an illness that must be managed with drug therapy, a disease, a complaint, a question, or a new condition that has developed.

The patient's idea of the primary reason for the encounter is vital information in the assessment of drug-related needs and is often documented directly in the patient's words.

> **Example** For the assessment of a patient with multiple active medical conditions, who is being treated by several physicians with numerous medications, and who asks you to attempt to simplify her complex medication schedule, you may want to note her description of "I need help to figure out if I really need to take all of these pills they have me taking." In this example, the patient's view of the reason for the encounter can be used to direct the practitioner to try to eliminate unnecessary or duplicate medications from her regimen. Simplifying the patient's drug regimen so she needs to take fewer doses less often throughout the day may also meet her needs.

The patient's primary concern is the focus of the assessment. The portion of your patient's medication experience that is the primary cause for the present encounter is what your patient is most concerned about today, and you must give it your first and full attention. This is the most current information that you have available. Other past information may also be valuable, but the truly current information is found in the patient's description of the primary reason for seeking your help today.

The history of the present problem can yield the most essential data you will need in your identification of the patient's drug therapy problems. Again, it is important to emphasize that the patient and the patient's view of his or her situation frequently serve to guide the assessment and identification of drug therapy problems. This is similar to the physician's assessment of a patient to determine the medical problem or diagnosis. The wealth of information that can be contained in your patient's *story* of the present problem includes its severity, context, location, quality, timing, modifying factors, and associated signs and symptoms.[4]

Early in your assessment as you explore the primary reason for the encounter, you will want to understand how important resolving this problem or condition is for your patient. You will need to determine when it began, previous attempts to treat it, and the results or outcomes of any previous therapeutic approaches. You will always need to explore fully what self-care steps your patient has taken in an attempt to control or resolve his/her problem. If your patient has had limited success in the past, you will want to discover how much faith your patient has in drug therapy, so you can determine if you can confidently recommend continuation. On the other hand, if your patient has attempted to treat his/her condition with little or no positive results, you must recognize that repeating this same drug therapy or recommending continuation of that same medication will have a negative influence on the therapeutic relationship and probably result in poor compliance.

This is a good time to consider the important connections that the practitioner must make throughout the assessment process. The presenting signs and symptoms form the basis for goals of therapy in the care plan. These goals of therapy will then be compared with outcomes to judge effectiveness of drug therapies during the follow-up evaluation step. Figure 6-1 describes these relationships.

> **Example** A patient who is diagnosed with major depression and who has experienced the signs and symptoms of irritability, difficulty sleeping, depressed mood, loss of energy, disappointment in self, and diminished interest in usual activities over the past 3–4 four weeks is started on a selective serotonin reuptake inhibitor (SSRI) to treat his depression. Improvement in these clinical signs and symptoms within an appropriate time frame form the goals of therapy, and outcomes related to the SSRI therapy will be evaluated based on the evidence of improvement in these same signs and symptoms at follow-up evaluation.

The information describing your patient's presenting signs and symptoms, illness, condition, or problem will focus much of the remaining assessment. Your patient's primary complaint, question, or illness serves as the *beginning* and the *ending* of the assessment. It will focus your inquiry and initiates connections with other patient-specific data you might need to gather later in the assessment. Furthermore, to conclude the assessment you must provide your patient with your clinical judgments about his/her primary presenting problem or question.

The following is a set of open-ended questions to help gather a complete, efficient, description of the patient's reason for the encounter:

- How long have you felt this way?
- How often does it occur?

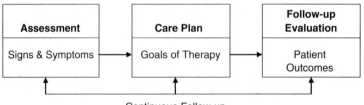

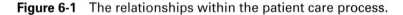

Figure 6-1 The relationships within the patient care process.

- When did it start?
- What do you mean when you say your medication makes you feel tired?
- What do you think is the cause?
- Why do you feel your medication is not working?

It is important to understand that during an assessment interview, all of the relevant information should be obtained, but the clinician rarely conducts an assessment in a strict section-by-section order. Patients provide information in the order and depth that makes the most sense to them. The clinician must be flexible enough to pursue a topic with the patient and later in the interview, return to obtain any additional information that might be required. This is why it is necessary for every pharmaceutical care practitioner to be completely familiar with all the components of the Pharmacotherapy Workup.

The most efficient way to do this is to allow patients to tell you their story—the medication experience—in their own words. This uncovers the information you will use to provide pharmaceutical care within the patient's understanding and relevance. The practitioner must help to guide the story-telling to include the necessary clarity, completeness, and detail to make drug therapy decisions. Practitioners are often tempted to take total control of the assessment interview, but this invariably leads to the practitioner not analyzing factors that are important to the patient.

If you are talking, your patient is not talking. If your patient is not talking, you are not gaining new information. As a student practitioner you are learning a new way of thinking and of making decisions in the best interest of patients regarding their diseases and their medications. Learning new methods of thinking and acting can be frustrating at times. As you gain more knowledge and experience, you will become more confident and more efficient. Experience requires learning at every opportunity and integrating what you have learned with what you already know. Take every opportunity with a patient to learn the most you can from his or her unique medication experience: what was effective, what failed, what they liked, what they did not like, and why. Adding the information from their stories to your clinical experience is difficult at first, but it begins with the assessment interview.[5]

Patient Demographics

The individual characteristics of each patient create the context for all of your clinical activities. Patient demographic information is needed to see each patient as a unique individual. The purpose of the patient demographic portion of your assessment is to determine who your patient is and to provide a description of him or her at the time of the assessment. Your goal is to observe and elicit information describing the personal characteristics of the patient that are relevant to making drug therapy decisions.

Your patient's demographic data consists of the information that allows you to treat him or her as a unique individual. Who is this patient? How does he or she appear? Does the patient live alone or with family members or friends? What makes this person unique and therefore have different drug-related needs than the last patient you met? Relevant information includes all of the data that will be useful to select and individualize drug therapies, doses, and instructions, establish goals of therapy, construct care plans, and suggest life style changes. This information will also be used to determine the optimal timing, methods, and intensity of follow-up evaluations to analyze actual positive and negative outcomes of drug therapies.

The patient demographics portion of your assessment can vary from requiring a few pieces of vital statistics to in-depth collection and analysis of information that personalizes your clinical decisions concerning the patient's drug-related needs. The initial patient demographic information most often includes age, gender (to assess risk factors including pregnancy), height, weight, and ethnicity/cultural origin.

Age of the patient Age is a vital statistic when providing pharmaceutical care as it is often applied to both the discovery of the indication for drug therapy as well as the appropriate choice of pharmacotherapy to manage the disease or illness. The patient's age is also required for selecting appropriate products and dosage forms suitable for his or her age group, and for dosing guidelines (pediatric, geriatric). The appropriate approach to drug therapy for pneumonia is different in a 7-week-old patient, a 7-year-old patient, and a 70-year-old patient. Age is best identified and documented as birth date, so that age can be continuously updated as you provide care year after year.

Height and weight Each patient's height and weight should be documented so it can be used for dosage individualization. In many situations observational estimates of body weight are sufficient, but for extremely obese patients, or infants and children, and when using medications that require precise dose to body weight determinations, the exact weight of your patient must be known.

Much of the drug dosing literature considers a normal or average adult body weight to be 70 kg and a body surface area of 1.73 m^2. Lean or ideal body weight is often a better determinant for drug dosage than total or actual body weight, especially in obese patients. A patient is considered to be overweight if his/her body mass index (BMI) is 25–29.9 kg/m^2 and obese if the BMI is $\geq$30 kg/m^2.[7] Lean body weight can be estimated for dosage individualization of specific medications. There are simple methods to estimate lean body weight, BMI, or body surface area using equations based on height and weight measurements (Table 6-3).[6–8]

Living situation   The patient's living situation is often a key factor in determining drug-related needs. Who lives with the patient and who cares for the patient? Does your patient have children who live at home, and are their ages important to consider for safety purposes (child-proof tops, storage of medications)? Does the patient live with his/her parents, spouse, or significant other? Does he or she live alone? Who is responsible for administering medications and making health care decisions? Do other family members have a history of certain diseases, illnesses, or other risk factors (smoking, alcohol use, eating disorder) that may negatively affect your patient's drug therapy outcomes (coronary artery disease, depression, allergies)?

Family background, health insurance, and other special needs that might require specific accommodations are also helpful to gather during the assessment.

Questions to help you understand more about your patient might include the following:

- Can you tell me a little about yourself?
- Can you describe your typical day?
- How would describe your family situation?
- What type of work do you do?
- Is anyone else at home also ill?
- How much assistance with taking your medications do you receive from other family members?
- What arrangements for transportation do you have to make to come to these appointments?
- Is there anything you would like me to do that will help you to understand and remember the instructions for your medications?
- What issues or problems do you have with insurance coverage for the medications that you need?

Table 6-3   Estimates for adult body weight, mass, and surface area

Ideal body weight males (kg) = 50 kg + [2.3 × inches > 5'0"]
Ideal body weight females (kg) = 45 kg + [2.3 × inches > 5'0"]
Body mass index (kg/m^2) = (weight in kg)/(height in meters)^2
Body surface area (m^2) = ((height in cm) × (weight in kg/3600))$^{1/2}$

Your patient's occupation and socioeconomic status can have a dramatic influence on drug-related needs and subsequent outcomes. Does your patient's occupation put him/her at risk for certain diseases, injuries, or drug therapy problems? Drowsiness from antihistamines often found in cough and cold products might have a different impact on your patient if he or she is a commercial airline pilot or over the road truck driver, as opposed to your next patient who is a studio musician or a librarian.

Pregnancy and breast-feeding   Practitioners are often confronted with inquires concerning the safety of medication use in pregnant or breast-feeding patients. The decisions in these situations involve weighing the therapeutic benefits of the drug to the mother against its risk to the developing fetus or infant.

When conducting an assessment of a pregnant patient, the practitioner should record the due date. Most pregnant women know their due date, and this allows the practitioner to determine which trimester the patient is in during any subsequent evaluations. Risk to the fetus is difficult to predict, however exposure to harmful drugs during the first trimester is most dangerous.

We often lack sufficient data and clear answers about the use of most medications during pregnancy or breast-feeding because the outcomes of such use are rarely studied and are difficult to collect. The amount of new information on drug effects on the fetus continues to grow. The risks that a drug poses to the fetus have been assigned to a risk factor level of A, B, C, D, or X. In this system, which is used by the U.S. Food and Drug Administration, the lowest level of risk is noted as risk factor A which is felt to be safely used during pregnancy, while the risk factor designated as X indicates that there is strong evidence of fetal abnormalities caused by the drug.[9,10] Each category is described in Table 6-4.

In general, substances of low molecular weight diffuse freely across the placenta due primarily to the concentration gradient. The vast majority of substances used for therapeutic purposes can pass from the mother to the fetus. The safety of medications used by mothers who are breast-feeding infants must also be assessed for the potential risk to the infant. In patients who are breast-feeding, the risks from a specific medication are usually much clearer, although we often must infer risk and benefit from data generated on related drug products. If the drug is generally safe to give directly to the infant, then it is generally thought to be safe to give to the mother during lactation.[10] Table 6-5 lists the pregnancy risk factor levels for commonly used medications.

Before discussing the patient's medication experience, it is important to review the demographic information elicited during the assessment.

Table 6-4 Risk factors: drug use during pregnancy[9,10]

Category A:	Controlled studies in women fail to demonstrate a risk to the fetus in the first trimester (and there is not evidence of a risk in later trimesters), and the possibility of fetal harm appears remote.
Category B:	Either animal-reproduction studies have not demonstrated a fetal risk, but there are not controlled studies in pregnant women, or animal reproduction studies have shown an adverse effect (other than a decrease in fertility) that was not confirmed in controlled studies in women in the first trimester (and there is no evidence of a risk in later trimesters).
Category C:	Either studies in animals have revealed adverse effects on the fetus (teratogenic, embryocidal, or other) and there are no controlled studies in women or studies in women and animals are not available. Drugs should be given only if the potential benefit justifies the potential risk to the fetus.
Category D:	There is positive evidence of human fetal risk, but the benefits from use in pregnant women may be acceptable despite the risk (e.g., if the drug is needed in a life- threatening situation or for a serious disease for which safer drugs cannot be used or are ineffective).
Category X:	Studies in animals or human beings have demonstrated fetal abnormalities, or there is evidence of fetal risk based on human experience or both, and the risk of the use of the drug in pregnant women clearly outweighs any possible benefit. The drug is contraindicated in women who are or may become pregnant.

Table 6-6 provides a review of the important variables and the influence each can have on your drug therapy decisions.

Understanding the Patient's Medication Experience

The patient's medication experience is the personal context for all of your patient-specific clinical decisions. The better you understand it, the better your decisions will be. A detailed description of the medication experience can be found in Chapter 5. You will be expected to know more about the patient's medication experience than any other member of the health care team.

The patient's description   No two patients have exactly the same medication experience. Even patients who have never taken any medications have some attitudes or beliefs concerning drug therapy that they acquired from

Table 6-5   Pregnancy risk factor ratings for commonly used medications[a]

Commonly used medications	Risk factor rating	Commonly used medications	Risk factor rating
Acetaminophen	B	Gabapentin (Neurontin)	C
Albuterol	C	Glipizide (Glucotrol)	C
Amlodipine (Norvasc)	C	Guaifenesin	D
Amoxicillin	B	Heparin	C
Ampicillin plus clavulanate potassium (Augmentin)	B	Ibuprofen	B
Atenolol	C	Imipramine	D
Atorvastatin (Lipitor)	X	Lansopraxole (Prevacid)	B
Azithromycin (Zithromax)	B	Levothyroxine	A
Captopril	C	Metformin (Glucophage)	B
Celecoxib (Celebrex)	C	Olanzapine (Zyprexa)	C
Cephalexin	B	Omerprazole (Prilosec)	C
Chlorpheniramine	B	Oxycodone	B
Cimetidine	B	Paroxetine (Paxil)	C
Ciprofloxacin	C	Phenytoin	D
Claritin (Loratadine)	B	Ranitidine	B
Codeine	C	Risperidone (Risperdal)	C
Digoxin	C	Simvastatin (Zocor)	X
Diltiazem (Cardizem)	C	Sertraline (Zoloft)	C
Fluoxetine (Prozac)	C	Warfarin	D
Furosemide	C		

[a]Manufacturers do not always submit new findings that change the risk factor ratings; therefore, it is important to check other sources such as Briggs Drugs in Pregnancy and Lactation.[10]

friends, family, or the media. The patient's medication experience is the most specific information you have available to make an assessment of your patient's drug-related needs. It includes the patient's preferences, attitudes, general understanding of his or her drug therapy, concerns about it, expressed expectations of desired outcomes, and the patient's medication taking behavior. An initial objective of the assessment is to make clinical judgments about the patient's preferences and attitudes concerning medications and to what extent they influence the decision-making process. Your patient has to decide if and how to use medications.

Table 6-6 A summary of demographic information and their influence on drug therapy decisions

Variable	Description of the pharmacological relevance of the information to decision-making
Age	• The risk of diseases changes with age. • The risk of exposure to various drugs is different among patients of different ages. • Dosage requirements vary greatly with age. • Absorption, metabolism, and elimination of most drugs changes with age. • Patients within different age groups have different medical problems and often have different goals of therapy. • Frequency and severity of drug therapy problems change with age. • In general, for pharmacotherapy decisions, patient ages are grouped as infants (birth to 12 months), children (1–2 up to 11–12 years), adolescents (11–19 years), adults, and elderly (65 and older). For example: 7-year-old patients with rheumatoid arthritis are often treated differently than 77-year-old patients with rheumatoid arthritis.
Gender	• Gender can influence disease risk and frequency. • Hypothyroidism, anemia, and osteoporosis requiring drug therapy are more common in females. • Cardiovascular disorders requiring drug therapy management develop more often in adult males.
Pregnancy	• Many drug therapies are known to be harmful to the fetus if taken by the mother during pregnancy. These drugs are teratogenic and their use is considered to be contraindicated during pregnancy. • Pregnancy can also create additional needs for vitamins and other supplements. • Diabetes, hypertension, and other medical conditions requiring drug therapy management can develop during pregnancy. • Most medications taken by nursing mothers can be transferred to the infant via breast milk. Infant safety must be considered before adding any medication to a nursing mother's regimen. • Postpartum depression can require short-term management with medications.
Occupation	• Medications that can cause central nervous system depression, drowsiness, or confusion may interfere with patients' ability to concentrate or make judgments required in their jobs. • Some occupations restrict medications that employees are allowed to use to manage illnesses. Examples include airline pilots, police, and other safety officers.

(Continued)

Table 6-6   (*Continued*) A summary of demographic information and their influence on drug therapy decisions

Variable	Description of the pharmacological relevance of the information to decision-making
Living arrangements	• Others who live in the same household as the patient may be available to assist with drug therapy management. For example: A family member who acts as the patient's caregiver may assist with drug administration. • Others in the household can also be exposed to medications known to be potentially dangerous. For example: Young children in the house need to be protected from medications that could cause them serious harm. • Consider storage of all medications, childproof containers, and the availability of antidotes.

Your patient's expression of preferences, needs, expectations, and concerns will form the basis for the majority of what will follow in the assessment, care plan, and evaluation. It is important to remind yourself that these early patient impressions are most important because they reflect how the patient sees the situation. You may discover that some other issue is more important or more critical, but you must always return to your patient's initial impressions because that is the basis for his/her decision-making process. Your clinical decisions, impression, advice, and knowledge must be related to the patient's view of his/her medication experience. Remember, the more you understand the patient's medication experience, the more likely it is that you can positively influence it.

In order to have this positive influence, you will need to assess your patient's overall understanding of his/her medical conditions or illnesses and how they are or can best be managed by drug therapies. Discovering the patient's understanding will help you determine what additional information and education you must provide.

The information you discover while inquiring about your patient's medication experience will direct virtually all your subsequent thinking and questioning. In order to contextualize your decision-making you will need to make clinical judgments about several aspects of the patient's view of his or her personal medication experience.

During the assessment step of your assessment, you will need to inquire and make judgments about the following questions:

- What is your patient's level of understanding of his/her disease or illness, drug therapies, and therapeutic instructions?
- What concerns does your patient have about his/her health in general or medical conditions and drug therapies in particular?
- What concerns does your patient have about side effects, toxicities, adverse events, or allergies?
- What does your patient dislike about his/her drug therapies?
- Are your patient's expectations and goals realistic and achievable?
- To what extent does your patient want to be an active participant in his/her care?
- To what degree is the cost of drug therapy, clinic visits, hospitalizations, or treatment failures, a concern for your patient?

You will want to inquire as to what the patient expects to gain from his/her drug therapies. What are the patient's goals of therapy? You will also need to determine if the patient's expectations are realistic. Your clinical judgment concerning these important areas of inquiry will establish the scope of patient information necessary to familiarize you with your patient's medication experience and to begin to establish a strong and positive therapeutic relationship.

Example   What your patient wants from you and expects from his or her drug therapies serves as the basis for establishing the goals of therapy that will become part of the care plan. If your patient who has injured her ankle 2 days ago states "I really wish you could give me something that will control the pain in my ankle so I can get a full night's sleep. I don't think that aspirin or ibuprofen are strong enough to help this time," you may recommend some change in analgesic therapy, anti-inflammatory drug therapy, or some other pharmacotherapeutic approach. From her statement you know that her goal of therapy is to get a restful night of sleep, and she has little confidence in the potential for aspirin or ibuprofen to be effective. The patient will evaluate the success of the treatment from this perspective.

Medication history   Your comprehensive assessment of the patient's medication history will include immunization status, social drug use, allergies, adverse reactions and other special needs, and a history of relevant medication use.

Immunization record   Even to this day, most patient care documentation systems, and in fact many health care record systems in general, do not adequately address individual immunization records. In the United States, tracking vulnerable children to ascertain their immunization status is largely left to the school systems. However, because one of your primary responsibilities as a pharmaceutical care practitioner is prevention, an assessment of your patient's immunization history is an essential part of the assessment.

With the exceptions of clean water, sanitation, and nutrition, the most effective mechanism that modern health care has developed to prevent disease and human suffering is immunization. Diseases such as polio, mumps, diphtheria, tetanus, pertussis, rubella, and many forms of hepatitis and influenza can be effectively prevented if patients are properly immunized. Immunization standards vary throughout the world, but they are commonly designed to ensure adequate protection against diseases that can reach epidemic proportions. Ensuring that your patient is adequately immunized is certainly a health care priority and a primary patient care responsibility in pharmaceutical care practice. Immunization recommendations differ with age.

Figure 6-2 shows the current recommendations from the Center for Disease Control and Prevention for children from birth to 18 years of age and for adults.

Questions that can help to elicit immunization information include the following:

- What can you recall about your immunizations?
- When was your last tetanus shot?
- When was your last flu shot?
- When was your last pneumonia shot?

Social drug use   The definition of drug use in the context of pharmaceutical care is quite extensive and implies a therapeutic use. Knowing your patient's exposure to caffeine, nicotine, alcohol, and drugs of abuse will avoid detrimental drug interactions, dosage errors, and even toxic reactions. When providing pharmaceutical care, you will need to assess your patient's use or exposure to these ubiquitous agents and determine the impact this exposure may be having on the health and well-being of this individual.

Use of these drugs may be a habit that the patient would like to discontinue, and, if so, you can be an invaluable resource in meeting the patient's drug-related needs.

When inquiring about tobacco use, you can ask:

- Are you now, or have you ever been a smoker?
- Is this something you would find difficult to give up?
- How would you describe your attempts to cut down or quit in the past?

	Birth	1 mo	2 mos	4 mos	6 mos	12 mos	15 mos	18 mos	24 mos	4–6 yrs	11–12 yrs	13–18 yrs
Hepatitis B	Dose 1		Dose 2			Dose 3						
Diphtheria, Tetanus, Pertussis			1	2	3			4				
Haemonphilus influenzae Type b			1	2	3	4						
Polio-inactivated			1	2		3				4		
Measles, Mumps, Rubella						1				2		
Varicella (chicken pox)												
Pneumococcal			1	2	3	4						
Hepatitis A (children in high risk regions)									Hepatitis A Series			
Influenza (Children ≥6 with asthma, diabetes, HIV, sickle cell, cardiac disease)						Yearly						

	19–49 Years	50–64 Years	65 Years & older
Tetanus, Diphtheria (Td)	1 booster every 10 years	1 booster every 10 years	1 booster every 10 years
Influenza	1 dose annually for persons with medical or occupational indications or household contacts of persons with indications	1 annual dose	1 annual dose
Pneumococcal (polysaccharide)	1 dose for persons with medical or other indications (1 dose revaccination for immunosuppressive conditions)	1 dose for person with medical or other indications (1 dose revaccination for immunosuppressive conditions)	1 dose for unvaccinated persons 1 dose revaccination

Figure 6-2 Current recommendations for children from birth to 18 years of age and for adults (see http:///www.cdc.gov/nip for more information).

Effective smoking cessation programs and products are widely available and can have a positive influence on a patient's quality of life and outcomes. The pharmaceutical care practitioner can provide this service. Moreover, poor outcomes from comorbidities, especially respiratory and cardiovascular disorders, can often be prevented through a comprehensive assessment and management of the patient's smoking and/or alcohol use. Similarly, constant exposure to drugs of abuse and the associated addictive behaviors of tolerance, withdrawal symptoms, self-deception, loss of will power, and distortion of attention, can place your patient at risk to experience serious medical, financial, compliance, or other drug therapy problems. It is essential to maintain patient confidentiality when assessing social drug use. Only collect and document information that is relevant to the drug-related decisions you will be making.

Allergies and adverse reactions   An essential part of any assessment of a patient's drug-related needs is your patient's drug allergies and a history of adverse drug reactions. This information will help to manage your patient's risk and thus prevent future drug therapy problems. The reason to distinguish between a drug allergy and an adverse reaction is that how you define the situation will dictate how you make drug therapy decisions to resolve or prevent it.

> **Example**   If your patient has a history of an allergic reaction to penicillin, this usually implies that it is not safe to expose him or her to penicillin (or related products) ever in the future. Reexposing the patient who is allergic to penicillin to a penicillin-containing product can be life threatening. Doing so would likely place your patient at immediate risk of a known, severe, and possibly life-threatening allergic reaction. This might include an anaphylactoid or anaphylactic reaction.

An adverse drug reaction most commonly involves a negative or undesirable effect that your patient experienced with a specific drug product in the past. These types of reactions are important to document, so you and others who provide care for the patient can consider the risks and benefits of using that particular agent again. In most cases, an allergic reaction to a drug product requires that the patient not receive that drug or related agents in the future. However, if your patient has experienced an undesirable adverse effect caused by a drug product that was not deemed to be allergic in nature, in future decisions that product may be considered appropriate despite the past adverse reaction. Chapter 5 describes adverse drug reactions and drug allergies.

> **Example**   If your patient experienced nausea and gastric discomfort when taking erythromycin to treat a skin infection, then you need to consider that adverse reaction when selecting antibiotics for that patient in the future. However, this adverse reaction does not necessarily preclude you from using erythromycin or related macrolide antimicrobials to treat future infections in that patient. Erythromycin might certainly be considered a viable treatment in your patient who experienced nausea from erythromycin as long as the first episode was appropriately assessed and documented as an adverse effect, and not as an allergic response.

To make these important clinical distinctions between allergic reactions and other predictable adverse drug reactions, you will need to be familiar with the presentation, timing, and common drugs involved in allergic reactions. Similarly, you will need to be familiar with commonly encountered adverse reactions to drugs, especially those that can be successfully managed by dosage adjustments or other means without necessitating withholding that medication from your patient in the future.

In the case of adverse reactions to drug products, you must assess whether your patient could not tolerate the medication, or a particular dosage form, and what reservations your patient might have about being reexposed to this particular medication.

Questions that might help to elicit this important information include:

- What happened when you took that drug?
- What happened when you stopped taking the drug?
- Have you ever taken that same medicine again?

When caring for young patients, you will want to pay particular attention to allergic symptoms that are common during infancy and childhood. These include eczema, urticaria, perennial allergic rhinitis, as well as reactions to insect bites and stings.

Health alerts, health aids, and special needs   Many patients have some special or unique needs that must be identified and incorporated into the assessment of specific drug therapy requirements. These often include physical limitations such as sight and/or hearing impairment. This might require larger than usual print for instructions or written or face-to-face follow-up rather than telephone communications. Patients requiring contact lenses or eye glasses for vision correction may appreciate larger or bolder print for instructions, and may be very interested in new products or advances in contact lens technologies or lens care products as they become available.

Although the general description of the patient often includes observable physical characteristics such as age, gender, race, height, and weight, it may also be helpful to note any other noticeable, presenting characteristics such as nervousness and difficulties with speech, hearing, or sight. Being aware of language difficulties can be helpful when trying to explain complicated instructions to patients or other family members.

Such cultural contexts and language differences can become barriers to your ability to optimize the patient's medication experience and achieve positive therapeutic outcomes. Your patient may benefit from a translator who can help you to assess the patient's drug-related needs. The use of a trained translator may be preferred to a family member because familial relationships may interfere with the communication of necessary information.

Physical limitations, including requiring a cane, walker, or wheelchair, must be noted and might require home visits, delivery of services, or mail services for medications and supplies to ensure that the patient receives all of the support and care required.

History of relevant medication use   The drug therapies that patients have taken in the past, usually during the last 6 months, can provide useful information. The assessment of past drug treatments is conducted for two primary reasons. First, to determine if the present problem has been treated before with medications and if so, what was the outcome or result. The best information a practitioner can have is that a certain drug regimen has already been used and was effective for a similar episode. If it was effective before, it is likely to be effective again.

The other usefulness of past drug treatment information is to determine if the patient has experienced any treatment failures and unwanted side effects to medications used in the past. If so, then it is important to not reexpose the patient to those drug therapies that have already caused harm. Gathering a comprehensive medication history will help the practitioner avoid repeating mistakes, treatment failures, and side effects of the past.

To be most useful, past drug treatment information should include the indication for the drug, the drug regimen taken the response to that therapy, and why the therapy was discontinued if relevant. For drug therapies taken in the distant past, it is often difficult to ascertain the exact dose and dosing intervals, and sometimes exact dates are not known.

Questions that can help to elicit this information are given below:

- How well did that medication work for you in the past?
- What happened when you took that drug in the past?
- How would you feel about using the same medication again?
- How would you feel about using the same medication but changing the amount we use in order to get a better result this time?

Current medication record   In order to make sound, rational decisions about drug therapy, you must have assessed your patient's medical conditions and all current drug therapies. Your patient's medication record includes: (1) the indication for drug therapy; (2) all of the drug products your patient is taking for that indication; (3) specifically how the patient is actually taking them; and (4) the patient's response to the drug therapy.

Medications: prescription, nonprescription, herbals   A complete medication record is most useful if it includes all prescription medications, all nonprescription products, professional samples, medications obtained from friends or family members, vitamins, nutritional supplements, home remedies, traditional medicines, and natural and homeopathic remedies. Indeed, it includes all substances being taken by the patient for therapeutic purposes. A comprehensive assessment will involve inquiries into conditions that your patient might be treating or preventing with vitamins or minerals, nonprescription cough and cold preparations, laxatives, antacids, topical ointments, creams, or lotions, oral contraceptives, aspirin, acetaminophen, ibuprofen, and dietary or herbal supplements. As some of these products are used on such a routine basis, many patients do not consider them treatments and will need to be asked directly to have them considered in the comprehensive assessment.

Establishing the appropriate indication or *connection* between each drug product that your patient uses and the corresponding medical condition, disease, or illness is a necessity in the provision of pharmaceutical care. For many patients this will be the first time that any practitioner has put forth the effort to collect, organize, assess, and document *indications* and associated *drug therapies*. These data are invaluable, not only for you as a pharmaceutical care practitioner, but also to medical, nursing, emergency, and dental practitioners, as well as other health care providers.

The comprehensive medication record will become the information centerpiece for you to make clinical decisions concerning your patient's drug-related needs. To be most useful, the medication record should clarify the associations between the patient's indications for drug therapy, the drug product and dosage regimens, and the patient's response to each medication regimen. This is accomplished by establishing the fundamental connections between the three important categories of information in the pharmaceutical care process, that of patient, disease, and drug. All three types of information are necessary in order to make rational decisions about a patient's drug therapies.

Recall the four essential elements in the survey of current medical conditions are as follows:

- The active medical condition, illness, disease, signs, and/or symptoms being treated or being prevented by the use of medications (indication)
- The drug product your patient is taking
- The dosage regimen your patient is actually using
- How your patient is responding to the medication—what progress toward desired goals of therapy has been achieved to date

Example "My patient's hypertension has been adequately controlled for the past 4 months with chlorthalidone 25 mg daily."

"He takes 81 mg of aspirin each morning as prevention of a myocardial infarction or a stroke."

"He takes 20 mg of oral propranolol 2 hours before his public speaking engagements in order to prevent stage fright."

The associations that must be made between these variables is illustrated in Fig. 6-3.

Indication A drug without an indication is just a bottle of pills. Assessing all of a patient's medications requires adequate data and an organized, yet comprehensive, thought process. It is essential to establish and document the clinical indication for every medication your patient is taking. The concept of *indication* for drug therapy is intended to encompass all of the clinical reasons that drug therapy might be required by a patient. The concept of indication is broader than simply a diagnosis.

A diagnosis is a medico-legal term used primarily by physicians to describe his or her best medical judgment describing patient's pathology or illness. A diagnosis is established after the medical practitioner meets with the patient, conducts an interview and physical examination, collects and interprets all relevant laboratory test results, and sometimes confers with colleagues. We use drugs in a much broader scope within the health care system.

We often initiate drug therapy before a firm diagnosis is established. We may use medications to assist in establishing the diagnosis. Drug therapy is also used to provide comfort during other treatments. Many preventive medications are used before the signs and symptoms of the disease are present.

Therefore, indication reaches well beyond disease or medical diagnosis, and includes the following uses for drug therapy.[11]

- Cure a disease or illness;
- Prevent a disease or illness;

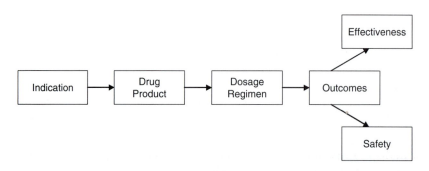

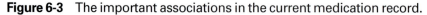

Figure 6-3 The important associations in the current medication record.

- Slow the progression of a disease or illness;
- Supplement nutritional, electrolyte, hormonal, or other deficiencies;
- Correct abnormal laboratory test results;
- Provide comfort or temporary relief from signs and symptoms of a disorder;
- Assist in the diagnostic process.

During the assessment, it is vital that the intended indication for each medication is identified, verified if necessary, and associated with the appropriate medication(s). This connection is required for all drugs in all patients. It is neither efficient nor safe to assume an indication.

Note   The effectiveness or safety of a drug product can only be assessed if you know the intended indication.

The clinical indication is necessary to establish goals of therapy, and goals of therapy are necessary to evaluate outcomes. Establishing and assessing the appropriateness of the indication directs the rest of the pharmaceutical care process. The care plan is dependent on the indication, as are all subsequent evaluations. Identifying and deciding whether the indication is clinically appropriate for the patient is the first clinical judgment you will make within the pharmaceutical care assessment.

Example   If the patient is taking ibuprofen to manage arthritis, the goals of therapy might include the reduction of pain and swelling in the affected joints. At a follow-up evaluation, the clinical outcome would be based on the presence or absence of the swelling and pain of the joints. However, if the patient was taking ibuprofen to manage migraine headaches, the goals of therapy would be quite different and might include the shortening of the duration of the headache and reduction in the severity of the headache pain.

Table 6-7 lists the 25 most common indications for drug therapy in patients who receive pharmaceutical care.

Source of medications   All of the drug products that your patient is taking—or is expected to take—are included in the medication record, whether the medication is a prescription filled at a pharmacy, received from mail-order, a nonprescription product purchased at a store, or a nutritional supplement or home remedy provided by a friend. All of these drug products must be considered in the medication record in order for you to make a comprehensive assessment of your patient's unique drug-related needs.

Table 6-7 Twenty-five most common indications for drug therapy[a]

1. Hypertension	14. Sinusitis
2. Hyperlipidemia	15. Menopausal symptoms
3. Osteoporosis	16. Otitis media
4. Diabetes	17. Anxiety
5. Vitamin/dietary supplement	18. Insomnia
6. Allergic rhinitis	19. Headache pain
7. Depression	20. Cardiac dysrhythmias
8. Esophagitis	21. Streptococcal throat
9. Pain (general)	infections
10. Hypothyroidism	22. Osteoarthritis
11. Asthma	23. Back pain
12. Arthritis pain	24. Angina pectoris
13. Bronchitis	25. Gastritis

[a]In 20,761 patients who have received pharmaceutical care (see Chapter 2 for a detailed description of the sample and methods used to generate these data).

Although prescription medications are a major source of drug therapies, patients also frequently self-medicate. The sources of these products vary and include purchasing nonprescription (over-the-counter or OTC) products, using physician samples, and obtaining medication directly from friends or family members. Samples and drug products provided by friends and family members represent approximately 5% of the products patients use to manage their health (refer to Chapter 2).

You will need to assess the appropriateness of the entire drug therapy including the drug product, dosage form, the dosage regimen your patient is expected to take, the dosage the patient is actually taking, the method of administration, and the duration of therapy. You will assess when the patient started the particular drug regimen, and, if applicable, when it was or should be discontinued is also important to consider and document in the medication record.

The medication record also contains a brief description of the clinician's impression of any evidence as to the effectiveness of each drug regimen, as well as any associated side effects. For every indication and medication combination you must assess the status of both positive and negative outcomes. In most situations the single most influential determinant a practitioner will use in clinical decision-making is direct, patient-specific evidence as to the actual effectiveness, or toxicity, of a particular drug regimen(s). Therefore, each assessment you conduct of a patient's drug-related needs must consider and document any evidence of drug therapy outcomes, be they successes or failures.

A comprehensive medication record which is organized by therapeutic indications, including clinical evidence of outcomes, rarely exists in any other place in the health care system. It is a valuable instrument, not only for you as a pharmaceutical care practitioner, but also for other health care practitioners who care for your patient. Also, patients express thanks and voice appreciation when you provide them with a copy of this type of clear, organized information about all of their medications. Our experience is that patients respond very positively when this record is made available to them as part of their personalized pharmaceutical care plan.

Other Clinical Information

Medical history   The primary purpose of the past medical history portion of the assessment is to describe and make appropriate connections between what you think your patient needs today and the influence of relevant past health events. The past medical history contains information about past serious illnesses, hospitalizations, surgical procedures, pregnancies, deliveries, accidents, or injuries. Data about important past medical conditions can lend useful information to the comprehensive assessment.

Any information in the patient's history or background that suggests a high risk or predisposition to develop a serious condition, or that would represent a contraindication to future drug therapies, should be described as part of the patient's past medical history. It is important to note that past successful or failed drug therapies are often the best predictors of future drug therapy outcomes for individual patients.

> **Example**   Patients who have a history of peptic ulcer disease are at higher risk of gastrointestinal erosion from nonsteroidal anti-inflammatory agents than are patients with no past history of peptic ulcer disease.

In order to make an appropriate transition from inquiring about your patient's current needs to questions about past medical history, you will find it helpful to guide your patient with the following:

- Ok, I think I understand what has been happening over the last few weeks; now, tell me about your health in the past.
- Tell me about any serious illnesses or medical problems you have had in the past.
- How has your health been in the past?

Gathering information about your patient's past medical history is often one of the most challenging for new practitioners. These data are usually well understood by the patient due to the fact that they have already occurred, and your patient has developed a full understanding of these past events. Your patient feels comfortable with this section of the *story*. This portion of the patient's explanations can become quite lengthy and may not add new relevant information to the assessment of current needs. Another challenge to keep in mind is that your patient is here for today's drug-related needs and drug therapy problem(s). There is a tendency, especially on the part of practitioners in their early stages of skill development, to over-collect and sometimes even over-interpret the importance of some historical data.

Before you finish the assessment and determine if drug therapy problems exist, you need to be certain that you have been comprehensive in your fact finding. A brief, but systematic, review of systems will serve that purpose.

Review of systems   An efficient review of systems is organized around body systems. Some practitioners begin with the head and work anatomically through the body. Beginning practitioners will find it useful to consult a list of relevant questions or illnesses so as to not miss an important finding. Positive responses by your patient need to be explored by more focused questions.

A review of systems is a survey of various bodily systems to uncover significant symptoms or problems (drug-related) that have not already been revealed during the assessment interview.[4]

The review of systems is designed to function as a screen for a large number of potential drug therapy problems that the patient may have or be at risk to develop. You will want to explain to the patient that this is a separate part of the assessment and helps you make certain that nothing important is omitted.

You will want to direct the patient to report common, recurrent, or particularly troubling symptoms.

- I need to ask you a series of standard questions to help make sure we do not miss any important information about how well your medications are working for you or any trouble they may be causing.

You will be examining and establishing connections between actions of the medications the patient is taking and signs and symptoms reported. The review of systems is therefore an excellent opportunity to check with the patient for any common side effects he/she may have, but did not associate with any drug therapies.

> **Example** By asking your patient if he or she has experienced any stomach discomfort, diarrhea, or vomiting during the past 2 weeks, you can make a clinical judgment as to whether he or she has experienced any bothersome gastrointestinal side effects from his or her antibiotic therapy or from any other medication.

The review of systems is used to organize new findings, and your interpretation of any abnormal or unexpected results ensures that a comprehensive review has been conducted. For each new finding in your review of systems, you will constantly be asking yourself "Is this something that is being caused by a drug, or is this something that I can treat with a drug?" As described earlier, patients will not always have the ability to identify or describe all of their drug-related needs, and you will need to systematically investigate and assess the patient's medical conditions, complaints, and concerns. When recording your findings in the review of systems, include not only the objective, empirical data but your interpretation of the clinical significance of the result.

> **Example** You can establish and document cause and effect relationships such as an elevation in blood glucose caused by an antihypertensive agent taken by the patient. Similarly, if your patient suffers from confusion and is going to be started on a particular drug that is known to cause cognitive difficulties, then this baseline status will be pertinent in order to evaluate the impact this new medication has on your patient.

The review of systems also allows you to explore in more depth any positive findings from earlier portions of the assessment. The length of the review of systems depends on what information you have gathered up to this point. It should require no more than a few minutes for most patients. The actual order of inquiry is not important, however most clinicians begin with the patient's vital signs.

For each portion in the review of systems we have developed key questions, or areas of inquiry, that are useful. All positive findings should be documented to permit efficient retrieval at a later date, either by you when initially providing care for your patient or by colleagues who subsequently participate in the patient's care. These questions are by no means exhaustive, but are designed to serve as examples of important probes focused on identifying additional drug-related needs at the patient-specific level. The list of questions that you will find helpful to establish your review of systems techniques is shown in Table 6-8.

Table 6-8   Pharmacotherapy Workup—Review of systems

Assessment questions:
- Are there deviations from normal which could be due to drug therapy?
- Are there deviations from normal which should be incorporated into the plan for follow-up evaluations of drug therapy?

Vital Signs
- Temperature: Heart Rate: Blood Pressure: Respiratory Rate:

Eyes, Ears, Nose & Throat
- Do you have any problems with your eyes or eyesight?
- Do you need to wear glasses or contacts?
- Any troubles with your contacts?
- Are you being treated for glaucoma, eye infections, ear infections, cold sores, or dental pain?
- Are you experiencing coughs, colds, sore throats, sinus infections, or seasonal allergies?

Cardiovascular
- Have you had any trouble with your heart; any abnormal rhythms (dysrhythmias), chest pain, dizziness, blood pressure problems?
- What was your blood pressure the last time it was measured?
- Have you ever had your cholesterol checked? What are your cholesterol levels?

Pulmonary
- Are you having any problems with your lungs?
- Do you experience shortness of breath that bothers you?
- Are you now or have you ever been treated for pneumonia, bronchitis, influenza, chronic obstructive pulmonary disease (COPD), pulmonary emboli, or chest pain?

Digestive
- Are you experiencing trouble with your stomach, heart burn, gastritis, or ulcers?
- Any stomach pain, trouble with your bowels, nausea, diarrhea, or vomiting?

Skin
- Are you having any problems with your skin?
- Are you bothered by itching, rashes, acne, eczema, or sores?
- Do you use any topical medications like ointments, creams, or salves?

Endocrine
- Do you have any thyroid problems?
- Have you ever had your blood sugar checked?
- Have you ever been told you have high blood sugar or diabetes?

Genitourinary
- Are you having any problems urinating?
- Any pain or urine discoloration?
- Are you experiencing yeast infections, dysmenorrhea, or urinary tract infections?
- What are you doing to prevent osteoporosis?
- Have you had a prostate test recently?
- Some people who use this medication experience some change in their sexual function; have you noticed any changes?

(*Continued*)

Table 6-8   (*Continued*) Pharmacotherapy Workup—Review of systems

Kidney
- Have you had any problems with your kidneys?
- Have you ever been told you have kidney disease?

Liver
- Have you noticed any signs of jaundice such as yellowing of the eyes or skin?

Hematological
- Do you bruise easily?
- Have you ever been told you have anemia?
- Do you take a multivitamin with iron?
- Do you take a folic acid supplement?

Musculoskeletal
- Do you have any problems with your joints or muscles?
- Do you exercise regularly?
- Any pain, swelling, or tenderness?
- Do you have any arthritis or arthritis-like pain?
- What medications do you use for relief of minor pain or discomfort?

Neurological
- Any problems with weakness, numbness, tingling, balance, or walking?
- Have you had trouble with seizures?
- Any difficulty with memory?

Psychiatric
- Any problems with anxiety, mood, depression, panic disorder, or attention deficit disorder?
- What do you do to relieve stress in your life?

The review of systems may include physical findings, descriptions and experiences offered by your patient, and laboratory values, in addition to baseline information required for later comparison to evaluate effectiveness and safety.

Example   An assessment for a patient with a seizure disorder will contain considerably more information in the neurological section of the review of systems than the gastrointestinal section.

Every patient has a temperature, a pulse, a systolic and diastolic blood pressure, and a respiratory rate. These data are always available, can be collected at very little or no cost, and are often important in drug therapy decision-making. Your interpretation transforms these data into information that can be useful in the provision of pharmaceutical care. Remember, many of the most commonly used medications can cause undesirable increases or decreases in your patient's vital signs. Additionally, these most important monitoring parameters are used to evaluate the outcome of drug therapies in almost all patients.

> **Example** Is the headache your patient has had for the past 3 days being caused by the ketoprofen she is taking for her tendonitis? Are your patient's myalgias being caused by atorvastatin (Lipitor) he is taking to manage his hyperlipidemia? Is the cough the patient has asked for help to treat being caused by the captopril he is taking to manage his hypertension?

The discipline that is required of you as a pharmaceutical care practitioner demands that each section of the review of systems be considered in order to avoid errors of omission. Only with this type of professional discipline and serious attention to detail can patients be confident that all of their drug-related needs are being addressed.

At this point in your assessment you will be establishing your clinical impressions of your patient's drug-related needs and how you can best meet them. However, up to now, you have been gathering information from your patient, primarily in response to information he or she has offered to tell you. You have been listening intently and creating a comprehensive list or mental picture of your patient's drug-related needs, wants, expectations, concerns, and understanding. It is now time to make the clinical decision of whether or not your patient has a drug therapy problem.

THE PHARMACOTHERAPY WORKUP

Now that you have a pharmacologically relevant understanding of your patient, you have the context in which to make patient-specific decisions. Individualized, logical, and systematic drug therapy decisions represent your professional contribution to patient care. It is drug therapy problem identification, resolution, and prevention that will serve as your unique contribution to your patient. Because drug therapy problems interfere with the patient's ability to reach his/her goals of therapy, it is of the utmost importance that you acquire the hypothetical-deductive reasoning skills and knowledge necessary to identify, resolve, and prevent drug therapy problems in order to have a positive impact on their health and welfare.

Standard of Care 2: Assessment of Drug-related Needs

STANDARD 2: THE PRACTITIONER ANALYZES THE ASSESSMENT DATA TO DETERMINE IF THE PATIENT'S DRUG-RELATED NEEDS ARE BEING MET, THAT ALL THE PATIENT'S MEDICATIONS ARE APPROPRIATELY INDICATED, THE MOST EFFECTIVE AVAILABLE, THE SAFEST POSSIBLE, AND THE PATIENT IS ABLE AND WILLING TO TAKE THE MEDICATION AS INTENDED.

Measurement criteria

1. The patient-specific data collected in the assessment are used to decide if all of the patient's medications are appropriately indicated.
2. The data collected are used to decide if the patient needs additional medications that are not presently being taken.
3. The data collected are used to decide if all of the patient's medications are the most effective products available for the conditions.
4. The data collected are used to decide if all of the patient's medications are dosed appropriately to achieve the goals of therapy.
5. The data collected are used to decide if any of the patient's medications are causing adverse effects.
6. The data collected are used to decide if any of the patient's medications are dosed excessively and causing toxicities.
7. The patient's behavior is assessed to determine if all his or her medications are being taken appropriately in order to achieve the goals of therapy.

If the patient's drug-related needs are not being met, then a drug therapy problem exists. Identifying drug therapy problems requires professional judgment, discipline, a thorough understanding of the patient as a whole person, drug and disease knowledge, communication skills, and a systematic approach to the patient care process. It is unique to pharmaceutical care practice that both the empirical problem, as well as your patient's perception of the problem, becomes the focus of all of your deductive energies.

The Pharmacotherapy Workup   There is considerable information to be learned about patients, pathophysiology, and pharmacotherapy, but in order to understand how to apply this information to help an individual patient, you need an organizing framework. You need a framework in which to think about your patient-specific information, your knowledge of patients, diseases, and drug therapy, and the decisions you have to make. This is called the Pharmacotherapy Workup, and you will use it for making drug therapy decisions each time you care for a patient.

All patients have basic drug-related needs, and your aim is to see that they are met at all times. Every patient needs each of his/her medications to be appropriately indicated for the condition being treated; the most effective drug therapy available; the safest drug therapy possible; and with all these in place, he/she must be willing and able to take the medication as directed.

During the Pharmacotherapy Workup you will systematically and repeatedly consider the questions dealing with indication, effectiveness, safety, and compliance. This disciplined way of examining patient-disease-drug findings is central to learning how to become successful at making sound decisions as to the optimal pharmacotherapy for any clinical situation. The Pharmacotherapy Workup is designed so that your decision-making is always completed in the rational order of (1) indication, (2) effectiveness, (3) safety, and (4) compliance. In other words, you assess a patient's drug therapy first, and only then do you assess the patient's behavior.

There is a tendency to pass judgment on whether a patient is being compliant before it is determined that the medication is appropriately indicated, effective, and safe. This is not logical. There is little reason for a patient to take a medication that is not appropriately indicated, effective, or safe for him/her.

The Pharmacotherapy Workup represents the cognitive work involved in pharmaceutical care. When the framework is built, you will have a complete assessment of your patient's drug-related needs.

Evaluating the Appropriateness of the Indication for the Patient's Drug Therapy

Figure 6-4 introduces the most basic structure of the Pharmacotherapy Workup and the first step of the decision-making that must occur. This basic structure illustrates the connections that must be established to determine if each drug product the patient is taking has an indication that is appropriate for the patient's medical problem and if each indication that requires drug therapy is being treated appropriately.

You must first make the connections between the indication (medical condition), the drug product, the dosage regimen, and the outcome. For

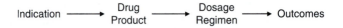

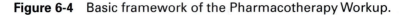

Figure 6-4 Basic framework of the Pharmacotherapy Workup.

each medication being taken by the patient, consider if there is a medical condition or illness present. What drug product is being used to manage the condition? What dosage is actually being taken? What has the patient's response been? This is the organization and meaning you bring to the patient's current medication record. This very basic series of connections lets you determine if the patient is taking any unnecessary drug therapy.

If there is not a clinical indication requiring the drug therapy, then the drug therapy is unnecessary. If there are any therapeutic indications that are not presently being treated, the patient needs additional drug therapy. During this step of the Pharmacotherapy Workup, you are constantly asking yourself if the patient's problem is caused by drug therapy or if the problem is something that can be treated with drug therapy.

Establishing that the patient has a clinically appropriate indication for the medication is of prime importance. It is virtually impossible to provide rational, personalized, valuable recommendations concerning a patient's drug therapy if you cannot identify the indication. Assuming what the indication might be from knowing only the drug product is dangerous and often leads to misleading and confusing decisions. You cannot optimize drug therapy if you do not know what is to be accomplished. The intended use of the medication is the starting point in drug therapy problem identification. In the case of nonprescription drug product use, the patient (or the patient's family member or care giver) has an indication in mind. The best method to gather this information is to ask the patient directly for what purpose he/she is using the product and what he or she is trying to achieve.

In the case of drug therapies that require a prescriber to initiate therapy, it is most helpful if you can educate the patient to ask why the prescriber is initiating this drug therapy. If your patient is not certain of the clinical intent of the medication, it is your responsibility to determine the intent of the prescriber. This can be accomplished through direct communication between you and the prescriber or by instructing the patient to ask the prescriber at the next office visit.

It is helpful for prescribers to write the indication within their dosing instructions. For example, "Take one tablet every morning to control blood pressure." Or "Take one capsule each week to prevent osteoporosis." Asking a prescriber to incorporate the intended use within the instructions can be extremely valuable. There is always an intended use (indication) for a drug prescribed by a practitioner who is licensed to prescribe drugs. The intended use is best known at the time the decision is made to prescribe a drug. Similarly, the patient always has an intended use in mind when he/she decides to self-initiate drug therapy that does not require a prescription. In

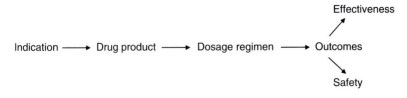

Figure 6-5   Outcome determinants of the Pharmacotherapy Workup.

any case, the indication is a vital piece of information in the identification and resolution of drug therapy problems.

If the patient has an indication that is appropriate for each medication and if each of the patient's medical problems is being treated or prevented with drug therapy, then you are ready to evaluate the patient's medications for effectiveness.

> **Note**   If the patient has an inappropriate indication or needs drug therapy, then you have identified a drug therapy problem.

Figure 6-5 introduces the two main determinants of drug therapy outcomes: effectiveness and safety. Whenever a medication is used, its results can be described by determining the effectiveness and the safety experienced by the patient. To be responsible for the outcomes of drug therapies means that you accept the responsibility to evaluate and make clinical judgments about both the effectiveness and safety of all of your patient's drug therapies.

Determining the Effectiveness of the Drug Regimen

Figure 6-6 introduces the information you will need to evaluate the effectiveness of your patient's medications. Drug therapy is effective if it is achieving the intended goals of therapy. Effectiveness is determined by evaluating the patient's response compared to the desired goals of therapy for each indication. In today's health care system these are not explicitly stated. To evaluate effectiveness you must establish *goals of therapy* based on the *signs and symptoms* experienced by patients, or from the abnormal *laboratory values* associated with the underlying disorder.

By comparing the desired goals with actual patient status at this time you can judge whether the drug therapy is being effective or not or if the drug therapy is failing to treat the condition.

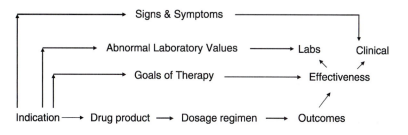

Figure 6-6 Effectiveness parameters of the Pharmacotherapy Workup.

Note If the patient's drug therapy is effective because the patient is taking the best product at an effective dosage, then the patient's drug-related need for effective drug therapy is met.

When the drug therapy is not effective for the patient, the practitioner will consider two of the most frequent reasons: "Is this the wrong product for this patient condition?" or "is the dosage regimen too low to produce the desired effects?" If the drug therapy is ineffective, then a drug therapy problem exists. Once again ask yourself "Is this problem caused by a [ineffective] drug or is this a problem I will resolve with [more] drug therapy?

The next objective is to determine if your patient is experiencing any safety issues secondary to drug therapy. In order to make this clinical judgment, we will introduce more criteria in the Pharmacotherapy Workup.

Establishing the Safety of the Drug Regimen

Drug products and dosage regimens can cause adverse drug reactions and/or toxicities in patients. *Adverse drug reactions* are either (1) undesirable or unintended responses to the known pharmacology of the drug product or (2) idiopathic effects experienced by the patient. *Toxicities* are the result of dosages that are too high for your patient.

The first safety consideration is reflected in the following question: "Is this undesirable effect the patient is experiencing caused by a drug he/she is taking?" The next safety consideration is whether the undesirable effect is related to (or proportional to) the dosage of the drug the patient took. Within the Pharmacotherapy Workup, practitioners must make clinical judgments as to whether an unwanted effect is dose-related or not. If the patient's drug therapy problem is related to the dosage of the product, then the resolution is to continue to use the same product, but to reduce the dosage regimen. The dosage regimen can be reduced by giving the patient a smaller dose or by instructing the patient to take the dose less frequently. Most drug therapy problems caused by taking too much of the correct drug product are predictable because they are simple extensions of the known pharmacology of the drug product. In general, dose-related problems are resolved by lowering the dose, while those reactions not dependent on the amount of a drug the patient takes are resolved by switching to another drug product.

Figure 6-7 illustrates how safety decisions are made within the Pharmacotherapy Workup.

Each arrow represents a decision on your part. When your decision is positive, the patient's drug-related needs are being met. When your decision is negative, a drug therapy problem exists.

Safety is established by evaluating clinical parameters (signs and symptoms) or laboratory values to determine if any are associated with the unwanted effects of the drug therapy. Practitioners constantly ask: "Is this problem caused by too much of a drug?" Or "Am I going to resolve this problem with a different drug?"

If the patient's drug therapy is safe in your clinical judgment, then the patient's drug-related need for safety is met, and you are ready to evaluate the patient's compliance with the medication.

Note If you have identified a medication or dosage of the medication that is unsafe, a drug therapy problem exists.

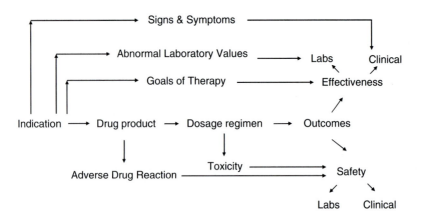

Figure 6-7 Effectiveness and safety parameters of the Pharmacotherapy Workup.

Understanding Patient Compliance

The disciplined thought process that is described in the Pharmacotherapy Workup requires pharmaceutical care practitioners to make clinical decisions about indication, effectiveness, and safety issues before they evaluate the patient's compliance.

> **Note**   Although we are aware of the controversy surrounding the term "compliance," we have chosen to continue its use. There is no concensus on alternative wording (adherance, concordance), and the term is used here specifically to mean compliance with a dosage regimen, not compliance with the orders of a paternalistic or authoritarian figure.

In pharmaceutical care practice noncompliance is considered a problem only after the drug therapy is deemed to be clinically indicated, judged likely to be effective in achieving the goals of therapy, and safe in that it is not causing or likely to cause any harm to the patient.

Noncompliance represents a distinct category in that it describes the behavior of the patient, not the drug therapy. Effective pharmacotherapy requires the medication be consumed in a particular dosage, at specified times, and for a specific period of time. Therefore, patients who are exhibiting a drug therapy problem of noncompliance need to be cared for in the context of altering their behavior. Identifying and resolving compliance problems are important responsibilities of every pharmaceutical care practitioner. Some clinicians and research articles refer to patient compliance behavior as adherence and define nonadherence as the lack of following treatment instructions. For the purposes of understanding drug therapy problems, the term *compliance* is used.

In the practice of pharmaceutical care, a noncompliant patient refers to someone who is not able or willing to take an appropriate, effective, and safe medication as intended. Your patient has a rational reason for the decisions he/she has made about whether or not to take the medication. Your responsibility is to discover that reason so you can help to optimize the patient's medication experience.

DRUG THERAPY PROBLEM IDENTIFICATION

In the process of assessing your patient's drug-related needs, it is possible that you will identify a situation where things are not as they should be. Perhaps your patient may be taking a medication, but there is no indication for it. Perhaps your patient is not benefiting from the medication he/she is taking. Your patient may be experiencing a side effect from one or more medications. Or, perhaps your patient cannot afford the medication that was prescribed, so he/she is not taking it. When you discover that your patient's medications are not appropriately indicated, as effective as they need to be, safe, or taken as indicated, you have identified a drug therapy problem.

The last standard of care that prescribes appropriate practitioner behavior refers to the identification of drug therapy problems.

Standard of Care 3: Identification of Drug Therapy Problems

STANDARD 3: THE PRACTITIONER ANALYZES THE ASSESSMENT DATA TO DETERMINE IF ANY DRUG THERAPY PROBLEMS ARE PRESENT.

Measurement criteria

1. Drug therapy problems are identified from the assessment findings.
2. Drug therapy problems are validated with the patient, his/her family, caregivers, and/or health care providers, when necessary.
3. Drug therapy problems are expressed so that the medical condition and the drug therapy involved are explicitly stated and the relationship or cause of the problem is described.
4. Drug therapy problems are prioritized, and those that will be resolved first are selected.
5. Drug therapy problems are documented in a manner that facilitates the determination of goals of therapy within the care plan.

Figure 6-8 illustrates where drug therapy problems can exist throughout the decision-making framework. This figure makes it clear that drug therapy problems can occur at each step of the medication use process. It should not come as a surprise then that almost half of all patients taking medications have a drug therapy problem that is interfering with achieving the goals of therapy.[11–15]

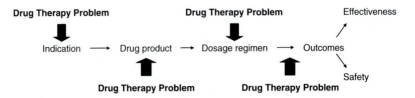

Figure 6-8 Drug therapy problem identification.

Each time a drug therapy problem occurs, the goals of therapy are compromised and cannot be met. Therefore, it is necessary to resolve these drug therapy problems before positive outcomes can be expected. This is the reason why the identification, resolution, and prevention of drug therapy problems is the most important responsibility of the pharmaceutical care practitioner.

The stating, identification of cause, prioritization, and resolution of drug therapy problems are discussed in detail in the next chapter.

SUMMARIZING THE ASSESSMENT

At the end of the assessment, you will want to summarize your findings, remaining questions, and clinical decisions. Summarizing and describing your findings with the patient up to this point serves several purposes. First, you can verify that you have an appropriate understanding of the patient's story, concerns, problems, and wants. Validating the assessment with the patient's knowledge helps the practitioner to be confident that he or she has interpreted the patient's information in a way that makes sense and is consistent with how he or she views the situation. Also, the act of summarizing with the patient lets the patient add additional information that might not yet have been considered during the assessment interview. This step also allows the patient to ask any questions that the practitioner has not dealt with during the assessment. Summarizing can also bring closure to this portion of the interview.

DOCUMENTING THE ASSESSMENT

It is essential that you document each visit and each encounter with every patient. In health care "if you did not document it, you did not do it." Your actions, interventions, advice, warnings, and drug therapies are all designed to impact another person. You are professionally obligated to keep a record of the care you provide for patients. At first, this task can seem labor-intensive and monotonous, but all of the time and effort spent documenting your initial assessment will yield great dividends at all follow-up evaluation visits.

Recording the findings from your assessment is best done at the time you see the patient or shortly thereafter. Waiting for a more convenient time to record essential patient information, clinical findings, and decisions will only lead to errors of omission or confusion in your documentation. In this section, we will describe the basic elements of your assessment that need to be documented. When learning this skill, it is often useful to create a written paper record. This allows you to learn what information you use to make your clinical decisions and how to make the appropriate connections between patient, disease, and drug information. When caring for many patients it is very difficult to maintain accurate and up-to-date records using a paper system. Computerized documentation systems have been developed to support busy practitioners and are discussed in Chapter 12.

The information you will find useful to record includes name, address, and contact information for the most common forms of communication including telephone, cell phone, and e-mail. Correct spelling of your patient's name is important and demonstrates respect. Some patients may change their names when married or divorced. Obviously, your patient's name is a personal characteristic that you must value whenever you speak with your patient, communicate in writing, or for record keeping purposes.

Contact information is used to mail, telephone, or e-mail information to your patient. These are not clinical data and can be collected by support personnel or simply supplied by the patient or a family member. You may need the patient's address to mail drug supplies or health information to the patient or for billing purposes. The patient's preferred telephone numbers, or parent(s)' in the case of pediatric patients, may be useful in order to conduct convenient follow-up evaluations in the future or to contact the patient with new or additional information. Many of your patients might prefer to be contacted using e-mail, and if that is their preferred method of routine communication, then you will want to accommodate them by recording an e-mail address in the pharmaceutical care chart.

Patient demographic information usually does not change too much and need only be recorded at the first encounter. Age is best recorded using birth date, so all care providers can determine the patient's correct age at any future visit. Weight changes can be noted as some drug dosing guidelines are based on body weight, usually in kilograms. Pregnancy status is essential to note as drug safety becomes an overriding issue in all pregnant and breast-feeding patients. Health insurance information changes so frequently that it is difficult to use the patient's health care record to keep current plan and policy numbers and eligibility.

The patient's primary reason for the encounter should hold a prominent place in the assessment record. Each visit may be for a different reason and therefore new or additional information may be required.

Your record of the patient's description of his/her medication experience is often best described in the patient's own words. This reduces your chances of over or under-interpreting patient comments or descriptions of concerns or beliefs about using medications to manage health. This is helpful to note if you need to attend to any specific or unique patient needs that are revealed in your patient's description of his/her medication experience. The immunization status can simply be noted as to any vaccinations your patient needs to receive or to update it if that is the case. Drug allergies warrant thorough description as to the offending agent, the timeframe of the reaction, the sequelae, and any treatment that was required. Some record systems place the drug allergy documentation in the very front in a bright color to notify all health care practitioners of this important risk factor.

Your record of your patient's current medical conditions and associated drug therapies can be considered the center piece of the assessment documentation. This will often be the first and only place in which all of your patient's medical conditions or illnesses, the drug products and dosages actually being used are gathered and organized in the same place. This record has five components for every medical condition: indication, drug product, dosage regimen, length of therapy, and response. The dosage regimen to be recorded is that actually taken by your patient. If it is different from that prescribed, note the difference. The responses to be documented include both positive results and any side effects experienced by the patient. Drug therapies are organized and grouped by medical condition. Tobacco, alcohol, and other social drug use are documented in terms of amounts or frequency of use.

Your pharmaceutical care record should also document relevant past medical events including surgeries, illnesses, accidents, and special dietary needs/restrictions if they contribute to your drug therapy decision-making.

You will need to record all pertinent findings from the review of systems. Positive findings as well as relevant negative findings are briefly noted. The absence of side effects or expected drug actions should be noted here.

Documenting your drug therapy decisions requires a clear record of the patient's problems or medical conditions, the drug therapy that is involved, and the relationship (cause and effect) between the two. Noting the cause of the drug therapy problem in the assessment is most valuable as it will guide future changes in your patient's drug therapies whether they are implemented by you or other clinicians.

It is often useful to write a brief, two to three sentence summary of the assessment in the record to summarize the most important information and findings.

A comprehensive record that includes the description of your patient, his or her medication experience, the medical condition(s), associated drug therapies, actual dosages, and the results as of the present visit is required to contribute in a consistently positive way to the patient's health.

Figure 6-9 is an example of an assessment documentation form.

Pharmacotherapy Workup© **NOTES**		**ASSESSMENT**			

<table>
<tr><td rowspan="6">CONTACT INFORMATION</td><td colspan="5">Name</td></tr>
<tr><td>Address</td><td>City</td><td></td><td>State</td><td>Postal Code</td></tr>
<tr><td>Telephone (h)</td><td>(w)</td><td>(cell)</td><td colspan="2">e-mail</td></tr>
<tr><td colspan="2">Pharmacy Name</td><td colspan="3">Clinic Name</td></tr>
<tr><td colspan="2">(tel)</td><td colspan="3">(tel)</td></tr>
</table>

<table>
<tr><td rowspan="7">DEMOGRAPHICS</td><td>Age</td><td>Date of Birth</td><td>Gender: M/F</td></tr>
<tr><td>Weight</td><td>Height</td><td>Lean Body Weight</td></tr>
<tr><td>Pregnancy status: Y/N</td><td>Breast Feeding: Y/N</td><td>Due Date</td></tr>
<tr><td colspan="3">Occupation</td></tr>
<tr><td colspan="3">Living Arrangements/Family</td></tr>
<tr><td colspan="3">Health Insurance (coverage issues):</td></tr>
</table>

REASON FOR THE ENCOUNTER

<table>
<tr><td rowspan="10">MEDICATION EXPERIENCE</td><td>What is the patient's general attitude toward taking medication?</td><td colspan="2">Needs attention in care plan</td></tr>
<tr><td></td><td>Y</td><td>N</td></tr>
<tr><td>What does the patient want/expect from his/her drug therapy?</td><td colspan="2">Needs attention in care plan</td></tr>
<tr><td></td><td>Y</td><td>N</td></tr>
<tr><td>What concerns does the patient have with his/her medications?</td><td colspan="2">Needs attention in care plan</td></tr>
<tr><td></td><td>Y</td><td>N</td></tr>
<tr><td>To what extent does the patient understand his/her medications?</td><td colspan="2">Needs attention in care plan</td></tr>
<tr><td></td><td>Y</td><td>N</td></tr>
<tr><td>Are there cultural, religious, or ethical issues that influence the patient's willingness to take medications?</td><td colspan="2">Needs attention in care plan</td></tr>
<tr><td></td><td>Y</td><td>N</td></tr>
</table>

Figure 6-9 Assessment documentation form (© 2003 The Peters Institute of Pharmaceutical Care).

	Birth	1 mo	2 mos	4 mos	6 mos	12 mos	15 mos	18 mos	24 mos	4–6 yrs	11–12 yrs	13–18 yrs
Hepatitis B	Dose 1	Dose 2			Dose 3							
Diphtheria, Tetanus, Pertussis			1	2	3		4					
Haemophilus influenzae Type b			1	2	3	4						
Polio-inactivated			1	2		3				4		
Measles, Mumps, Rubella						1				2		
Varicella (chicken pox)												
Pneumococcal			1	2	3	4						
Hepatitis A (children in high risk regions)									Hepatitis A Series			
Influenza (children ≥ 6 with asthma, diabetes, HIV, sickle cell, cardiac disease)					Yearly							

CHILDHOOD IMMUNIZATIONS*

___ Current on all childhood immunizations

	19–49 Years	50–64 Years	65 Years & older
Tetanus, Diphtheria (Td)	1 booster every 10 years	1 booster every 10 years	1 booster every 10 years
Influenza	1 dose annually for persons with medical or occupational indications or household contacts of persons with indications	1 annual dose	1 annual dose
Pneumococcal (polysaccharide)	1 dose for persons with medical or other indications (1 dose revaccination for immunosuppressive conditions)	1 dose for person with medical or other indications (1 dose revaccination for immunosuppressive conditions)	1 dose for unvaccinated persons 1 dose revaccination

ADULT IMMUNIZATIONS*

___ Current on all adult immunizations

*see http://www.cdc.gov/nip for more information

Substance	History of Use	Substance	History of Use
Tobacco __No tobacco use	__ 0–1 packs per day __ >1 packs per day __ previous history of smoking __ attempts to quit	Alcohol __No alcohol use	__ < 2 drinks per week __ 2–6 drinks per week __ > 6 drinks per week __ history of alcohol dependence
Caffeine __No caffeine use	__ < 2 cups per day __ 2–6 cups per day __ > 6 cups per day __ history of caffeine dependence	Other recreational drug use	

SOCIAL DRUG USE

Figure 6-9 (*Continued*)

		Medication Allergies (drug, timing, reaction—rash, shock, asthma, nausea, anemia)
ALLERGIES & ALERTS		Adverse reactions to drugs in the past
		Other Alerts/Health Aids/Special Needs (sight, hearing, mobility, literacy, disability)

	INDICATION	DRUG PRODUCT	DOSAGE REGIMEN dose, route, frequency, duration	START DATE	RESPONSE effectiveness/safety
CURRENT MEDICAL CONDITIONS AND MEDICATIONS					

	INDICATION	DRUG THERAPY	RESPONSE	DATE
PAST DRUG THERAPIES				

PAST MEDICAL HISTORY (RELEVANT ILLNESSES, HOSPITALIZATIONS, SURGICAL PROCEDURES, INJURIES, PREGNANCIES, DELIVERIES)

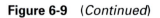

Figure 6-9 (*Continued*)

NUTRITIONAL STATUS (NOTE DAILY INTAKE OF CALORIES, CALCIUM, SODIUM, CHOLESTEROL, FIBER, POTASSIUM, VITAMIN K)			
calories	K⁺	cholesterol	Vitamin K
calcium	Na⁺	fiber	

OTHER FOOD OR DIETARY RESTRICTIONS/NEEDS

Vital signs: BP _____/_____   HR _____bpm   Resp Rate _____   Temp____

		y/n				y/n
REVIEW OF SYSTEMS	General Systems	Poor appetite		GU/Reproductive	Dysmenorrhea/ menstrual bleeding	
		Weight change			Incontinence	
		Pain			Impotence	
		Headache			Decreased sexual drive	
		Dizziness (vertigo)			Vaginal discharge or itching	
	EENT	Change in vision				
		Loss of hearing			Hot flashes	
		Ringing in the ears (tinnitus)		Kidney/Urinary	Urinary frequency	
		Bloody nose (epistaxis)			Bloody urine (hematuria)	
		Allergic rhinitis			Renal dysfunction	
		Glaucoma		Hematopoietic Symptoms	Excessive bruising	
		Bloody sputum (hemoptysis)			Bleeding	
	Cardiovascular	Chest pain			Anemia	
		Hyperlipidemia		Musculoskeletal	Back pain	
		Hypertension			Arthritis pain (osteo/rheumatoid)	
		Myocardial Infarction			Tendonitis	
		Orthostatic hypotension			Painful muscles	
	Pulmonary	Asthma		Neuropsychiatric	Numb, tingling sensation in extremities (parasthesia)	
		Shortness of breath				
		Wheezing				
	Gastrointestinal	Heartburn			Tremor	
		Abdominal pain			Loss of balance	
		Nausea			Depression	
		Vomiting			Suicidal	
		Diarrhea			Anxiety, nervousness	
		Constipation			Inability to concentrate	
	Skin	Eczema/Psoriasis			Seizure	
		Itching (pruritis)			Stroke/TIA	
		Rash			Memory loss	
	Endocrine Systems	Diabetes		Infectious Disease	HIV/AIDS	
		Hypothyroidism			Malaria	
		Menopausal Symptoms			Syphilis	
	Hepatic	Cirrhosis			Gonorrhea	
		Hepatitis			Herpes	
	Nutrition/Fluid/ Electrolytes	Dehydration			Chlamydia	
		Edema			Tuberculosis	
		Potassium deficiency				

Figure 6-9 (*Continued*)

DRUG THERAPY PROBLEMS TO BE RESOLVED

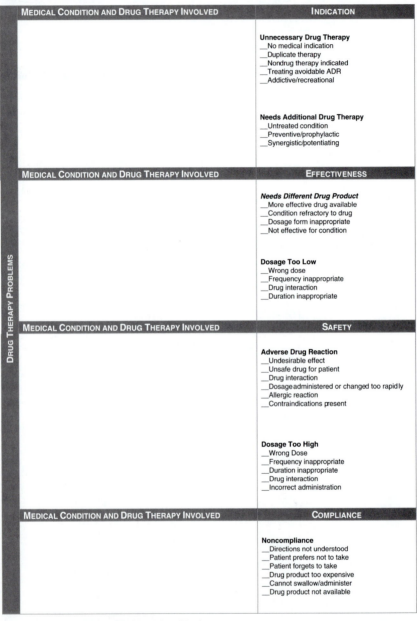

DRUG THERAPY PROBLEMS	MEDICAL CONDITION AND DRUG THERAPY INVOLVED	INDICATION
		Unnecessary Drug Therapy __No medical indication __Duplicate therapy __Nondrug therapy indicated __Treating avoidable ADR __Addictive/recreational **Needs Additional Drug Therapy** __Untreated condition __Preventive/prophylactic __Synergistic/potentiating
	MEDICAL CONDITION AND DRUG THERAPY INVOLVED	EFFECTIVENESS
		Needs Different Drug Product __More effective drug available __Condition refractory to drug __Dosage form inappropriate __Not effective for condition **Dosage Too Low** __Wrong dose __Frequency inappropriate __Drug interaction __Duration inappropriate
	MEDICAL CONDITION AND DRUG THERAPY INVOLVED	SAFETY
		Adverse Drug Reaction __Undesirable effect __Unsafe drug for patient __Drug interaction __Dosage administered or changed too rapidly __Allergic reaction __Contraindications present **Dosage Too High** __Wrong Dose __Frequency inappropriate __Duration inappropriate __Drug interaction __Incorrect administration
	MEDICAL CONDITION AND DRUG THERAPY INVOLVED	COMPLIANCE
		Noncompliance __Directions not understood __Patient prefers not to take __Patient forgets to take __Drug product too expensive __Cannot swallow/administer __Drug product not available

____No Drug Therapy Problem(s) at this time

Figure 6-9   *(Continued)*

SUMMARY

Patient care requires time, commitment, knowledge, skills, and compassion. The assessment step will require most of your time and energy. The assessment is the most important step in the care process because it establishes the direction, urgency, and resources that will be committed to a patient's drug-related needs.

Understanding a patient's medication experience depends on the quality of the therapeutic relationship established between you and your patient. The patient's medication experience is the personal basis on which your patient makes drug therapy decisions. You will use the Pharmacotherapy Workup to make your drug therapy decisions, but the more you understand and pay attention to your patient's past experience, preferences, and concerns about medications, the more likely you will have a positive impact on the outcomes of drug therapies.

As a pharmaceutical care practitioner you bring new knowledge and skills to patient care. You will contribute in many ways, but essentially you are adding and verifying the clinical appropriateness of the indication for every medication, the medication's effectiveness and safety, and the patient's compliance. This simple, straightforward approach places all of your patients' drug therapies into a rational context and greatly increases the probability of positive outcomes.

EXERCISES

6-1 Select two individuals who will engage in a 30–40 minutes discussion regarding their drug therapies. Do not choose members of your family or close friends as these relationships may interfere with the patient care process. Complete an assessment of each individual's drug-related needs, and document the completed assessment on the documentation form provided at the end of Chapter 6.

6-2 Consider how *relevant* information changes depending on the type of patient being cared for, his/her diseases, and the drug therapy being taken.

What information might you need from an 86-year-old patient compared to a 2-year-old patient? What information might you need from someone who has chronic asthma as compared to someone with an acute urinary tract infection? And what information might you need from someone who is taking an antibiotic to reduce acne compared to someone who is using insulin therapy for diabetes?

6-3 The assessment process begins before a word is spoken. Explain how this occurs.

6-4 Describe the rationale behind the assessment process of the Pharmacotherapy Workup. Explain why order is important when assessing appropriateness, effectiveness and safety of a patient's medication as well as the compliance behavior of the patient.

REFERENCES

1. Lipkin, M.J., Putman, S.M., Lazare, A. *The Medical Interview: Clinical Care, Education, and Research*. New York: Springer; 1995.
2. Billings, J.A., Stoeckle, J.D. *The Clinical Encounter: A Guide to the Medical Interview and Case Presentation*. Year Book Medical Publishers, Inc. Chicago, 1989.
3. Coulehan, J.L., Block, M.R., Biblis, M.M. (ed), *The Medical Interview: Mastering Skills for Clinical Practice*. Philadelphia, PA: F.A.Davis Company; 2001.
4. Cole, S.A., Bird, J., Schmitt, W. (ed), *The Medical Interview: The Three-Function Approach*. St. Louis, MO: Mosby Inc.; 2000.
5. Savett, L., *The Human Side of Medicine*. Westport Connecticut: Auburn House; 2002.
6. Anderson, P.O., Knoben, J.E., Troutman, W.G., *Handbook of Clinical Drug Data*, 10th ed. New York: McGraw-Hill; 2002.
7. Lacy, C.F., Armstrong, L.L., Goldman, M.P., Lance, L.L., *Lexi-Comp's: Drug Information Handbook–APhA*, 11th ed. Hudson, OH: Lexi-Comp Inc.; 2003.
8. Ansel, H.C., Stoklosa, M.J., *Pharmaceutical Calculations*, 11th ed. Philadelphia, PA: Lippincott Williams & Wilkins; 2001, p. 79.
9. *Drug Facts and Comparisons,* 8th ed. St. Louis, MO: Wolters Kluwer Health; 2004, p. 1127.
10. Briggs, G.G., Freeman, R.K., Yaffee, S., *Drugs in Pregnancy and Lactation: A Reference Guide to Fetal and Neonatal Risk*, 2nd ed. Baltimore, MD: Williams & Wilkins; 1986.
11. Cipolle, R., Strand, L.M., Morley, P.C., *Pharmaceutical Care Practice*. New York: McGraw Hill; 1998.
12. Espejo, J., Fernandez-Llimos, F., Machuca, M., Faus, M.J., Drug-related problems: definition and proposal for its inclusion in the international classification of primary care (ICPC) from WONCA. *Pharm Care Espana* 2002; 4(2):122–127.
13. Chicano Pia, P. Identification and resolving of drug-related problems: experience in a health center. *Pharm Care Espana* 2002; 4(5):300–313.
14. Tuneu Valls, L., Garcia-Pelaez, M., Lopez Sanchez, S., Serra Soler, G., Alba Aranda, G., Irala Andart, C., Ramos, J., Tomas Sanz, R., Bravo Jose, P., Bonal de Falgas, J. Drug-related problems in patients who visit an emergency room. *Pharm Care Espana* 2000; 2(3):177–192.
15. Mant, A., *Thinking About Prescribing: A Handbook for Quality Use of Medicines*. Sydney, Australia: The McGraw-Hill Companies, Inc.; 1999.

DRUG THERAPY PROBLEMS

Key Concepts

[1] *Identifying, resolving, and preventing drug therapy problems is the unique contribution of the pharmaceutical care practitioner.*

[2] *Identifying a drug therapy problem is a clinical judgment that requires that the practitioner identify an association between the patient's medical condition and the patient's pharmacotherapy.*

[3] *Drug therapy problems can occur at every step of the medication use process.*

④ *There are seven distinct categories of drug therapy problems.*

⑤ *How the practitioner describes the drug therapy problem influences the selection of interventions to resolve the problem.*

⑥ *A correctly stated drug therapy problem includes (a) a description of the patient's condition or problem; (b) the drug therapy involved; (c) the specific association between the drug therapy and the patient's condition.*

⑦ *Drug therapy problems should be evaluated for their severity, acuteness, and significance to the patient to determine how quickly the resolution of the problem must occur.*

⑧ *When multiple drug therapy problems exist, prioritize them and begin with the problem that is most important to the patient and/or is critical to the health of the patient.*

⑨ *Patients who have no drug therapy problems still require a care plan and follow-up evaluation to ensure that the goals of therapy continue to be met and no new drug therapy problems develop.*

Drug therapy problems are the clinical domain of the pharmaceutical care practitioner. The purpose of identifying drug therapy problems is to help patients achieve their goals of therapy and realize the best possible outcomes from drug therapy. In this chapter, we will describe drug therapy problems and their central importance to the practice of pharmaceutical care.

DRUG THERAPY PROBLEMS: TERMINOLOGY

The identification of drug therapy problems is the focus of the assessment and the last decision made in that step of the patient care process. Although drug therapy problem identification is technically part of the assessment process, it represents the truly unique contribution made by pharmaceutical care practitioners. Therefore, a separate chapter has been devoted to describing drug therapy problems so that you can learn to identify, resolve, and most importantly, prevent drug therapy problems in your practice.

Drug therapy problems are a consequence of drug-related needs that have gone unmet. They are central to pharmaceutical care practice.

Definition A drug therapy problem is any undesirable event experienced by a patient which involves, or is suspected to involve, drug therapy, and that interferes with achieving the desired goals of therapy.[1,2]

Every health care practitioner is responsible for helping patients with problems that require a certain level of professional sophistication to identify, prevent, or resolve. Societies have made dentists the primary health care practitioner responsible for identifying and resolving dental problems. Not all dental problems require the sophistication of a licensed dentist to resolve, but those dental problems that an individual patient cannot identify (diagnose) or resolve on his/her own require the knowledge and skills of a dentist.

Identifying drug therapy problems is to pharmaceutical care what making a medical diagnosis is to medical care. It is the most important contribution you can make. Drug therapy problems represent the major responsibility of the pharmaceutical care practitioner.

Pharmaceutical care practitioners use the term *problem* to denote an event associated with or caused by drug therapy that is amenable to detection, treatment, or prevention. A drug therapy problem is a clinical problem, and it must be identified and resolved in a manner similar to other clinical problems.[2] Patients have drug therapy problems—drug products do not have drug therapy problems and practitioners do not have drug therapy problems. It must be emphasized here that the most important role for the pharmaceutical care practitioner is to *prevent* drug therapy problems from occurring. This is surely the most valuable service a practitioner can provide his or her patient.

Components of a Drug Therapy Problem

To identify, resolve, and prevent drug therapy problems, the practitioner must understand how patients with drug therapy problems present in the clinical setting. The patient's drug therapy problem always has three primary components:

1. An undesirable event or risk of an event experienced by the patient. The *problem* can take the form of a medical complaint, sign, symptom, diagnosis, disease, illness, impairment, disability, abnormal laboratory value, or syndrome. The event can be the result of physiological, psychological, sociocultural, or economic conditions.[1,2]
2. The *drug therapy* (products and/or dosage regimen) involved.
3. The *relationship* that exists (or is suspected to exist) between the undesirable patient event and drug therapy. This relationship can be

   (a) the consequence of drug therapy, suggesting a direct association or even a cause and effect relationship, or

   (b) to require the addition or modification of drug therapy for its resolution or prevention.[1]

Stating the problem and identifying the cause requires that all three components be known. This step involves clinical judgment by the practitioner. There is no "right answer" as to whether or not a drug therapy problem exists. There is only the practitioner's clinical judgment and rationale for the decision. This is the reason pharmaceutical care can contribute uniquely to patient care. No other practitioner can identify and resolve drug therapy problems as routinely and comprehensively as the pharmaceutical care practitioner.

> **Example**   "Mr. M.'s elbow pain is not being effectively controlled because the dosage of ketoprofen he has been taking for the past three days is too low to provide relief."
>
> "My patient is experiencing orthostatic hypotension with mild to light headaches each morning because the 2 mg dose of risperidone she takes in the morning is too high."
>
> "My patient has lost her ability to taste secondary to her captopril therapy."
>
> "Mrs. W. requires additional calcium supplements in order to prevent osteoporosis."

Having one set of standard definitions and one set of distinct categories for all drug therapy problems helps to define a fixed and manageable set of professional responsibilities for the pharmaceutical care practitioner.

All patient problems involving medications can be categorized into one of seven types of drug therapy problems. These include any and all side effects, toxic reactions, treatment failures, or the need for additive, synergistic, or preventive medications, as well as noncompliance. The seven categories of drug therapy problems are described in Table 7-1.

Practitioners frequently perceive that an infinite number of drug therapy problems exist given the rapidly expanding array of drug products available, the growing number of diseases being recognized and diagnosed, and the growing numbers of patients entering our health care system. The existence of an endless list of possible drug therapy problems might seem logical due to the fact that, during 2002, there were 3.3 billion prescriptions dispensed from community pharmacies throughout the United States[3] and over 44,000 hospitalized patients die each year resulting from medical errors.[4] Although there are many thousands of drug

Table 7-1 Description of drug therapy problem categories

1. The drug therapy is unnecessary because the patient does not have a clinical indication at this time.
2. Additional drug therapy is required to treat or prevent a medical condition in the patient.
3. The drug product is not being effective at producing the desired response in the patient.
4. The dosage is too low to produce the desired response in the patient.
5. The drug is causing an adverse reaction in the patient.
6. The dosage is too high, resulting in undesirable effects experienced by the patient.
7. The patient is not able or willing to take the drug therapy as intended.

products available, billions of prescriptions dispensed each year, and numerous acute and chronic diseases managed with drug products, there are only seven different categories of drug therapy problems.

These seven categories should not be confused with the traditional criteria for categorizing medication errors which describe the correct drug, correct dose, correct route, correct frequency, and correct duration. This approach establishes the prescribing and delivery of the drug product and not the patient's clinical condition as the focus of the problem. Drug products do not cause toxicity until they are taken by a patient. Drug products cannot prevent diseases unless they are taken at the appropriate time and at the appropriate dosage by patients. Drug products cannot cure a disease unless and until a sufficient dosage is taken by the patient. Drug therapy cannot be considered to have failed to manage a disease unless it was actually taken by the patient. Therefore, drug therapy problems always involve the patient, the drug, and the medical problem that connects them.

This categorization of drug therapy problems was first defined, described, and developed in 1990 by the research group at the Peters Institute of Pharmaceutical Care at the University of Minnesota.[2] The seven categories of drug therapy problems have been examined, critiqued, and applied to practices in a variety of settings, cultures, and languages.[5–8]

Knowing that there are only seven basic categories of drug therapy problems is a powerful concept for students and practitioners. These categories define the set of problems that might be caused by drugs and/or that can be resolved by drug therapy and therefore describe the scope of responsibilities of the pharmaceutical care practitioner. Note that the first two categories of drug therapy problems are associated with the INDICATION. The third and fourth categories of drug therapy problems are associated with EFFECTIVENESS. The fifth and sixth categories of drug therapy problems are associated with

SAFETY. The seventh category deals with patient COMPLIANCE. This order is significant in that it describes the rational decision making process of the Pharmacotherapy Workup (Table 7-2).

You will note that the first six categories of drug therapy problems describe clinical problems that the patient experiences resulting from the *actions of drug therapy* on his/her health. These six categories are differentiated from the seventh in a unique and important way. The seventh category, noncompliance, results from the *actions the patient* makes concerning his/her willingness or ability to use the medication as instructed.

These categories of drug therapy problems are not specific to pharmacological class, area of practice specialty, medical service, or level of practitioner education or training. Drug therapy problem categories are also not specific to a unique patient group based on age, disease state, or health care plan. Hospitalized patients do not have different categories of drug therapy problems than ambulatory patients. The categories apply across all patient, practitioner, and institutional variables.

All practitioners who provide pharmaceutical care must be able to identify, prevent, and resolve any and all of the seven types of drug therapy problems for a given patient. When the practitioner concludes that a patient has a drug therapy problem, he/she is obligated to resolve that problem.

Categorizing drug therapy problems into seven categories can be an empowering process for a number of reasons. First, categorizing drug therapy problems can serve as the focus for developing a systematic process of problem solving whereby the practitioner contributes significantly to the overall positive health outcomes of patients. A systematic process will not only aid the practitioner in achieving successful outcomes on an individual patient basis, but could also aid pharmacoepidemiologists in the development of a national or even international database concerning drug therapy problems.[2] Second, these categories help to clarify and demarcate the professional responsibilities and accountability of the pharmaceutical care

Table 7-2 Drug therapy problems as unmet drug-related needs

Drug-related needs	Categories of drug therapy problems
INDICATION	1. Unnecessary drug therapy
	2. Needs additional drug therapy
EFFECTIVENESS	3. Ineffective drug
	4. Dosage too low
SAFETY	5. Adverse drug reaction
	6. Dosage too high
COMPLIANCE	7. Noncompliance

practitioner. This is most helpful in a team-oriented health care delivery system. Few practicing physicians, nurses, health care administrators, or payers need to be convinced that these problems are important, their prevention necessary, and their resolution in need of an expert.[7] Third, this process illustrates how adverse drug reactions are but one category of drug therapy problem, and it also puts noncompliance into an appropriate clinical perspective. It becomes clear that practitioners must proactively identify, resolve, prevent drug therapy problems of all types in order to ensure that each patient experiences effective and safe pharmacotherapy.

The fourth function of this categorization is to provide the clinical work of the pharmaceutical care practitioner with a vocabulary consistent with that used by other healthcare professionals. By defining the practitioner's function in terms of identification, resolution, and prevention of drug therapy problems, his/her function is placed in a patient-care context consistent with the responsibilities of other healthcare practitioners. Recall, in the practice of pharmaceutical care, the patient—and not the drug product—is the major focus of the practitioner's energies, skills, knowledge, decisions, and actions.

The development of new drug products and the generation of new pharmacological knowledge are based on the same set of fundamental pharmacological principles as drug therapy problems: clinical indication, effectiveness, safety, and compliance. When a new drug product is developed for commercial use, numerous rigorous research studies must be conducted in order to demonstrate the *safety* and *efficacy* when used to treat a specific *indication*. Therefore, the wealth of information generated in populations of patients during the drug development process can be applied directly in the provision of pharmaceutical care to individual patients.

Drug therapy problems can and do occur at any stage of the patient's medication use process (Figure 7-1). Therefore, the practitioner must anticipate drug therapy problems in order to prevent them.

As described in the assessment chapter (Chapter 6), the sequence of how drug therapy problems are identified is important. The order in which you

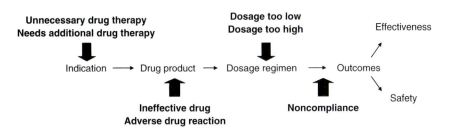

Figure 7-1 Drug therapy problem identification.

make decisions is of the utmost importance to ensure that your assessment is comprehensive and your clinical decisions are rational. Remember, in the practice of pharmaceutical care, decisions concerning an INDICATION are made first, then, decisions concerning EFFECTIVENESS can be established, followed by SAFETY considerations. These categories of drug therapy problems describe the action that the drug therapy is having on the patient. Finally, COMPLIANCE problems represent the willingness and ability of the patient to take the medication as intended.

CATEGORIES AND COMMON CAUSES OF DRUG THERAPY PROBLEMS

As with most clinical problems, drug therapy problems cannot be resolved or prevented unless the cause of the problem is clearly understood. It is necessary to identify and categorize not only the drug therapy problem, but also its most likely cause. Only then can the practitioner proceed with confidence to its resolution or prevention. The common causes of drug therapy problems are summarized in Table 7-3.

Table 7-3 Categories and common causes of drug therapy problems

Drug therapy problem	Common causes of drug therapy problems
Unnecessary drug therapy	• There is no valid medical indication for the drug therapy at this time. • Multiple drug products are being used for a condition that requires single drug therapy. • The medical condition is more appropriately treated with nondrug therapy. • Drug therapy is being taken to treat an avoidable adverse reaction associated with another medication. • Drug abuse, alcohol use, or smoking is causing the problem.
Need for additional drug therapy	• A medical condition requires the initiation of drug therapy. • Preventive drug therapy is required to reduce the risk of developing a new condition. • A medical condition requires additional pharmacotherapy to attain synergistic or additive effects.

(Continued)

Table 7-3   (*Continued*) Categories and common causes of drug therapy problems

Drug therapy problem	Common causes of drug therapy problems
Ineffective drug	• The drug is not the most effective for the medical problem. • The medical condition is refractory to the drug product. • The dosage form of the drug product is inappropriate. • The drug product is not an effective product for the indication being treated.
Dosage too low	• The dose is too low to produce the desired response. • The dosage interval is too infrequent to produce the desired response. • A drug interaction reduces the amount of active drug available. • The duration of drug therapy is too short to produce the desired response.
Adverse drug reaction	• The drug product causes an undesirable reaction that is not dose-related. • A safer drug product is required due to risk factors. • A drug interaction causes an undesirable reaction that is not dose-related. • The dosage regimen was administered or changed too rapidly. • The drug product causes an allergic reaction. • The drug product is contraindicated due to risk factors.
Dosage too high	• Dose is too high. • The dosing frequency is too short. • The duration of drug therapy is too long. • A drug interaction occurs resulting in a toxic reaction to the drug product. • The dose of the drug was administered too rapidly.
Noncompliance	• The patient does not understand the instructions. • The patient prefers not to take the medication. • The patient forgets to take the medication. • The drug product is too expensive for the patient. • The patient cannot swallow or self-administer the drug product appropriately. • The drug product is not available for the patient.

A pharmaceutical care practitioner should have a tacit understanding of the common causes of drug therapy problems because their identification is the essence of pharmaceutical care practice. By identifying the cause of the drug therapy problem, the practitioner and patient can rationally construct a care plan to resolve that drug therapy problem, thereby making it possible for the patient to achieve his/her goals of therapy.

Drug Therapy Problem 1: Unnecessary Drug Therapy

The drug therapy is unnecessary because the patient does not have a clinical indication at this time.

The following is a list of common causes of drug therapy problems involving patients who are taking unnecessary drug therapies. These common causes of drug therapy problems are listed in order of frequency of occurrence in practice:

- There is no valid medical indication for the drug therapy at this time.
- Multiple drug products are being used for a condition that requires single drug therapy.
- The medical condition is more appropriately treated with nondrug therapy.
- Drug therapy is being taken to treat an avoidable adverse reaction associated with another medication.
- Drug abuse, alcohol use, or smoking is causing the problem.

The Pharmacotherapy Workup guides the practitioner to be thorough and to consider if the patient is taking unnecessary drug therapies.

Example   The patient is taking three different laxative products in an attempt to treat his constipation.

Patients receiving care from clinicians trained and experienced in providing pharmaceutical care have drug therapy problems of all types. Our sample of 5136 patients received pharmaceutical care from January 1996 through December 2002, in over 26,238 encounters (see Chapter 2 for details). Within this group of 5136 patients, several patients were taking unnecessary drug therapies. The most frequent causes were that no valid therapeutic indication was present (242 patients, 4.7%), or the patient was taking duplicate drug therapies (241 patients, 4.7%).

Drug Therapy Problem 2: Needs Additional Drug Therapy

Additional drug therapy is required to treat or prevent a medical condition or illness from developing.

The following is a list of common causes of drug therapy problems involving patients who require additional drug therapies to meet their needs:

- A medical condition requires the initiation of drug therapy.
- Preventive drug therapy is required to reduce the risk of developing a new condition.
- A medical condition requires additional pharmacotherapy to attain synergistic or additive effects.

Prevention is a major objective of pharmaceutical care practice. As new and innovative drug regimens are designed and demonstrated to be efficacious at preventing many diseases, it is important that patients receive appropriate preventive medications. We now have confirmed evidence that daily, low dose aspirin use can prevent heart attacks (myocardial infarction) and/or strokes in patients with certain risk factors. There are numerous trials demonstrating that fractures and other injuries can be minimized by the use of daily calcium supplements to slow or prevent bone loss (osteoporosis) in women. Safer and more efficacious immunizations are constantly being developed to prevent serious infectious diseases including measles, mumps, rubella, influenza, and hepatitis. Table 7-4 lists several examples of drug therapies commonly used to prevent disease or illness.

> **Example**   The patient is at high risk to contract pneumonia and therefore requires a pneumococcal vaccine.

The delivery of a comprehensive level of pharmaceutical care requires the practitioner to provide proactive care rather than simply react to prescriptions, changes in drug orders, or questions from patients or other care providers. Not only does this patient-specific, drug therapy problem identification method facilitate providing preventive care, but the patient remains the focus of all inquiries and investigations. This exemplifies a major difference between pharmaceutical care practice as a rational approach to identifying and resolving drug therapy problems and most traditional methods that are based on a review of a list of medications, often referred to as a drug profile.

A patient-centered focus must be established and maintained if the practitioner is to adequately identify potential risk factors or problems,

Table 7-4 Pharmacotherapy as prevention

Preventive drug therapy	Clinical indication
Aspirin	Prevention of heart attack and/or stroke
Calcium supplements	Prevention of osteoporosis
Folic acid supplement (during pregnancy)	Prevention of neural tube defects
Pneumococcal vaccine	Prevention of pneumococcal pneumonia
Neupogen (filgrastim)	Prevention of infection in selected patients receiving anti-cancer drug therapies
Sunscreens	Prevention of sun-induced skin disorders
Dimenhydrinate	Prevention of motion sickness
Oral contraceptives	Prevention of pregnancy
Amoxicillin	Endocarditis prophylaxis in dental patients with cardiac lesions or prosthetic heart valves.
Colchicine	Prophylactic therapy for patients with frequent attacks of gouty arthritis

especially those for which no drug has yet been prescribed or recommended. If the practitioner's efforts are limited simply to reviewing a list of medications which has already been prescribed for, or consumed by, the patient, then there is little chance that all the potential problems that the patient might be at a high risk to develop will be identified, and certainly not prevented.

In the same group of 5136 patients receiving pharmaceutical care, 1947 (37.9%) patients required additional drug therapy to be initiated as treatment and/or prevention at some time during their care. Frequent causes for this drug therapy problem include an untreated medical condition (1009 patients, 19.6%), the prevention of a medical condition (809 patients, 15.8%), and the addition of drug therapies to achieve an additive or synergistic effect (680 patients, 13.2%). It is clear that pharmaceutical care practitioners are commonly required to initiate preventive therapy.

Drug Therapy Problem 3: Ineffective Drug

The drug product is not being effective at producing the desired response.

The following is a list of common causes of drug therapy problems involving patients who are taking drugs that are not effective:

- The drug product is not the most effective for the indication being treated.
- The medical condition is refractory to the drug product.

- The dosage form of the drug product is inappropriate.
- The drug is not effective for the medical problem.

Example   JT's hypertrigylceridemia is not being effectively treated with Colestid (colestipol) 8 grams two times daily because this drug is not effective at reducing high levels of triglycerides.

Choosing the drug regimen that will be the most effective for an individual patient involves an important set of clinical decisions. Effectiveness can only be realized if an appropriate drug product is selected, and the dosage used is sufficient to produce the desired outcome.

It is important to keep in mind that if a drug product has been demonstrated to be efficacious in 75% of patients with a certain medical condition, then it is likely that 25% of your patients with that same condition will not respond positively. Therefore, even if a drug product is thought to be the first line therapy or the "drug of choice," it will not be effective for all patients.

The concept of the drug of choice is an overly-simplistic view of clinical pharmacology and pharmacotherapeutic principles. New agents are developed constantly and some are shown to be more efficacious than previously existing drug products. Entire approaches to therapy can change over time. As an example, in the 1970s, the drug therapy of choice for peptic ulcer disease was antacids. This changed to H2-inhibitors, such as cimetidine and ranitidine during the next decade. In the 1990s many ulcer patients were found to respond to combination antibiotic therapy due to *H. pylori* involvement. By 2002, the third and fourth leading prescription drug sales in the United States were Prevacid (lansoprazole) and Prilosec (omeprazole), both proton pump inhibitors used to treat and prevent peptic ulcer disorders.[3] Selecting a drug product for a patient that is likely to be effective requires a thorough understanding of the pathophysiology of the patient's disorder and the pharmacology of the drug product being considered. The pharmaceutical care practitioner must keep up to date with new products and the primary literature to ensure the best choices are being made for a particular patient. In the 5136 patients receiving pharmaceutical care, 715 (14%) were assessed to be taking an ineffective drug product.

Drug Therapy Problem 4: Dosage Too Low

The dosage is too low to produce the desired response.

The following is a list of common causes of drug therapy problems involving patients whose dosage regimens are insufficient to produce the desired effects:

- The dose is too low to produce the desired response.
- The dosage interval is too infrequent to produce the desired response.
- A drug interaction reduces the amount of active drug available.
- The duration of drug therapy is too short to produce the desired response.

Example The patient's 10 mg daily dose of glipizipe (Glucotrol) is too low to provide adequate control of her blood glucose.

The second type of drug therapy problem associated with lack of effectiveness is seen in patients who receive a dosage regimen of a product that is not sufficient to produce the desired pharmacological result. A dosage regimen has multiple parts and includes the drug product, the dose, the dosing interval, and the duration of therapy. All of these components must be appropriate for your patient in order to produce the desired outcome. Too often patients are given a drug product that is considered to be efficacious, but the dosage regimen is not sufficient to benefit the patient.

People like to use safe drug therapies. *It is easy to make drug therapies reasonably safe, simply under-dose everyone.* If the patient takes too little of the right drug, there is only a small likelihood of experiencing any undesirable effects. On the other hand, there is virtually no chance that the patient will benefit from an insufficient dosage regimen.

Allopathic practitioners do not intentionally provide insufficient doses for a patient. However, published dosing guidelines are often so conservative that patients suffer through ineffective drug therapy because they are instructed to take the "recommended" dose. The tools, knowledge, and successful approaches to the dosing of drugs based on patient-specific parameters play an important role in the provision of pharmaceutical care. Clinical pharmacists developed many useful and successful guidelines to improve our ability to ensure that each and every patient receives a dosage regimen that is based on individual clinical parameters, in the broadest sense, and therefore can be maximally effective.[9]

There are also many instances in which patients are started on drug therapies using a very low or conservative dosage regimen in order to "see what happens." This logical and often nontoxic approach requires that the practitioner is fully committed to follow-up at scheduled intervals to evaluate the patient's status and make any necessary dosage adjustments. Without this critical follow-up evaluation step, the patient is destined to suffer unnecessary periods of inadequate treatment and continued illness because the dosage received is too low to produce the desired outcomes.

Similarly, patients may not be taking the dose of a drug product often enough to fully realize the benefit. If the dosing interval is too prolonged, the beneficial effects of the drug may disappear before the effects of the next dose appear. Adjusting the dosing interval is a common intervention to resolve some effectiveness drug therapy problems.

Drug therapy problems resulting from under-dosing medications are among the most frequently encountered problems in clinical practice. In our sample of patients seen between 1996 and 2002, 1436 patients (28%) of patients with drug therapy problems were receiving too low a dosage to be of benefit. Drug therapy problems that prevent patients from receiving effective therapy have a negative impact in terms of health and costs. Treatment failures result in prolonged suffering and additional health care costs. These data from pharmaceutical care practices reveal that one out of every five patients incurred the costs of medical care, the costs of drug therapy, and the risks associated with their medications, but did not receive any of the benefit. The most common causes for under-dosing patients were that the dose was insufficient and that the dosing interval was incorrect. The dose was assessed to be too low in 807 (15.7%) while the dosing interval needed to be changed in an additional 373 (7.3%) of patients.

Drugs do not have doses, people have doses.[10] Making certain that patients are taking an adequate dosage of their medications to produce the desired effects is a responsibility of the practitioner. One size does not fit all, and one dose does not work for all patients. Student practitioners need to understand that published dosing guidelines are usually generated through highly controlled research studies and therefore can only be used as initial guidelines for drug dosing. Patients will require varying amounts of medications in order to produce the desired pharmacological effects.

Drug Therapy Problem 5: Adverse Drug Reaction

The drug is causing an adverse reaction.

The following is a list of common causes of drug therapy problems involving patients who are taking drug products that are not safe:

- The drug product causes an undesirable reaction that is not dose-related.
- A safer drug product is required due to risk factors.
- A drug interaction causes an undesirable reaction that is not dose-related.
- The dosage regimen was administered or changed too rapidly.

- The drug product causes an allergic reaction.
- The drug product is contraindicated due to risk factors.

Example The patient has developed a rash covering his upper torso and arm caused by the cotrimoxazole he was taking to treat a wound infection.

If the patient has a negative reaction to a drug product it is considered an adverse drug reaction. The resolution calls for discontinuing that product and identifying one that would likely be effective and would also be safer for the patient. Compare this type of drug therapy problem with those undesirable events that are caused by the patient receiving too high a dose. In these cases, the remedy is most often to reduce the dosage regimen. It is important for pharmaceutical care practitioners to distinguish between undesirable events that are dose-related and those that are not. One thousand one hundred and seventy-two (22.8%) patients experienced an adverse drug reaction during some time of their course of therapies. Eight hundred and thirty-four (71%) of these patients experienced the undesirable effect that was not dose-related, while 180 (15.4%) patients required a drug product to be discontinued because it was unsafe for the patient due to individual risk factors or the presence of comorbidities. Fourteen percent of the patients in this sample had an adverse drug reaction identified at their first encounter with the pharmaceutical care practitioner. This emphasizes the need for continued follow-up evaluations to ensure all of a patient's drug therapies are safe as well as effective.

The lack of a uniform definition and the collective inability of the health care system to create and support an effective infrastructure to identify, document, resolve, and report adverse drug reactions (ADRs), has resulted in an amazingly sparse amount of practical information that practitioners can apply to protect patients from serious and life-threatening experiences. The need for a uniform definition is clearly illustrated in the list of terms used to describe various types of undesired reactions to medications. Table 7-5 lists terms commonly used to describe adverse drug reactions.[1] The category of "safety" in drug therapy problems finally provides a standard vocabulary for and approach to adverse drug reactions in patients.

Drug Therapy Problem 6: Dosage Too High

The dosage is too high, resulting in undesirable effects.

The following is a list of common causes of drug therapy problems involving the patient whose dosage regimen of a drug is too high and is therefore resulting in unacceptable risk or harm:

Table 7-5   Terms used to describe adverse drug reactions

Adverse event	Excessive therapeutic effects
Adverse drug reactions	Erroneous use and accidents
Adverse reactions	Iatrogenic disease
Complications	Iatrogenic illness
Drug-induced illness	Negative therapeutics/effect
Drug-induced disease	Pathological reaction
Drug-induced injury	Prescribing errors
Drug intolerance	Side effect
Drug-interaction	Super infection
Drug misadventuring	Unwanted pharmacological effects

- Dose is too high.
- The dosing frequency is too short.
- The duration of drug therapy is too long.
- A drug interaction occurs resulting in a toxic reaction to the drug product.
- The dose of the drug was administered too rapidly.

Example   The patient developed bradycardia and second degree heart block resulting from a 0.5 mg daily dose of digoxin used for congestive heart failure. This dose was too high for his advanced age and declining renal function.

Drugs often exert their pharmacological activities at many different sites in the body or within several organ systems or enzymatic pathways at the same time. Some of these known pharmacological activities will be considered beneficial for the specific indication of the patient. The other known, but undesirable, pharmacological actions are considered side effects. However, *drugs do not know why we sell them, or why we use them.* Drugs merely exert their pharmacology on the patient; sometimes the results are beneficial, sometimes they are not. Therefore, it is important for the pharmaceutical care practitioner to have an extensive and in-depth understanding of the pharmacology of the drugs his/her patient is taking. Most side effects are predictable, and therefore often preventable, extensions of the known pharmacology of the drug.

In approximately 6% of patients, the practitioner determined that the unwanted effects were dose-related and could be resolved by adjusting the dosage regimen downward. Distinguishing dose-related effects from adverse drug reactions that cannot be resolved by reducing the dosage is important. These data also demonstrate the great need to evaluate patients for the negative outcomes of drug therapies as well as the intended positive outcomes.

Drug Therapy Problem 7: Noncompliance

The patient is not able or willing to take the drug therapy as intended.

The following is a list of common causes for patients not to adequately comply with the drug therapy instructions. The causes are listed from most frequently to least frequently encountered in practice:

- The patient does not understand the instructions.
- The patient prefers not to take the medication.
- The patient forgets to take the medication.
- The drug product is too expensive for the patient.
- The patient cannot swallow or self-administer the drug product appropriately.
- The drug product is not available for the patient.

Example   The patient is not able to remember to instill her timolol eye drops twice daily for her glaucoma.

When pharmaceutical care practitioners conclude that a patient is being noncompliant they mean the following:

Definition   Noncompliance is defined as the patient's inability or unwillingness to take a drug regimen that the practitioner has clinically judged to be appropriately indicated, adequately efficacious, and able to produce the desired outcomes without any harmful effects.

When a practitioner decides that the patient's drug therapy problem is a compliance problem, he/she must be certain that the patient's medication regimen has been judged to be therapeutically indicated, effective, and safe. Recall, the term *compliance* is used to mean compliance with a dosage regimen, not with the orders of a paternalistic or authoritarian figure. There is a reason for all noncompliance, and it is the practitioner's responsibility to discover that reason. The cause, or reason, for noncompliance determines the interventions and care that are necessary to alter or improve the patient's behavior. Keep in mind if the patient stops taking a drug because it was not being effective, it is an effectiveness problem—not a compliance problem. Similarly, if your patient stopped taking her medication because it was making her too dizzy to stand up, it is likely a safety problem and not a compliance problem. Less than 20% of all drug therapy problems are compliance problems. Our research and clinical experience indicates that the majority (>80%) of drug therapy problems, involve problems with indication, effectiveness, and/or safety.

Noncompliance among patients receiving prescription medications has been studied quite extensively.[7,11] This common drug therapy problem has most often been examined from the point of view of the practitioner rather than from the more influential attitude of the patient. Considerable efforts have been expended to identify the social characteristics of patients that might be indicators of who will and who will not comply with a given medication regimen. Most social factors, including age, sex, race, social class, marital status, and religion have proven to be of low value in identifying compliant and noncompliant patients.[11]

In order to successfully follow any set of instructions, patients must first understand them. Practitioners often use language and terminology that is unclear to, or not understood by, the patient. Sometimes patients have different definitions of terms, and these differences can result in misunderstandings, confusion, and noncompliance.

Patients can have very different interpretations of common phraseology used in prescription directions, such as "two times a day." What message are you trying to send to your patient with instructions such as "take this medicine twice a day?" Most often the intended message is two doses, taken about 12 hours apart. However, without being explicit about these instructions, patients may interpret "two times a day" quite differently. Consider what timeframe is intended when common activities such as telephoning a friend or checking your e-mail twice a day are described.

Not only are patients capable of making rational decisions, they actually make numerous decisions concerning their own health and well being throughout the various stages of the diagnostic and therapeutic processes. Each patient decides whether to be concerned about signs, symptoms, or the discomfort present and decides to agree, or not to agree, with the diagnosis that is presented. Furthermore, patients decide whether they believe that the proposed therapy is likely to achieve their desired outcome.

Patients decide how they will comply with medications. Patients tend not to take medications that they do not understand. They usually do not take drug therapies that they believe will not benefit them. Patients also do not take drugs if they have safety concerns about the product.

Similarly, people do not begin taking a medication without their own preconceived ideas, nor do they enter a health care system without such preferences. They have their own health care beliefs, ideas about medications, and most importantly, they have ideas about what they want and when they want it. Patients weigh the advantages and disadvantages of drug therapy, the risks and benefits, and the possible discomfort of changing their own behavior against the likelihood of a positive outcome.

As with any person who is asked or expected to follow a set of directions, the patient must determine for him/herself whether doing what the practitioner has recommended is really going to be in his/her best interest. If patients believe that it will be, then they are likely to do their best to comply with the instructions. On the other hand, patient package inserts and coaching by clinicians will be of little value if patients do not perceive that a condition can cause harm or discomfort, or if they do not believe that the recommended therapy will reduce the threat or discomfort caused by the ailment.

When patients choose not to take a medication as intended, they have what they consider to be a good reason for not accepting advice and complying with their prescription instructions. Practitioners must internalize the fact that patients' perceptions and health care belief systems discovered during the assessment process (see Chapter 5) are major driving forces that ultimately influence the decision to seek care or not, and to follow instructions and advice or not.

Patient behavior in taking medications has a significant impact on pharmacotherapy outcomes. The last category of drug therapy problems describes patient actions when they do not or cannot adhere to the instructions.

The rate of noncompliance among patients receiving pharmaceutical care is low. This category of drug therapy problem is resolved through interventions such as making the instructions clearly understandable to the patient, providing the patient with a daily medication diary, medication administration reminders, calendars, pill boxes, and access to free medication programs or price reduction programs offered by some manufactures or governmental agencies.

In our sample of 5136 patients, less than 17% were determined to be noncompliant during their care. Of the patients who had problems complying with the instructions for their medications, four causes for noncompliance were among the most frequently encountered. Five hundred and eighty-two (11.3%) reported that they did not understand the instructions that they were given as to how to properly take or administer their medications. This was the cause identified in 46% of the cases of noncompliance. Both prescription and nonprescription products were involved.

In 247 encounters (13.3% of total encounters in which noncompliance was a problem), patients explained that they understood the rationale for the treatment but preferred not take the medication. In these situations, the practitioners intervened with some alternate form of drug therapy that the patient agreed to use. Two hundred and forty-five (4.8%) patients found that their drug therapies were too costly and therefore did not follow the instructions. Less expensive products were identified and substituted in these cases. The fourth most common cause of noncompliance was that the patient forgot to take the medication. Two hundred and nineteen (4.3%) of patients did not remember to take their drug therapies as intended.

Many patients receiving pharmaceutical care have to manage multiple drug therapies. More than 50% of patients require five or more different drug regimens, several of which require multiple doses each day. Simplifying a patient's drug regimens can have a dramatic impact on the patient's ability to follow all of the instructions properly.

In sum, patients have drug therapy problems of all types that involve medications of all types and that interfere with achieving the goals of therapy for medical conditions of all types. Table 7-6 categorizes the 11,726 drug therapy problems that were identified and resolved among the 5136 patients receiving pharmaceutical care. These drug therapy problems were identified and resolved in over 26,238 encounters between January 1996 and December 2002.

These practice-based results create an interesting picture of how medications are presently being used within the health care system. Far more people can benefit from additional drug therapies to prevent or treat illnesses than are presently recognized. Drug therapies are frequently used at dosages not sufficient to provide effective therapy. Patients often have not been adequately instructed on the optimal way to use their medications. These problems occur at a frequency sufficient to keep many pharmaceutical care practitioners busy helping patients achieve the results they want from their medications.

Table 7-6 A summary of the drug therapy problems identified and resolved in 5136 patients who had 26,238 pharmaceutical care encounters

Drug therapy problem category	Count	%
1. Unnecessary drug therapy	688	6
2. Needs additional drug therapy	3,246	28
3. Ineffective drug	882	8
4. Dosage too low	2,328	20
5. Adverse drug reaction	1,704	14
6. Dosage too high	602	5
7. Noncompliance	2,276	19
Total	11,726	100

STATING DRUG THERAPY PROBLEMS

When you identify and describe a patient's drug therapy problem, you are adding new and unique information about the patient's case. Therefore, it is important to describe your patient's drug therapy problem in a concise, accurate, and informative manner.

A statement describing the patient's drug therapy problem(s) consists of three components:

1. A description of the patient's medical *condition*
2. The *drug therapy* involved
3. The specific *association* between the drug therapy and the patient's condition

How the drug therapy problem is described by the practitioner is of paramount importance. In the context of an individual patient, the identification of a drug therapy problem establishes the practitioner's responsibilities to that patient. This will not only determine the solution employed, but often dictates other components of the care plan, including clinical and laboratory parameters to be evaluated and the schedule for follow-up visits.

The way in which a drug therapy problem is stated or described can greatly influence the care of a patient. Simply stating that a patient is experiencing "toxicity" from drug therapy is not very useful. The type of toxicity (i.e., nephrotoxicity, leucopenia, thrombocytopenia, pseudomembranous colitis, diarrhea, bleeding) and the specific drug associated with this undesirable event are essential to know. Also, describing if the patient is experiencing a dose-related or nondose-related reaction should be identified as part of the description of the patient's drug therapy problem.

Experienced practitioners are mindful of the benefit of stating drug therapy problems in a format that is most useful and with an appropriate level of specificity for the patient's condition at the time of intervention.

> **Example** It is not very useful to describe the patient's drug therapy problem as "the drug she is taking for her high cholesterol is not working."
>
> Describing all of the components of your patient's drug therapy problems is more useful. "The Lipitor (atorvastatin) therapy that she has been taking for the past 3 months for hyperlipidemia has only resulted in a 5% reduction of her total cholesterol using an aggressive dosage of 80 mg daily."

The terminology used to describe a drug therapy problem can also greatly influence how a patient or other health care practitioners perceive and resolve the problem. Terminology that implies cause and effect must be differentiated from terminology that implies a weaker association. Consider the different interventions that might be initiated to resolve drug therapy problems stated through the following pairs of examples:

- The 29-year-old patient is having continued breakthrough seizures due to subtherapeutic phenytoin concentrations.
  This drug therapy problem requires an increase in the patient's phenytoin dosage.
- This 29-year-old patient is noncompliant with phenytoin therapy as she forgets to take her medication, and she is experiencing continued seizure activity.
  This drug therapy problem would be resolved by providing the patient with a daily medication reminder device or a medication diary to help keep track of her medication use.

- The 61-year-old male business executive is experiencing gastrointestinal bleeding caused by aspirin therapy.
  This drug therapy problem would be resolved by determining the clinical indication for his aspirin therapy and substituting another medication that is less likely to cause gastrointestinal bleeding.
- This 61-year-old male patient, who is presently taking low dose aspirin as prophylaxis to prevent a second myocardial infarction, has a history of several episodes of gastrointestinal bleeding from peptic ulcers.
  This drug therapy problem would be prevented by using an enteric-coated aspirin product and frequently evaluating him for any gastrointestinal symptoms.

- The 43-year-old female patient, who is being treated for pneumonia with gentamicin therapy, has poor renal function.
  This drug therapy problem would be prevented by adjusting her dose and interval to provide desired peak and trough gentamicin serum concentrations and by determining her individual pharmacokinetic parameters for gentamicin.
- This 43-year-old female patient with pneumonia has acute renal failure secondary to gentamicin therapy.
  This drug therapy problem can be resolved by discontinuing the gentamicin therapy treating the pneumonia with a different antibiotic that is not harmful to the kidneys.

These examples illustrate the importance of clarity when stating or describing drug therapy problems. The description of the patient's drug therapy problem directly influences the changes that will be made in the patient's pharmacotherapy regimens.

PRIORITIZING DRUG THERAPY PROBLEMS

Once identified, each drug therapy problem can be prioritized as to the urgency with which it needs to be addressed. This prioritization depends upon the extent of the potential harm each problem might inflict on the patient, the patient's perception of the potential harm, and the rate at which this harm is likely to occur. If multiple drug therapy problems are to be dealt with sequentially, the patient should be involved in the decision as to the priority given to each drug therapy problem.

Using organized intelligence is the best approach to problem solving.[12] The same logic is applied to identify, prioritize, and resolve drug therapy problems in complex patients. In patients with multiple drug therapy problems, some problems are identified but are considered to be of a lower priority, and the effort to resolve it is delayed until drug therapy problems with a higher priority are first addressed. However, it remains essential to document those drug therapy problems assigned a lower priority, so they eventually receive the attention required and are not forgotten.

Prioritizing drug therapy problems is an essential skill because of the high frequency with which you will encounter patients who have more than one drug therapy problem at the same time. Our research shows that approximately 21% of patients have multiple drug therapy problems when initially assessed by the pharmaceutical care practitioner.

Once the list of drug therapy problems is prioritized according to risk to the patient, the list is reviewed and the following issues addressed:

1. Which problems must be resolved (or prevented) immediately and which can wait
2. Which problems can be resolved by the practitioner and patient directly
3. Which require the interventions by someone else (perhaps a family member, physician, nurse, or some other specialist)

Patients will help to prioritize drug therapy problems appropriately and they can also help you identify them initially.

Obviously, pharmaceutical care practitioners hold a great deal of the responsibility for identifying drug therapy problems. Much of this responsibility stems from their special knowledge and experience in the fields of pharmacology, pharmacotherapy, pathophysiology, and toxicology. However, patients often identify their own drug therapy problems. This occurs through self-diagnosis, self-examination, and introspective comparisons with previous states of health, or the condition of friends, colleagues, acquaintances, and family members.

When a patient has, or at least feels he/she has, identified a drug therapy problem, it must receive the full attention of the clinician. When a patient self-identifies a drug therapy problem, the practitioner must make it a priority. One might ask in a patient-centered practice: "Who better to recognize drug therapy problems than the patient?"

An example of the potential impact of patients' perception of what is and what is not a drug therapy problem can be found in the evidence that indicates many elderly patients reveal that they will discontinue taking prescribed medications, without seeking the advice of a health care professional, if they perceive they are not experiencing the beneficial effects of the drug.[13] In other words, if patients assess that their drug therapy is ineffective, they will discontinue exposing themselves to the potential harmful and costly effects of that therapy. This may be considered to be "rational noncompliance".[14]

> **Example**   Consider a 57-year-old male patient who feels the medication he is taking for his back pain is not being effective (acetaminophen 1000 mg three times daily). This patient is taking a daily dose of 0.200 mg of levothyroxine (Synthroid) to manage hypothyroidism. He is also taking 81 mg of enteric-coated aspirin each morning as primary prevention of heart attack.
>
> Your assessment will include all of these drug therapies and their associated indications. However, you will have to give priority to the primary drug therapy problem recognized by the patient, that of ineffective analgesic therapy for back pain.

PATIENTS WITH NO DRUG THERAPY PROBLEMS

It is the practitioner's responsibility to identify any and all drug therapy problems that the patient could have. Or, the practitioner may conclude, with substantive evidence, that the patient does not have any drug therapy problems at the present time. A conclusion that no drug therapy problems exist means that all the patient's drug therapies are clinically indicated, the dosage regimens are producing the desired results, and they are not causing any intolerable side effects. A finding that there are no drug therapy problems present will also be interpreted as the patient understands, agrees with, and is compliant with all of his/her drug regimens and instructions. Finally, the decision that the patient has no drug therapy problems at this time indicates that all of the patient's drug-related needs are being met, and no adjustments in drug products or drug dosage regimens are required.

In cases when the patient does not have a drug therapy problem, the pharmaceutical care practitioner focuses on assuring that the goals of therapy are being met and that the patient is not at risk of developing any new problems. Providing continuous care requires the assurance of progress toward achieving and maintaining the desired goals of therapy. Patients who have no drug therapy problems at this time still require a care plan and follow-up evaluation to ensure that goals of therapy continue to be met and no new drug therapy problems develop. Therefore, care plans and follow-up evaluation activities continue even when no drug therapy problems are found (see Chapters 8 and 9).

DOCUMENTING DRUG THERAPY PROBLEMS

The standard for documenting the patient's drug therapy problems is that each problem identified is added to the patient's record and includes the medical condition, illness, or complaint involved, the drug therapy or therapies involved, and the likely cause of the drug therapy problem. Drug therapy problems are most efficiently documented within the care plan for each medical condition involved (see Chapter 8). The interventions required to resolve the drug therapy problem will also be associated with that care plan. The action that was taken (increase dosage, discontinue drug therapy, add preventive drug to regimen) also needs to be recorded. Although it is not always necessary, some practitioners also record the individuals involved in resolving the drug therapy problem (patient, family, physician, nurse).

It is sometimes useful to document the economic impact of identifying and resolving a drug therapy problem at the time the service is provided. Recording instances in which clinic, specialist, or hospitalization visits were avoided because the drug therapy has been improved, can help to justify the cost of a new or expanding pharmaceutical care service. These additional service management records can be maintained separately from the patient's personal care records and summarized quarterly or annually. The Assurance Pharmaceutical Care system maintains records that facilitate information retrieval and data consolidation, as well as providing the summary reports needed to evaluate the practitioner's services and support improvements and expansion in that service (see Chapter 2).

Figure 7-2 is an example of a paper (manual) record to document drug therapy problems and their causes.

DRUG THERAPY PROBLEMS TO BE RESOLVED

MEDICAL CONDITION AND DRUG THERAPY INVOLVED	INDICATION
	Unnecessary Drug Therapy __No medical indication __Duplicate therapy __Nondrug therapy indicated __Treating avoidable ADR __Addictive/recreational **Needs Additional Drug Therapy** __Untreated condition __Preventive/prophylactic __Synergistic/potentiating
MEDICAL CONDITION AND DRUG THERAPY INVOLVED	EFFECTIVENESS
	Needs Different Drug Product __More effective drug available __Condition refractory to drug __Dosage form inappropriate __Not effective for condition **Dosage Too Low** __Wrong dose __Frequency inappropriate __Drug interaction __Duration inappropriate
MEDICAL CONDITION AND DRUG THERAPY INVOLVED	SAFETY
	Adverse Drug Reaction __Undesirable effect __Unsafe drug for patient __Drug interaction __Dosage administered or changed too rapidly __Allergic reaction __Contraindications present **Dosage Too High** __Wrong dose __Frequency inappropriate __Duration inappropriate __Drug interaction __Incorrect administration
MEDICAL CONDITION AND DRUG THERAPY INVOLVED	COMPLIANCE
	Noncompliance __Directions not understood __Patient prefers not to take __Patient forgets to take __Drug product too expensive __Cannot swallow/administer __Drug product not available

(Left vertical label: DRUG THERAPY PROBLEMS)

___No Drug Therapy Problem(s) at this time

Figure 7-2 Drug therapy problem documentation form.

SUMMARY

The centrality of drug therapy problems to the practice of pharmaceutical care cannot be overemphasized. It is essential that practitioners who intend to provide pharmaceutical care understand the descriptions and identification of each type of drug therapy problem as well as their common causes. The discipline and thought required to practice pharmaceutical care guide the practitioner to first make certain that all of the patient's indications for drug therapy are being appropriately treated and that no unnecessary drug therapy is being taken. Then, the practitioner can logically consider product selection and/or dosage adjustment to maximize the effectiveness of the medication. The practitioner must then make certain that all drug therapies will be as safe as possible for the patient. It is important to reemphasize that only after these first three primary pharmacotherapy principles have been fully addressed, are compliance and cost issues considered.

The data generated from patients seen in practice present interesting observations. It is instructive to note that compliance problems are not those most frequently associated with drug therapies seen in clinical practice. Patients requiring the practitioner to provide appropriate drug therapies for preventive and treatment purposes occur most frequently. Also, it is important to note that in today's health care system, patients are under-dosed three to four times more frequently than they are over-dosed. Providing patients with drug therapies at doses that are not sufficient to produce a clinical benefit is a major error in the care of many.

The responsibility to identify, resolve, and prevent drug therapy problems is the unique contribution that pharmaceutical care practitioners make to a patient's health care. It serves as a "gyroscope" to focus the practitioner's clinical activities in cases that involve patients with numerous, complex, and difficult therapeutic dilemmas. Constant referral to the seven categories of drug therapy problems ensures that a consistent, rational, comprehensive, and effective care plan can be established for even the most complicated patient.

EXERCISES

7-1   Discuss the differences between drug therapy problems and medical problems.

7-2   Explain what is meant by the phrase, "the patient has no drug therapy problems at this time."

7-3   Describe your criteria for prioritizing drug therapy problems.

7-4 Describe the drug therapy problem in each of the following scenarios:

    (a) D.S. is a 57-year-old female patient with seasonal allergic rhinitis (hay fever). She has no drug or food allergies. Two weeks ago her allergic rhinitis became really bothersome due to constant sneezing and nasal congestion. She bought two bottles of Afrin nasal spray (oxymetazoline hydrochloride). She has been using two sprays in each nostril twice daily the past 2 weeks. She does not seem to be getting any better. She comes to you today to get some expert advice. What is her drug therapy problem?

    (b) M.S. is a 24-year-old male who was prescribed penicillin VK 500 mg orally three times daily for 10 days for streptococcal pharyngitis (Strep throat) 1 day ago. Today, M.S. comes to you with a rash on his arms and torso. He has never reacted like this before to any medications. He wants your advice on this matter. What is his drug therapy problem?

    (c) J.H. is a 15-year-old high school student. She has no significant past medical history or drug allergies. Last Tuesday night she had a gymnastic competition. During her competition on the balance beam, she fell and twisted her ankle. The pain was not bad, so she got back up on the beam and finished her routine. After her performance, she iced her ankle because it was stiff. Two days later her ankle was still painful and swollen. She came to you to find out what else she should do for her ankle so she can be back to normal by Saturday for her next big competition. What is her drug therapy problem?

    (d) J.H. is a healthy 24-year-old female graduate student who has no significant past medical problems. She currently takes no medications on a regular basis. She came to you last week to get a pain reliever for her headache. You recommended that she take two tablets of Tylenol (acetaminophen) 325 mg every 4 hours as needed for headache pain. J.H. bought a bottle of Tylenol. She decided to take one tablet twice daily as needed. One week later, she is back to see you claiming that the Tylenol did not help her. What was her drug therapy problem?

REFERENCES

1. Cipolle, R., Strand, L.M., Morley, P.C., *Pharmaceutical Care Practice*. New York, NY: McGraw Hill; 1998.
2. Strand, L.M., et al., Drug-related problems: Their structure and function. *DICP Ann Pharmacother* 1990; 24:1093–1097.

3. Vaczek, D., *Top 200 Drugs of 2002*; 2002, www.pharmacytimes.com.
4. Kohn, L.T., Corrigan, J.M., Donaldson, M.S. (eds), *To Err is Human: Building a Safer Health System*. Washington, DC: National Academy Press; 2000, p. 26.
5. Rovers, J.P., et al., *A Practical Guide to Pharmaceutical Care*. 2nd ed. Washington, DC: American Pharmaceutical Association; 2003.
6. Tuneu Valls, L., et al., Drug related problems in patients who visit an emergency room. *Pharm. Care Espana* 2000; 2(3): 177–192.
7. Mant, A., *Thinking about prescribing: A handbook for quality use of medicines*. Sydney, Australia: The McGraw-Hill Companies, Inc.; 1999.
8. Hepler, C.D., Segal, R. *Preventing medication errors and improving drug therapy outcomes: A management systems approach*. Boca Raton, FL: CRC Press; 2003.
9. Dipiro, J.T., et al., *Pharmacotherapy—A Pathophysiologic Approach*, 5th ed. New York, NY: McGraw-Hill; 2002.
10. Cipolle, R., Drugs don't have doses people have doses. *Drug Intell Clin Pharm*, 1986; 20(11):881–882.
11. Sackett, D.L., Haynes, R.B., *Compliance with Therapeutic Regimens*. Baltimore, MD: The Johns Hopkins University Press; 1976.
12. Descartes, R., *The Formulation of a Rational Scheme of Knowledge in Discourse on Method and the Meditations*. Harmondsworth, England: Penguin Classics; 1968, pp. 27–91.
13. Ziegler, D.K., et al., How much information about adverse effects of medication do patients want from physicians? *Arch Intern Med* 2001; 161:706–713.
14. Conrad, P., The meaning of medications: another look at compliance. *Soc Sci Med*, 1985; 20:29–37.

EIGHT

THE CARE PLAN

Key Concepts

1. *A care plan is developed for each of the patient's medical conditions being managed with pharmacotherapy.*

2. *A goal of therapy is the desired response or endpoint that you and your patient want to achieve from pharmacotherapy.*

3. *The key to a successful care plan is clear, measurable goals of therapy which include a parameter, desired value(s), and a time-frame for achieving them.*

4 *The care plan includes interventions to resolve the drug therapy problems, interventions to achieve goals of therapy, and any necessary interventions to prevent drug therapy problems.*

5 *Pharmacotherapy interventions include initiating new drug therapy, discontinuing drug therapy, or changing the product and/or dosage regimen.*

6 *Additional interventions to achieve the goals of therapy can include patient education, medication compliance reminders/devices, referrals to other health care providers, or monitoring equipment to measure outcome parameters.*

7 *The last activity in the care plan is scheduling a follow-up evaluation with the patient to determine the outcomes of pharmacotherapy at a clinically appropriate time.*

8 *Documentation of the care plan establishes the relationships between the goals of therapy, and interventions designed to achieve the goals.*

PURPOSE, ACTIVITIES, AND RESPONSIBILITIES

The purpose of the care plan is to determine, with the patient, how to manage his or her medical conditions or illnesses successfully with pharmacotherapy and includes all the work that is necessary to accomplish this. The activities and responsibilities involved in care planning are described in Table 8-1.

Table 8-1   Care planning activities and responsibilities

Activities	Responsibilities
Establish goals of therapy	Negotiate and agree upon endpoints and timeframe for pharmacotherapies. Inform patients of their responsibilities to accomplish goals.
Determine appropriate interventions to: resolve drug therapy problems achieve goals of therapy prevent new problems	Consider therapeutic alternatives and select patient-specific pharmacotherapy, patient education, and other nondrug interventions.
Schedule follow-up evaluation	Establish a schedule for follow-up evaluation that is clinically appropriate and convenient for the patient.

Standard of Care 4: Development of Goals of Therapy

There is a standard for each of the activities in the care plan. The first of these follows:

STANDARD 4: THE PRACTITIONER IDENTIFIES GOALS OF THERAPY THAT ARE INDIVIDUALIZED TO THE PATIENT.

Measurement criteria

1. Goals of therapy are established for each indication for drug therapy.
2. Desired goals of therapy are described in terms of the observable or measurable clinical and/or laboratory parameters to be used to evaluate effectiveness and safety of drug therapy.
3. Goals of therapy are mutually negotiated with the patient and health care providers when appropriate.
4. Goals of therapy are realistic in relation to the patient's present and potential capabilities.
5. Goals of therapy include a timeframe for achievement.

The care plan allows you to work with the patient, who may have different expectations or understanding of his or her medication. Most often the care plan serves as a negotiated agreement or a *joint venture* between the practitioner and the patient. In the case where care is provided using a team approach, the team functions as a single entity when negotiating a care plan. When family members, guardians, friends, or other caregivers act on the patient's behalf or in conjunction with the patient, it is helpful if this patient is represented by a single voice when negotiating the details of a care plan with a practitioner. The structure of a care plan functions as a framework for the cooperative efforts of all those involved in the management of a patient's medications especially regarding the goals of therapy.

In the ambulatory setting, care plans and goals of therapy must be communicated and understood by several individuals including patients, family members, physicians, and pharmacists. Organizing care plans and clearly stating goals of therapy can benefit all patients in all settings. Recent evidence in intensive care units (ICU) revealed that the daily use of a "goals" form reduced the length of stay in the ICU by 50%.[1] In the ICU, the team includes physicians, nurses, respiratory therapists, and pharmacists. To manage the work required to care for patients in an ICU, the entire care team must agree upon the goals of therapy, the tasks to be performed, and the communications plan.

In most clinical practices, care plans are organized by *medical condition*. In pharmaceutical care, care plans are organized by *indications* for drug therapy (i.e., pain management, sinusitis, prevention of osteoporosis). This structure allows the practitioner to be constantly aware of the indications the patient has for drug therapies and how best to manage each of them.

It is important to note that patients often have multiple medical conditions requiring drug therapy. Some conditions are acute and can be resolved with effective drug therapy, while many are chronic disorders requiring long-term pharmacotherapy management plans. Therefore, the pharmaceutical care practitioner constructs a separate care plan for each indication. This allows for more organized decision-making and facilitates follow-up evaluations. Keeping separate care plans for separate indications facilitates record keeping in that changes in one or two drug therapies can be noted in the appropriate care plan, while not affecting or confusing the information in the plans treating the patient's other disorders. This organization of care plans by indication becomes more important as patient complexity increases. Being responsible for the outcomes of drug therapies in a patient with 8 medical conditions and 11 separate drug therapies requires strict organization to avoid confusion, mistakes, and errors of omission.

Multiple drug therapies for the same indication are grouped together within the same care plan. This allows you to evaluate the impact of the entire pharmacotherapeutic approach for each condition and thus make rational decisions about changes that might be required. Our data indicate that it is very common for patients to require multiple drug therapies at the same time. Pharmaceutical care practitioners in the ambulatory setting provide care for patients taking from one to as many as 20 or more medications. The average is more than five medications at the same time when prescription, nonprescription, herbal, and vitamin supplements are taken into account (see Chapter 2).

Common things are common. As a new practitioner, it is helpful to become familiar with the most common drug-related needs your patient will have. In ambulatory practices, several indications for drug therapy occur frequently. Table 8-2 lists the most frequent indications for drug therapy in patients receiving pharmaceutical care in ambulatory practice settings. This list can serve as an excellent study guide because patients with combinations of these conditions will be encountered numerous times throughout your practice career. These twenty-five indications represent 70% of all the indications treated in this patient sample.

Table 8-2   Common indications for pharmacotherapy[a]

1. Hypertension	14. Anxiety
2. Hyperlipidemia	15. Pain (general)
3. Diabetes	16. Cardiac dysrhythmias
4. Osteoporosis prevention	17. Headache pain
5. Vitamin/dietary supplements	18. Ischemic heart disease
6. Allergic rhinitis	19. Osteoarthritis
7. Esophagitis	20. Myocardial infarction
8. Depression	21. Angina pectoris
9. Menopausal symptoms	22. Constipation
10. Arthritis pain	23. Stroke/CVA
11. Hypothyroidism	24. Back pain
12. Insomnia	25. Congestive heart failure
13. Asthma	

[a]Data generated from all 26,238 encounters with the 5136 patients described in Chapter 2.

The major questions you must consider to construct a successful care plan are:

1. What goals of therapy are you and your patient trying to achieve with pharmacotherapy?
2. What are you going to do, or how are you going to intervene, to resolve any drug therapy problems identified during the assessment?
3. What interventions (drug therapies, devices, patient education) are you going to provide to ensure that your patient achieves the desired goals of therapy?
4. When are you going to follow-up with your patient to determine the actual outcomes of drug therapies and other interventions?

ESTABLISHING GOALS OF THERAPY

Goals of therapy are necessary in order to produce and document positive outcomes. For each medical condition, you and the patient must agree upon clear and concise goals of therapy. Establishing goals of therapy is an essential step toward ensuring a patient will maximally benefit from drug therapies.

Goals of therapy allow all those involved in a patient's drug therapy to participate constructively. When goals of therapy are agreed upon and described explicitly, not only can the patient work toward achieving them, but so can supportive family members and other health care providers.

The goals of drug therapy are to:

1. Cure a disease
2. Reduce or eliminate signs and/or symptoms
3. Slow or halt the progression of a disease
4. Prevent a disease
5. Normalize laboratory values
6. Assist in the diagnostic process

Most drug therapies are used to manage chronic diseases which are not curable with our existing drug products. Examples of chronic disorders that are not yet curable with drug therapy include diabetes, arthritis, hypertension, hyperlipidemia, and hypothyroidism. The goals of therapy for these disorders will include reducing or eliminating the patient's signs and symptoms, the normalization of laboratory values, and slowing the progression of the disease. Table 8-3 contains examples of common disorders and the category of goals of therapy that most frequently apply.

Goals of therapy have a specific structure and always include

1. clinical *parameters* (signs and symptoms) and/or laboratory values which are observable, measurable, and realistic;
2. a desired *value* or observable change in the parameter;
3. a specific *timeframe* in which the goal is to be met.

Goals of therapy have the qualities of being realistic, observable, measurable, and describable by the patient and/or the practitioner. Patient-specific goals of therapy also must be associated with a timeframe describing when each goal should be achieved. This timeframe is important to your patients as it lets them know *what* to expect and *when* to expect it. The time-course for achieving patient-specific goals of therapy also serves as a guide to establishing an appropriate schedule for you and your patient to evaluate the impact or outcomes of drug therapy (Fig. 8-1). It is not very useful to say your goal is for the patient to feel better soon. What is meant by *feel better*? When is *soon*? A goal of therapy might be stated as "The patient's elbow pain will be eliminated within 24 hours," or "The patient's diastolic blood pressure will be below 85 mmHg within 30 days," or "The patient will have no more than two episodes of seizures within the next month," or

Table 8-3   Examples of medical conditions for the goals of therapy

Goal of therapy	Medical condition
Cure a disease	Streptococcal pneumonia Otitis media Diarrhea
Reduce or eliminate signs and/or symptoms	Major depression Allergic rhinitis Common cold
Slow or halt the progression of disease	Diabetes Congestive heart failure Ischemic heart disease
Prevent a disease	Osteoporosis Myocardial infarction Pneumococcal pneumonia
Normalize laboratory values	Hypokalemia Anemia

Assist in the diagnostic process	Anxiety associated with MRI
	  procedures
	
	Intraocular pressure tests
	  for glaucoma

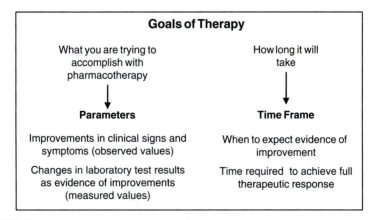

Figure 8-1   Components of goals of therapy.

"The patient's serum potassium will increase to between 3.5 and 4.5 meq/L within 48 hours."

The patient's presenting signs and symptoms most often form the foundation for the patient-specific goals of therapy within the care plan.

> **Example**　For a patient who suffers from allergic rhinitis and presents with nasal congestion, runny nose, and eye itching, but no cough or loss of taste, the patient-specific goals of therapy might include the relief of the patient's complaints of nasal congestion, runny nose, and eye itching in a timeframe of 48 hours.

Given this type of patient-specific goal, a rational approach to pharmacotherapy is possible. Patient-specific goals should be realistic and observable or measurable. They include your patient's presenting concerns, problems, complaints, signs, symptoms, and/or abnormal laboratory test results. Eliciting goals of therapy and obtaining agreement with the patient can be facilitated with the following discussion questions.

- What would you like to achieve with your medications?
- What are your goals for this therapy?
- How do you feel about trying to achieve ... with a new drug therapy?

There are generalized goals of therapy that have been established for many medical conditions by groups of practitioners and researchers who specialize in the treatment of a particular disorder. These general guidelines (see Table 8-4) have been established in the literature and verified in practice and can be used as initial goals until patient-specific goals of therapy can be negotiated and agreed upon by those involved in the care of the patient.[2–5] These include such published parameters as goals for blood pressure in patients with hypertension,[6] goals for serum lipids in patients with hyperlipidemia,[7] and recommended goals for glycemic control in patients with diabetes.[8] To optimize each patient's medication experience, patient-specific goals must be established, agreed upon, and documented in the patient's individualized care plan(s).

As a blueprint to achieve positive outcomes, the care plan includes your decisions as to how specific goals of therapy will be achieved and when this should be accomplished. All of the activities that you perform are called interventions. These interventions may directly involve drug regimens, or they may utilize education, technology, exercise, or dietary instructions.

Table 8-4 Goals of therapy for common medical conditions

Medical condition	General guidelines for goals of therapy	Comments
Hypertension	Systolic 115–140 mmHg Diastolic 75–90 mmHg <130/80 for patients with diabetes or chronic kidney disease	The aim of reducing blood pressure is to minimize end-organ damage including heart disease (angina, myocardial infarction, heart failure), stroke, renal impairment, and/or retinopathy. Evaluate effectiveness of drug therapy monthly for the first 3–6 months following initiation or change in antihypertensive therapy.
Hyperlipidemia	Total cholesterol <200 mg/dL Low density lipoproteins (LDL) <100 mg/dL SI <2.5–3 mmol optimal and considered the goal in patients with coronary heart disease (CHD) and 2 additional risk factors <130 mg/dL (SI <4 mmol/L) in patients with 2 risk factors <160 mg/dL (SI <5 mmol/L) in patients without risk factors. High density lipoproteins (HDL) >40 mg/dL (SI < 1.04 mmol/L) Triglycerides <150 mg/dL (SI <3 mmol/L)	Goal of therapy varies depending on other patient risk factors including hypertension, smoking, family history of coronary heart disease (CHD), males >40 or female >45, and HDL <40 mg/dL. Peak effects on lowering lipids can be evaluated 4–6 weeks after starting or changing drug therapy. Statins can be expected to lower LDL 18–55% and triglycerides 7–30%. Niacin therapy can be expected to lower LDL 5–25% and triglycerides 20–50%. Once goals are achieved, continuous follow-up evaluation every 6 months to 1 year is recommended.

(Continued)

Table 8-4   (*Continued*) Goals of therapy for common medical conditions

Medical condition	General guidelines for goals of therapy	Comments
Diabetes	Blood glucose Fasting or preprandial 80–120 mg/dL (4–7 mmol/L) 2 hours postprandial 100–140 mg/dL (5–10 mmol/L) Glycosolated hemoglobin (HbA1C) < 7%	The aim of glycemic control is to reduce risk of microvascular complications including poor wound healing, retinopathy possibly leading to blindness, polyuria, polydipsia, polyphagia, and diabetic ketoacidosis. HbA1C is used to evaluate glucose control over the past 2–3 months.
Allergic rhinitis	Reduction or elimination of signs and symptoms which may include: rhinorrhea, sneezing, nasal congestion, postnasal drip, and/or conjunctivitis	Therapeutic benefits of nasal steroids can be seen within a few days, but may require 2–3 weeks to see maximum response. Antihistamines generally produce maximum benefit when administered a few hours before exposure to allergen.
Gastroesophageal reflux disease	Alleviate or eliminate patient's symptoms which often include esophagitis (heart burn), hypersalivation, belching, regurgitation after eating. Decrease frequency and duration of gastroesophageal reflux Heal the injured mucosa Prevent recurrence	Symptom relief generally observed within 2 weeks. However, prolonged treatment (8–16 weeks) required to achieve healing and minimize recurrence.

(Continued)

Table 8-4   (*Continued*) Goals of therapy for common
medical conditions

Medical condition	General guidelines for goals of therapy	Comments
Depression	Improvement of patient's target signs and symptoms identified before starting drug therapy including depressed mood, loss of interest and enjoyment, fatigue, reduced energy, reduction in self-confidence, appetite, disturbed sleep, reduced concentration and attention. Aim is to reduce symptoms and help patient return level of functioning present before the onset of illness.	Adverse effects of antidepressant drugs may occur immediately, while symptoms of depression may not improve for several weeks. Antidepressants typically require 1–4 weeks to begin to be effective. Full effect may take 6 weeks, and in some cases improvement may continue for several months. Some symptoms can improve quickly, with energy and interest improving within 10–14 days. Mood improvement often requires 2–4 weeks. Continuous follow-up evaluations every 6–8 weeks to ensure continued control.
Hypothyroidism	Achieve normal thyroid function, reverse any biochemical abnormalities, and provide relief of symptoms which may include lethargy, weakness, loss of ambition and energy, dry skin, cold intolerance, weight gain, constipation, coarse hair, periorbital puffiness, muscle cramps, myalgias, abnormal menses, decreased libido.	Initial response to drug therapy generally observed in 4–6 weeks. If dosage changes are required, allow 4–6 weeks to determine effectiveness of new therapy. Full effects require 4–6 months.

(Continued)

Table 8-4   (*Continued*) Goals of therapy for common
medical conditions

Medical condition	General guidelines for goals of therapy	Comments
	Thyroid stimulating hormone (TSH) The TSH is generally elevated in primary hypothyroidism. Goal is to reduce TSH to normal values of 0.3–5 mU/L	
	Free T_4 Generally decreased in primary hypothyroidism. Goal is to increase to 0.8–1.5 ng/dL	
Insomnia	Improvement in symptoms such as difficulty falling asleep, maintaining sleep, not feeling rested following sleep, daytime fatigue, and/or decreased ability to concentrate.	Sedation effects of drug therapy should be expected within 1–2 hours. Hypnotic effects of benzodiazepines can be maintained for 1 month with night use.
Asthma	Maintain normal activity levels. Prevent symptoms of wheezing, cough, dyspnea, and/or chest tightness. Maintain normal, or improve, spirometry. Spirometry goals vary with severity of asthma levels 1 through 4. Level 1 FEV_1 or PEF >80–85% of patient's personal best or predicted value Level 2 FEV_1 or PEF >80% of patient's personal best or predicted value Level 3 FEV_1 or PEF >60–80% of patient's personal best or predicted value	Early evaluation based on FEV_1 at 30 min after use of inhaled β_2-agonists is a useful predictor of outcome. Patient usage of inhaled β_2-agonists on a daily or weekly basis is used to evaluate effectiveness of pharmacotherapeutic plan. Use of short-term β_2-agonists on a daily basis indicates addition of inhaled corticosteroids therapy is needed. When inhaled corticosteroids are added for long-term control, improvements observed in 1–2 weeks with maximum effectiveness evaluated in 4–8 weeks.

(*Continued*)

Table 8-4   (*Continued*) Goals of therapy for common medical conditions

Medical condition	General guidelines for goals of therapy	Comments
	Level 4 FEV$_1$ or PEF >60% of patient's personal best or predicted value	Following a severe exacerbation requiring hospitalization, return to normal lung function may require 3–7 days.
		Once stable, patient's drug therapy should be evaluated every 3–6 months.

mmHg = millimeter of mercury; SI = systéme international; mg/dL = milligram/deciliter; mmol = millimole; mmol/L = millimole/liter; mU/L = milliunits/liter; ng/dL = nanograms/deciliter; FEV$_1$ = Forced expiratory volume in one second; and PEF = Peak expiratory flow.

INTERVENTIONS

The next standard of care for developing a care plan refers to the interventions that must be made to optimize the patient's medication experience.

Standard of Care 5: Statement of Interventions

STANDARD 5: THE PRACTITIONER DEVELOPS A CARE PLAN THAT INCLUDES INTERVENTIONS TO: RESOLVE DRUG THERAPY PROBLEMS, ACHIEVE GOALS OF THERAPY, AND PREVENT DRUG THERAPY PROBLEMS.

Measurement criteria

1. Each intervention is individualized to the patient's conditions, drug related needs, and drug therapy problems.
2. All appropriate therapeutic alternatives to resolve drug therapy problems are considered, and the best are selected.
3. The plan is developed in collaboration with the patient, his/her family and/or care-givers, and health care providers, when appropriate.
4. All interventions are documented.
5. The plan provides for continuity of care by including a schedule for continuous follow-up evaluation.

The patient's care plan is constructed by selecting the interventions that will help the patient to achieve the desired goals of therapy. These interventions will resolve any drug therapy problems identified during the assessment, optimize the patient's medication experience, and prevent drug therapy problems. Finally, all care plans must contain a scheduled plan for the follow-up evaluation.

Interventions to Resolve Drug Therapy Problems

The resolution of drug therapy problems is given highest priority within a pharmaceutical care plan. Drug therapy problems need to be resolved because they interfere with patients realizing their goals of therapy and meeting their drug-related needs.

> **Example**   If your patient is not realizing the full effectiveness from her prescribed antihistamine to manage seasonal allergic rhinitis because the dose is too low, the dosage regimen must be increased before there is any realistic hope of achieving a positive outcome.
>
> Similarly, if your patient is experiencing dose-related side effects from her antihistamine, the dosage regimen must be modified in order for her to receive appropriately indicated drug therapy that is both effective and safe.

The patient's drug therapy problems must be dealt with first in the care planning process. With the goals of therapy firmly in mind, you can decide how you will intervene on the patient's behalf in order to resolve the drug therapy problem. It is very difficult to resolve a drug therapy problem without a clear goal in mind.

Interventions designed to resolve drug therapy problems include the full spectrum of modifications in drug dosage regimens. These might include initiating new drug therapy, changing the drug product, altering the dose and/or the dosing interval, or discontinuing drug therapy. Each of these decisions is a balance between potential benefit to the patient (achieving goals of therapy) and potential harm to the patient through the selection of a specific drug product and/or dosage regimen. The drug product and/or dosage regimen determines the safety parameters you will evaluate at follow-up visits.

In clinical practice, drug therapy problems are considered resolved when the practitioner initiates or executes an intervention. Therefore, drug therapy problems are documented as being resolved at the time the intervention is initiated. After appropriate interventions have been chosen to resolve the patient's drug therapy problem, specific interventions and individualized drug therapies to achieve the goals of therapy can be designed and implemented to optimize the patient's medication experience.

It is important to include the patient at each step in your decision making process. The following questions can facilitate this discussion:

- How do you feel about making these adjustments in your medications?
- Is this a change that you think you can manage in your daily use of this medication?
- What do you think would be the best way to improve your therapy?

In pharmaceutical care practices, 75–80% of interventions to resolve drug therapy problems are negotiated and agreed upon directly between the patient and the practitioner. The original prescriber is involved in the remaining 20–25% either through direct contact or via preapproved protocols or collaborative practice agreements (see Chapter 2).

Once the drug therapy problem is fully addressed in the patient's care plan, the goals of therapy of the primary indication can again be considered. The intent of the goals of therapy is to provide direction to a variety of activities for the patient and the practitioner. The goals of therapy become the agreed upon target of the prescriber's drug therapy, the patient's nonprescription drug therapy, your interventions, the patient's interventions and compliance behavior.

Interventions to Achieve Goals of Therapy

The interventions portion of the care plan represents the creative portion of the clinical problem-solving process. Based on the patient's value system and his/her sense of what is important, you and your patient collaborate to establish a prioritized list of activities designed to effectively and efficiently address all drug-related needs. The interventions you select are grounded in patient preferences, selected according to patient needs, and limited by patient tolerance. Therefore, the higher the level of patient participation and the more creative you can become at individualizing the care plan to meet your patient's unique needs, the higher the success rate will be. This success is not only evaluated as compliant behavior but also in terms of patient outcomes that are positive when measured.

Interventions to achieve the goals of therapy can include the drug regimen(s) the patient should receive, changes in drug therapy that are required, patient-specific education or information, referrals to specialists, instructions on how to properly use prescription drug products, nonprescription drug products, and how to use other remedies, products, and devices.

The dispensing of drug products is an important intervention in a patient's care plan. A care plan is of little value if the patient is unable to acquire the medication, unable to afford the medication, unable to take the medication, or simply refuses to fill a prescription. All of these issues can cause additional drug therapy problems.

Interventions to Prevent Problems

Each pharmaceutical care plan must also address the need to prevent the development of new drug therapy problems. This is an area that can be confusing to some when first beginning to practice. Actions required to prevent a problem are in direct response to risk factors identified in the assessment of the patient's drug-related needs. These interventions are unique to each patient's situation.

In the course of clinical practice, practitioners always design drug therapies and patient education to avoid preventable side effects or risks known to be associated with certain drug therapies or diseases. If these are routine and standard practice then they do not necessarily become part of the patient's individualized care plan. Examples include initiating antihypertensive therapy with a minimal dosage to prevent orthostatic hypotension or warning patients about drowsiness associated with some antihistamine products. Practitioners also routinely recommend that patients take certain medications with food to avoid stomach upset. These types of interventions are due to the pharmacological or chemical properties of the drug and/or the disease but are not unique to the patient. These would be considered standard or routine instructions and would be provided for all patients taking those medications.

The types of preventive actions to be considered in this step are interventions that are necessary due to unique patient risk factors. What do you need to do because of your patient's specific circumstances to make certain that nothing harmful occurs while taking medications?

> **Example** If your 19-year-old female patient is pregnant, you may decide to make certain that she is getting enough folic acid and other vitamins during her pregnancy. Additionally, you may also need to suggest that she reduce consumption of caffeinated and alcoholic beverages during her pregnancy and not take prescription or nonprescription drug products without checking with you first.

Both of these interventions are preventive because she is pregnant. Neither would likely be considered if she was not pregnant. Only a comprehensive, disciplined assessment can identify patient risk factors that indicate the need for preventive interventions.

Preventive measures often are given a second priority status and do not always become fully integrated into a patient's care plan. This is certainly the case in health care systems where acute treatment and therapies designed to cure illness and reduce symptomatology are the primary focus. In the United States during the height of the health care industry's focus on high technology, and expensive, curative medical interventions, the immunization rate among young children against measles, mumps, rubella, polio, diphtheria, tetanus, and pertussis was approximately 50%.[9] During this time, the primary responsibility to ensure that children received proper immunizations was delegated to the school systems.

Prevention interventions are often avoided by patients because of the delay in observable positive patient outcomes and the cost of the preventive intervention itself. This is unfortunate because the cost of the disease itself is much greater. Interventions designed to prevent the development of a drug therapy problem can take the form of the initiation of drug therapies, vitamins, diets, immunizations, exercise programs, counseling (either directly to the patient or the patient's caregiver), or recommendations made on behalf of the patient to the prescriber (physician, dentist, nurse practitioner, and/or optometrists) (Table 8-5).[10]

Table 8-5   Preventive pharmacotherapy

Examples of common interventions designed to prevent the development of future drug therapy problems, new diseases or illnesses, include

- Calcium supplements in postmenopausal females;
- Subcutaneous heparin or low molecular weight heparin to prevent pulmonary emboli and deep vein thrombosis;
- Aspirin to prevent recurrent myocardial infarction;
- The use of lipid-lowering agents to prevent cardiovascular disease;
- Maternal folic acid supplements to prevent neural tube defects and congenital orofacial clefts;
- Misoprostol use to prevent gastrointestinal erosions and ulcers associated with nonsteroidal anti-inflammatory drugs;
- Need for allergy or *bee sting* kits for a patient with a history of severe allergic reactions;
- Smoking cessation approaches to prevent pulmonary disease, cardiovascular disease or cancer, and antibiotics used to prevent infections during surgical or dental procedures;
- Need to prevent the flu using influenza immunizations in an elderly patient with chronic diseases.

Therapeutic Alternatives

There is seldom, if ever, only one best intervention. You must decide what interventions you will select to resolve the patient's drug therapy problem, and you must decide what interventions you will select to ensure that your patient can achieve the goals of therapy. In addition, you must decide what other interventions your patient might require in order to prevent the development of drug therapy problems. Notice that for each set of clinical decisions you are making you must consider all of the reasonable alternatives available.

Clinicians train themselves to consider several options that might be useful for each patient. They will weigh these options in their minds or discuss them with colleagues and decide which are best for the patient. Here, practitioners apply the rational process of the Pharmacotherapy Workup (see Chapter 6). The clinician considers effectiveness as the first criterion when selecting therapeutic alternatives. The next consideration of therapeutic alternatives involves safety issues. This is when your pharmacotherapy knowledge base is applied to help individual patients. Which drug product in combination with what dosage regimen is most likely to achieve the goals of therapy? This is an important clinical decision-making process.

During the learning phase, it is useful to always identify at least three different therapeutic alternatives for every drug therapy decision you make with your patients. This helps you to learn about drugs that you may not otherwise encounter, and it helps you to learn to investigate, compare, and contrast the evidence supporting efficacy and safety of drug products used for similar indications. When you make recommendations to prescribers for changes in your patient's drug therapy, you will want to provide two alternatives that you consider acceptable. Always indicate which of the two is preferred and why.

Discussing options with your patient can be facilitated with the following questions.

- What is your preference given these approaches for treating your illness?
- There are several medications available to treat your illness, which would you prefer?
- Which therapy do you feel will work best for you?

Drug therapy alternatives constitute a unique knowledge base that the pharmaceutical care practitioner brings to the patient's case, whether practicing independently or as part of a team. In general, drug therapies are considered as viable therapeutic alternatives if there is evidence (in the literature and/or your own clinical experience) of efficacy in managing the patient's medical condition. The list of therapeutic alternatives is then assessed according to the safety risk to the patient. Practitioners must make these benefit-to-risk decisions continuously for their patients.

It is the responsibility of the clinician to consider all of the viable therapeutic alternatives. This list continuously expands. In the United States alone, the Food and Drug Administration approves a new drug product for use approximately every 10 days. A completely new drug entity is approved for use in general practice every 74 days.[11] The importance of therapeutic alternatives in your clinical decision-making process may be best exemplified by the fact that there are now more than two dozen different antidepressant medications available to treat patients with major depression. That is twice the number of therapeutic alternatives that were available when the first edition of *Pharmacotherapy: A Pathophysiological Approach* was published in 1989.[12]

Cost Considerations

Cost considerations should become important only after you have generated therapeutic alternatives based on effectiveness and safety. Any drug therapy that is ineffective for a patient or results in toxicity is too expensive.

Too often, if the differences between the clinical efficacies and/or safety of various drug therapy alternatives have not been well documented, they are considered to be the same. Not knowing the evidence as to whether one therapy is more efficacious than another, and assuming they are the same, is very different. This results in choosing the less expensive of the alternatives. Drug costs are easy to determine and require no clinical judgment. The rational decision-making process within the Pharmacotherapy Workup requires the practitioner discover and incorporate comparative efficacy data and safety data in order to make the optimal clinical decisions about drug therapies.

> **Note** Considering drug product costs before efficacy and safety considerations is not rational and can often be harmful and wasteful.

Cost is an important management issue, but effectiveness and safety always take precedence in the decision-making process of a clinician. After you have considered the evidence of efficacy and safety, then convenience and cost considerations can be applied. The least expensive drug therapy is the one that is effective and does not cause the patient harm.

SCHEDULE AND PLAN
FOR FOLLOW-UP EVALUATIONS

The last standard of care for care plan development refers to the follow-up evaluation that must be scheduled with each patient.

Standard of Care 6: Establishing a Schedule for Follow-up Evaluations

STANDARD 6: THE PRACTITIONER DEVELOPS A SCHEDULE TO FOLLOW-UP AND EVALUATE THE EFFECTIVENESS OF DRUG THERAPIES AND ASSESS ANY ADVERSE EVENTS EXPERIENCED BY THE PATIENT.

Measurement criteria

1. The clinical and laboratory parameters to evaluate effectiveness are established, and a timeframe for collecting the relevant information is selected.
2. The clinical and laboratory parameters that reflect the safety of the patient's medications are selected, and a timeframe for collecting the relevant information is determined.
3. A schedule for the follow-up evaluation is established with the patient.
4. The plan for follow-up evaluation is documented.

The final intervention that practitioners negotiate during the care planning process is the schedule and plan for follow-up evaluation. Every intervention in a care plan may have a positive impact on the patient, a negative impact, or no demonstrable impact at all. Only through a well-constructed comprehensive follow-up evaluation can the practitioner and the patient learn whether the pharmacotherapies, drug information, and other interventions have met the patient's drug therapy needs and resulted in the intended positive patient outcomes.

Detailed documentation communicates to all involved in the patient's care which parameters will be evaluated at follow-up to judge effectiveness and safety. Published guidelines such as those listed in Table 8-4 serve as initial desirable outcomes until patient-specific outcomes are known.

Interventions may also represent the work that needs to be performed at some later date to ensure the continued effectiveness and safety of drug therapies. The appropriate time for the patient and the practitioner to meet again must be established. At this time, the progress of the intervention, drug therapy regimens, changes in products and dosage regimens, devices, information, and referrals provided for the patient will be evaluated. It is important to be explicit. The more precise you are about when to have the next clinical encounter, the better. Being precise about the follow-up evaluation helps the patient understand your commitment to achieving the goals of therapy that the two of you have established.

The plan for the follow-up evaluation addresses three basic questions:

1. When should the follow-up evaluation be scheduled?
2. How will you determine if positive outcomes have occurred?
3. How will you determine if negative outcomes have occurred?

Bringing the care plan to a conclusion can be facilitated by asking the following questions:

- Your next follow-up evaluation should take place in 4-6 weeks. When would you like to schedule our next visit?
- How would you prefer to be contacted—by telephone, fax, or e-mail?
- Is there a best time to reach you?

When to Follow-up

Deciding *when* to see your patient again to determine the effectiveness and safety of the therapy is a clinical decision. The optimal timing for the next follow-up evaluation is often difficult for new practitioners to determine. Most textbooks do not provide precise timetables for scheduling the follow-up visit, as each patient's situation involves different combinations of drug therapies, comorbidities, and risk factors. The clinical decision as to the optimal time to schedule follow-up visits should be based on the most likely period for the desired benefits to manifest themselves, balanced with the most likely time for harm or side effects to appear.

Evaluating effectiveness requires an understanding and appreciation for the onset of action and the time to maximum effect of each of your patient's medications.

Evaluating safety requires an understanding and appreciation for what the side effects are and when they are likely to occur. Therefore, the clinical decision as to when to schedule the next follow-up evaluation becomes the balance between: "When am I likely to see the beneficial effects?" versus "When am I likely to see the adverse effects or toxicity?" A rule of thumb for student practitioners is: "Use whichever of these two occur sooner to schedule the next follow-up."

In general, the more evidence, experience, and confidence you have that the care plan will result in positive outcomes and not result in undesired toxicity, the longer the time interval between follow-up evaluations. On the other hand, the less supportive evidence, data, information, clinical experience, and confidence that you and/or your patient have in the care plan, the sooner and more frequent the follow-up evaluations should be scheduled.

> **Note**   During the learning phase, it is helpful to remember the adage: *Follow-up early and follow-up often.*

DOCUMENTING THE CARE PLAN

Documentation of the care plan is required. Recording the care plan(s) allow(s) you to organize even the most complex pharmacotherapeutic approaches into a format that patients and other practitioners can easily understand and follow. Care plans are documented separately by medical condition or illness. A patient who is managing two chronic conditions and one acute illness with five total medications will have three care plans.

The care plan document lists the indication and includes a brief summary of the signs and symptoms. Goals of therapy must be a prominent part of every care plan. One of the most valued additions that a pharmaceutical care practitioner makes to the patient's health records is explicitly stated goals of therapy.

Students may want to record two or three therapeutic alternatives which were considered for each indication to ensure that the most rational options have been considered. Practitioners do not often record alternatives considered but not selected.

The care plan needs to be complete and should follow the structure of drug product(s) and dosage instructions including dose, route, frequency, and duration. Any special dosing instructions that will help the patient maximally benefit from the drug therapy should be included in the care plan. If the drug therapy is a change from earlier regimens, it should be noted and dated in the care plan. Multiple drug therapies for the same condition are contained in the same care plan. Any changes in drug products, dosage regimens, or instructions should be recorded so that the patient's care plan is continuously current and includes all forms of pharmacotherapy the patient is receiving.

Other interventions to support the specific pharmacotherapy should also be recorded. These often include health advice, exercise, dietary changes, or instructions on the proper use of medication administration devices or drug monitoring devices.

The care plan should include the schedule for the next follow-up evaluation including effectiveness and safety parameters to be evaluated.

Figure 8-2 is an example of a care plan documentation form for each of your patient's medical conditions or illnesses requiring pharmacotherapy.

Pharmacotherapy Workup© **NOTES**   **CARE PLAN**

INDICATION _____
(Description and history of the present illness or medical condition including previous approaches to treatment and responses)

GOALS OF THERAPY(improvement or normalization of signs/symptoms/laboratory tests or reduction of risk)
1.

2.

DRUG THERAPY PROBLEMS to be resolved

____None at this time

Therapeutic Alternatives (to resolve the drug therapy problem)
1.

2.

PHARMACOTHERAPY PLAN (Includes current drug therapies and changes)

MEDICATIONS (DRUG PRODUCTS)	DOSAGE INSTRUCTIONS (DOSE, ROUTE, FREQUENCY, DURATION)	NOTES CHANGES

Other interventions to optimize drug therapy

SCHEDULE FOR NEXT FOLLOW-UP EVALUATION:

Figure 8-2 Care plan documentation form (© 2003 The Peters Institute of Pharmaceutical Care).

SUMMARY

In summary, the care plan is used to organize all of the patient's pharmacotherapies and other interventions to optimize the drug therapy. The foundation of each care plan is the goal of therapy. Drug, device, and educational interventions and all future follow-up evaluations are coordinated within the care plan to achieve the patient's goals of therapy. Goals of therapy are necessary and guide multiple practitioners to provide collaborative care. The patient and practitioner need to negotiate and agree upon goals of therapy, selected interventions including drug products, dosage regimens, instructions, and schedule for future follow-up evaluations. The patient must clearly understand which interventions the practitioner will be responsible for and which will be the patient's responsibility. Lastly, the patient needs to understand what improvements in signs and symptoms and what changes in laboratory tests can be expected from the drug therapies and how they will be used to evaluate effectiveness and safety at the next follow-up evaluation visit.

EXERCISES

Select two individuals who can set aside 30–40 min to discuss their drug therapies. Do not choose members of your family or close friends as these relationships may interfere with the patient care process. Complete an assessment of each individual's drug-related needs and document the completed assessment on the documentation form provided at the end of Chapter 6.

8-1 For each of the two patients, develop a care plan for each of the patient's active medical problems. Establish and record goals of therapy for each medical condition. Include the laboratory and/or clinical parameter(s) to be used, the desired value, and the timeframe for each goal of therapy.

Determine the appropriate interventions to resolve any drug therapy problems that you have identified.

Determine the appropriate follow-up evaluation timeframe for the two patients. Explain why you selected the designated timeframe.

8-2 Document the care plans developed in the previous exercise using the documentation form provided at the end of Chapter 8.

8-3 The prevention of drug therapy problems is one of the pharmaceutical care practitioner's responsibilities. Describe which criteria you will use to determine when to develop and include specific interventions in the care plan to prevent a drug therapy problem.

8-4 The amount of effort required to develop a care plan is inversely proportional to the amount of effort committed to the assessment that was completed. Explain why this is the case.

REFERENCES

1. Pronovost, P., Berenholtz, S., Dorman, T., Lipsett, P.A., Simmonds, T., Haraden, C. Improving communication in the ICU using daily goals. *J Crit Care* 2003; 18(2):71–75.
2. *National Guideline Clearinghouse. www.guideline.gov.* 2002.
3. Dipiro, J.T., et al., *Pharmacotherapy—A Pathophysiologic Approach*, 5th ed. New York: McGraw-Hill; 2002.
4. Gray, J. (ed), *Therapeutic Choices*. Canadian Pharmacists Association; Ottawa, Ontario Canada 2003.
5. Koda-Kimble, M.A., Young, L.Y., *Applied Therapeutics: The Clinical Use of Drugs*. Baltimore, MD: Lippincott Williams & Wilkins; 2001, p. 2–4.
6. National High Blood Pressure Education Program. The Seventh Report of the Joint National Committee on Prevention, Detection, Evaluation, and Treatment of High Blood Pressure. *Hypertension.* 2003 Dec; 42(6):1206–52.
7. National Cholesterol Education Program. Third Report of the National Cholesterol Education Program (NCEP) Expert Panel on Detection, Evaluation, and Treatment of High Blood Cholesterol in Adults (Adult Treatment Panel III). *Circulation.* 106(25):3143–3421; 2002 Dec. 17.
8. Canadian Diabetes Association. Clinical Practice Guidelines Expert Committee. Targets for Glycemic Control. *Canadian Journal of Diabetes.* Dec. 2003; 27(52):518–520.
9. Shalala, D.E., Giving pediatric immunizations the priority they deserve. *J Am Med Assoc* 1993; 269:1844–1845.
10. Bosker, G., *Pharmatecture: Minimizing Medications to Maximize Results*. St. Louis, MO: Facts and Comparisons; 1996.
11. Peteresen, M., New Medicines Seldom Contain Anything New, Study Finds. *The New York Times*; May 29, 2002.
12. DiPiro, J.T., Talbert, R.L., Hayes, P.E., Yee, G.C., Posey, L.M., *Pharmacotherapy: A Pathophysiologic Approach*. New York: Elsevier; 1988.

CHAPTER NINE

FOLLOW-UP EVALUATION

Key Concepts

1. *The purpose of the follow-up evaluation is to determine the patient's outcomes in relation to the desired goals of therapy.*

2. *Parameters that reflect both effectiveness and drug safety must be evaluated.*

3 *The evaluation of effectiveness of pharmacotherapy includes measurable improvement in clinical signs and symptoms and/or laboratory values.*

4 *The evaluation of the safety of pharmacotherapy includes evidence of adverse drug reactions and/or toxicity.*

5 *Patient compliance and its influence on outcomes are determined during the follow-up evaluation.*

6 *The outcome status of the patient's medical condition being treated or prevented with drug therapy is determined and described.*

7 *The patient is reassessed to determine if any new drug therapy problems have developed.*

8 *The follow-up evaluation is the step in which actual results and outcomes from drug therapies are documented.*

PURPOSE, ACTIVITIES, AND RESPONSIBILITIES

The purpose of the follow-up evaluation is to determine the patient's outcomes from drug therapy and to compare these results with the patient's goals of therapy. The follow-up evaluation activities and responsibilities are described in Table 9-1.

Table 9-1 Follow-up evaluation activities and responsibilities

Activities	Responsibilities
Elicit clinical and/or laboratory evidence of actual outcomes and compare them to goals of therapy.	Evaluate effectiveness of pharmacotherapy.
Elicit clinical and/or laboratory evidence of adverse effects or toxicity to determine safety of drug therapy.	Evaluate safety of pharmacotherapy.
Document clinical status and any changes in pharmacotherapy that are required.	Make a judgment as to the clinical status of the condition being managed with pharmacotherapy.
Assess patient for any new problems.	Assess patient compliance and identify if any new drug therapy problems have occurred.
Schedule next follow-up evaluation.	Provide continuous care.

Standard of Care 7: Follow-up Evaluation

THE PRACTITIONER EVALUATES THE PATIENT'S OUTCOMES
AND DETERMINES THE PATIENT'S PROGRESS TOWARD THE
ACHIEVEMENT OF THE GOALS OF THERAPY, DETERMINES IF
ANY SAFETY OR COMPLIANCE ISSUES ARE PRESENT, AND
ASSESSES WHETHER ANY NEW DRUG THERAPY PROBLEMS
HAVE DEVELOPED

Measurement criteria

1. The patient's outcomes from drug therapies and other interventions are documented.
2. The effectiveness of drug therapies is evaluated, and the patient's status is determined by comparing the outcomes within the expected timeframe to achieve the goals of therapy.
3. The safety of the drug therapy is evaluated.
4. Patient compliance is evaluated.
5. The care plan is revised, as needed.
6. Revisions in the care plan are documented.
7. Evaluation is systematic and ongoing until all goals of therapy are achieved.
8. The patient, family and/or care-givers, and health care providers are involved in the evaluation process, when appropriate.

No one cares how much you know, until they know how much you care.
Caring is demonstrated through the activities of the follow-up evaluation.
This is an essential activity in the provision of pharmaceutical care. It adds
new information to the patient's medication experience and potentially to
the practitioner's pharmacotherapeutic knowledge base. The only way to
know whether the drug therapy your patient is taking is effective and/or safe
is to conduct a follow-up evaluation.

Follow-up evaluation activities represent a new step in the health care
system that does not routinely occur with drug therapy when pharmaceutical care is not provided.

Note   You have not provided pharmaceutical care unless and until you
have followed-up with your patient to determine what has happened
as a result of your clinical decisions, drug therapy advice and care
planning.

Although all practitioners provide drug therapy advice and instructions
with the best of intentions, these well-meaning interventions do not always
have positive outcomes.

Your clinical decisions, drug therapies, and advice can produce any one of the following three outcomes:

- The intended positive clinical result
- A negative clinical result
- No demonstrable change

It is difficult to overemphasize the importance of the evaluation step in the patient care process. The follow-up evaluation is where and when practitioners gain *clinical experience*. Follow-up evaluations provide the evidence of effectiveness and safety.

Throughout the assessment and care planning steps of the Pharmacotherapy Workup, you have been assessing your patient's drug-related needs. You have been acting on what you think your patient's drug therapy problems are, and you have been intervening by doing what you think has the best probability of achieving your patient's goals of therapy. All of this rational clinical thinking produces actual (real) results (outcomes). Learning from real results, good or bad (effectiveness or safety), is the working definition of clinical experience. Observing what resulted from your clinical decisions constitutes clinical experience. New knowledge is gained during each follow-up evaluation. The follow-up evaluations are the most productive times for clinicians to learn which medications and which dosage regimens are most effective, and which cause harm.

The outcomes of drug therapies, drug therapy decisions, drug information, referrals, and other interventions are unknown until the practitioner conducts a follow-up evaluation with the patient. If the result is positive, you have learned that a certain drug regimen was effective in a specific clinical situation, and you will never forget. If the result is negative, you have learned that a certain drug regimen failed to produce the desired results. Either result provides the greatest learning that a student practitioner can experience. The same holds true for learning about adverse effects of drug therapies. If the patient experiences an adverse effect and describes that to you, or if you observe it at the follow-up evaluation, that information is added to your long-term clinical database. Dan Canafax, Pharm.D., a colleague for many years, commonly instructed students and residents on the University of Minnesota renal transplant service "If you want to learn about side effects, talk to your patients. They will teach you about side effects."

During the follow-up evaluation, the practitioner is looking for evidence of effectiveness, safety, and any new problems that may have occurred since the last visit. At each follow-up, the practitioner is looking for *good, bad*, and *new*. In general, the good (effectiveness) comes in the form of the disappearance of the signs and symptoms of the disease or illness. The bad (safety) comes in the form of adverse and harmful effects from drug therapies.

EVALUATING EFFECTIVENESS OF DRUG THERAPIES

During the follow-up evaluation, the practitioner and the patient compare the goals of therapy with patient outcomes. The most frequent parameters used to evaluate the clinical outcomes that result from a patient's drug therapy are clinical and/or laboratory parameters (Fig. 9-1).

Clinical Parameters—Improvement in Patient Signs and Symptoms

Changes in clinical parameters are frequently used to determine the effectiveness of drug therapy. Positive clinical outcomes are most often associated with the disappearance or diminution of the patient's presenting signs and symptoms. Clinical parameters of the disease or illness often include clinical manifestations such as levels of pain, anxiety, mood changes, inflammation, or frequency and severity of cough, seizures, bleeding, sleep disturbances, tremors, and shortness of breath. Changes in these parameters are determined by asking the patient to describe them at the follow-up evaluation and comparing the patient's response to what you

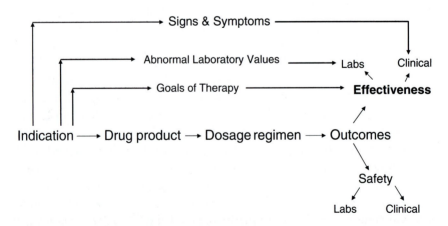

Figure 9-1 Pharmacotherapy Workup. See Chapter 6 for details.

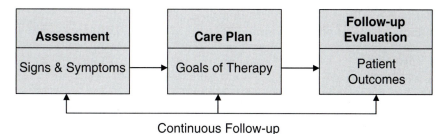

Figure 9-2 The relationships in the patient care process.

observed and documented during the assessment interview or the most recent patient encounter.

The practitioner's observational and clinical inquiry skills are applied during the follow-up evaluation in a similar manner to that of the assessment interview. The practitioner must have the clinical knowledge and ability to gather relevant information from the patient so that an evaluation of the clinical effectiveness of the patient's drug therapies can be made. The process of outcomes evaluation is straightforward. What clinical parameters were used to establish the goals of therapy? What is the status of those same parameters today? The practitioner establishes the relationships between (1) the original presenting signs and symptoms of the disease or illness; (2) the clinical parameters used to establish the goals of therapy; and (3) the improvement in those same clinical parameters at the time of follow-up (Fig 9-2).

Table 9-2 presents examples of common disorders in which effectiveness of pharmacotherapy is evaluated based on changes in clinical signs and symptoms.

Laboratory Parameters—Improvement in Laboratory Test Results

Outcome evaluations often rely on changes in laboratory values. In some diseases or conditions, there are few or no clinical manifestations, and outcome judgments are based primarily on improvements in laboratory test results. Hyperlipidemia is a common example in which measurements of the patient's serum lipids (cholesterol, low-density lipoproteins—LDL, high-density lipoproteins—HDL, and triglycerides) serve as the parameters to determine the effectiveness of drug therapy. Patients seldom exhibit clinical symptoms associated with hyperlipidemia. Therefore, *effectiveness* evaluations are often based on laboratory measurements (Table 9-3).

Table 9-2 Clinical signs and symptoms used to evaluate effectiveness of pharmacotherapy

Therapeutic indication	Clinical parameters
Back pain	Severity and frequency of pain, range of motion, ability to ambulate
Migraine	Headache pain, retro-orbital pain, nausea, vomiting, visual disturbances
Major depression	Mood changes, feelings of sadness, level of energy, interest or enjoyment in usual or favorite activities, insomnia, agitation, fatigue, ability to think or concentrate, thoughts of death
Anxiety disorder	Level of restlessness, concentration, irritability, muscle tension, sleep disturbance
Cough	Severity and frequency of cough, interruption of daily activities or sleep
Rash	Change in color and/or size, associated inflammation, itching
Osteoarthritis	Use-related pain in weight-bearing joints including knee, hip, spine, and hands. Stiffness after rest.

Pharmaceutical care practitioners must understand the impact that drug therapies have on specific laboratory tests in order to determine if they are effective. The timing of when to collect the sample for the laboratory test is an important clinical decision. Often the practitioner must decide if the question to be answered at the follow-up evaluation is: "Will this drug regimen have any beneficial effect for my patient?" In this case, the practitioner

Table 9-3 Laboratory test results used to evaluate effectiveness of pharmacotherapy

Therapeutic indication	Laboratory parameters
Hyperlipidemia	Cholesterol, low-density lipoproteins (LDL), triglycerides, high-density lipoproteins (HDL)
Anemia	Complete blood count (CBC), hemoglobin (Hb), hematocrit (Hct) , red blood cell count, mean corpuscular volume (MCV), reticulocyte index, serum ferritin, iron-binding capacity, serum iron, serum B_{12}
Cardiac dysrhythmias	Electrocardiogram (ECG, EKG)
Diabetes mellitus	Blood or plasma glucose, hemoglobin (A1C)

would want to know how soon any positive effect can be measured. The more common question is: "How much of an impact will this drug regimen have on my patient?"

>   **Example**   Most HMG CoA reductase inhibitors (statins) begin to improve serum lipid determinations within a few days (5–14 days), but generally several weeks (3 to 6) are required to see the full extent of the changes in serum lipids. Waiting only 1–2 weeks after initiating lipid-lowering pharmacotherapy to measure changes in serum lipids might provide information as to whether the selected therapy is likely to have any effect at all on the patient's lipid profile. However, waiting 6 weeks or longer is more likely to provide evidence as to the extent of the benefit the patient is likely to experience from the drug regimen. In the first case, the laboratory test is used to evaluate whether any effectiveness is likely and in the second case, the laboratory test result is used to determine the *extent or degree* of benefit the patient has received from the drug therapy.

Follow-up evaluations of patients with acute disorders can serve to evaluate the final patient outcomes. Follow-up evaluations for patients with chronic conditions serve to establish the present status of the patient's condition. Patients with chronic conditions require continuous follow-up which is initially designed to ensure that the drug therapy has in fact produced the desired effects (effectiveness), followed by less frequently scheduled evaluations designed to ensure that the patient remains stable and the drug therapy continues to benefit the patient. Typically, follow-up evaluation schedules are more frequent at first, until the goals of therapy are achieved (desired blood pressure, cholesterol, or level of pain), and then are scheduled less frequently (quarterly or semiannually) in order to determine that the maintenance drug therapy continues to effectively manage the patient's condition.

EVALUATING THE SAFETY OF DRUG THERAPIES

The follow-up evaluation requires proactive practitioner involvement. That is to say, it is here that practitioners assertively assume the responsibility to reach out to patients and demonstrate caring behavior. Experienced pharmaceutical care practitioners understand that it is their responsibility to determine if drug therapies are in fact safe for their patients, and the best way to ensure safety is to determine whether the patient is experiencing any negative effects.

It is unacceptable to wait for the patient to contact you if he/she has any side effects from the drug therapies that you provided. This type of passive approach is inconsistent with the value of pharmaceutical care and results in over $175 billion in drug-related morbidity and mortality in the United States each year.[1-3] To conduct a comprehensive, adequate follow-up evaluation requires active communication with each patient and feedback concerning any problems. Such feedback either validates the care plan or questions its appropriateness, thereby leading to improvements in the patient's medication experience.

Drug products are produced and made available for patient use because they possess a set of pharmacological actions. Most drugs exhibit several related pharmacological activities, some beneficial, some undesirable. Which are considered beneficial and which are considered undesirable depend upon the therapeutic indication (why we are using the drug). However, when you use a drug at doses high enough to exhibit its pharmacological activities, any and all of those pharmacological actions can and will occur. Those actions that are desirable help to achieve the goals of therapy. The undesired actions are most often called adverse effects or side effects.

> **Example**   Aspirin is known to have analgesic, antipyretic, and anti-inflammatory properties. It impairs prostaglandin biosynthesis. Aspirin inhibits cyclooxygenase-1 (COX-1) associated with gastrointestinal irritation, renal effects, and irreversible inhibition of platelet aggregation, and also inhibits cyclooxygenase-2 (COX-2) which provides aspirin anti-inflammatory properties. When a patient is treated with aspirin, all of these effects occur to varying degrees. If the intended therapeutic indication was to manage pain (analgesia), then the platelet inhibitory activities, which can aggravate bleeding, are undesirable and would be considered a side effect. On the other hand, if the patient is using aspirin as secondary prevention of a heart attack (MI) or stroke (CVA), then the platelet pharmacology is the desired action and renal and gastrointestinal activities would be considered negative consequences. *The aspirin does not know why you are using it. It just exerts all of its pharmacological activities.*

The practitioner and the patient need to know the intended therapeutic indication and evaluate it for effectiveness. At the same time the practitioner must expect drug therapies to exert all of their known pharmacological actions.

Clinical Parameters—Patient Signs and Symptoms as Evidence of Drug Safety Problems

Patients manifest undesirable actions of drugs in many ways. The practitioner's follow-up evaluation must include determining if any of the patient's clinical manifestations are due to adverse drug effects or due to toxic reactions related to excessive dosage of the medication. The vast majority of medications used in modern medicine are taken orally. Therefore, it is not surprising that gastrointestinal irritation is a common problem with medications. Nausea, vomiting, and diarrhea are often caused by the direct irritative effects of the drug on the gastrointestinal lining. Similarly, many undesirable drug effects manifest as skin eruptions or rashes. Drugs that exhibit some of their pharmacological activities within the central nervous system can cause patients to become drowsy, somnolent, dizzy, agitated, or confused.

The two major categories of undesirable effects are unpredictable adverse reactions associated with the product itself and those reactions related to the dosage of the drug. The unpredictable effects include allergic reactions, hypersensitivity reactions, or idiosyncratic adverse events. The substantially more frequent category of undesirable drug effects results from the predictable, pharmacological action of the drug regimen and is related to the dosage of the drug.

In general, adverse effects of drug therapies manifest as clinical signs or symptoms and/or as alterations in laboratory test results. The practitioner evaluates clinical parameters and/or laboratory parameters during each follow-up evaluation in order to determine the safety of the patient's drug therapy (Fig. 9-3).

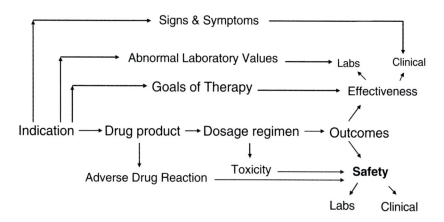

Figure 9-3   Pharmacotherapy Workup. (Refer to Chapter 6 for details)

Laboratory Parameters—Abnormalities in Laboratory Test Results as Evidence of Drug Safety Problems

It is common to require the measurement of specific laboratory tests as part of a follow-up evaluation to determine the safety of the patient's drug therapies. Drug toxicities can often be identified before severe or permanent harm is caused by evaluating laboratory tests parameters on a scheduled basis.

> **Example** Several of the drug products commonly used to manage hyperlipidemia can cause liver damage, including atorvastatin (Lipitor), simvastatin (Zocor), pravastatin (Pravachol), lovastatin (Mevacor). Tests to determine the presence and extent of hepatic damage are recommended at baseline and every 12 weeks as part of the follow-up evaluation of patients using these agents to lower cholesterol and other lipids. If the results of these hepatic injury tests become elevated to greater than 2 to 3 times normal, the drug therapy needs to be discontinued and different therapeutic alternatives need to be used to manage the patient's hyperlipidemia.
>
> Another example of using laboratory test results to evaluate risk of drug safety would be measuring serum potassium in patients receiving digoxin therapy. The cardiac toxicity of digoxin is more pronounced in the presence of hypokalemia, hypomagnesemia, and hypercalcemia. Risk of digoxin toxicity is reduced if serum electrolyte concentrations are evaluated at follow-up and maintained within the desired normal ranges.

It is important for the pharmaceutical care practitioner to know the laboratory test parameters that are most useful in detecting drug toxicity and to make certain that these tests are appropriately scheduled as part of the patient's follow-up evaluation. You can depend upon medical practitioners to focus on ordering and evaluating laboratory tests designed to determine the presence or absence of diseases, however, it is the responsibility of the pharmaceutical care practitioner to make certain that the tests required to ensure safety of all of the patient's drug therapies are properly obtained and evaluated.

In summary, the activities of the follow-up evaluation step of the care process include the collection, interpretation, and evaluation of clinical and laboratory parameters to judge effectiveness of the patient's drug therapy. Follow-up evaluation activities also include the collection, interpretation, and evaluation of clinical and laboratory parameters used to judge the safety of the drug therapy the patient is taking.

DETERMINING THE CLINICAL OUTCOME STATUS

Pharmaceutical care practitioners are responsible for the outcomes of drug therapies. To determine if this fundamental professional responsibility is being met, practitioners must make a clinical judgment about patient outcomes.

Each follow-up evaluation contains the practitioner's clinical judgment as to how effective the care plan and the associated drug therapies have been in achieving the goals of therapy for each of the patient's medical conditions. From the information gathered at the follow-up evaluation, the practitioner and the patient can evaluate the outcomes or results up to that point in time. The practitioner is responsible to document the progress (or lack of progress) in achieving the goals of therapy. The status of each medical condition being managed by medications is evaluated at each follow-up encounter. This provides a *picture* of the effectiveness of the patient's drug therapy over time.

For patients with acute disorders, the follow-up evaluation often serves as the determination of the final outcome. More commonly, for patients with chronic conditions, continual or serial follow-up evaluations over time serve to establish the improvement or decline in the status of the patient's condition being managed with drug therapy during that same timeframe.

The terminology used to describe clinical outcome status resulting from drug therapies is precise and represents both the decisions and actions on the part of the pharmaceutical care practitioner.

The standard pharmacotherapy outcome status terms describe two characteristics of the patient's drug therapy:

1. the progress, or lack of progress, in achieving the desired goals of therapy at the time of the follow-up evaluation; and
2. the action, if any, taken to adjust the patient's drug therapies.

In practice, many patients have multiple conditions and require drug therapy for both acute and chronic conditions simultaneously. Therefore, you will require a working vocabulary of terms that can be used to effectively describe and document the outcome and status of all of your patients' conditions that you are managing with medications. A standard set of definitions for pharmacotherapy outcomes has been established.[4] The descriptions below are designed to provide additional explanations of these terms.

Resolved   The patient's desired goals of therapy have been successfully achieved, and drug therapy can be discontinued. The use of the term *resolved* is intended to represent a final positive patient outcome, and is most often applicable to acute medical conditions or illnesses. The action taken, in this case discontinuing the drug therapy, should be documented in your patient's pharmaceutical care records along with the clinical and/or laboratory evidence of the positive outcome.

> **Example**   Consider the case of a successful treatment of a community acquired pneumonia in a 53-year male patient with a 10-day course of oral erythromycin therapy at a dosage of 500 mg four times each day. By the end of the 10 days of antibiotics, the patient's temperature is back to normal, he has stopped coughing, his white blood count is no longer elevated, and the infiltrates originally seen on his chest x ray have cleared. He does not require any further antibiotics past the original 10-day course of treatment. No additional follow-up is needed as his pneumonia has resolved.

Stable   The patient's goals of therapy have been achieved, and the same drug therapy will be continued to optimally manage the patient's chronic disease. This is most frequently the case when drug therapy is used to treat or prevent a chronic medical condition or illness. In these cases, stabilizing the patient's clinical condition and/or improving laboratory test results were the predetermined desired goals.

> **Example**   In order to stabilize a 63 year old female patient's blood pressure within a desired range of 110–120/70–80 within 2 months the practitioner initiates pharmacotherapy with 50 mg of hydrochlorothiazide every morning, a sodium restricted diet, and a low impact exercise program. At the 60-day follow-up evaluation, the patient's blood pressure was 112/80 and her hypertension was judged to be stable and no changes in hydrochlorothiazide dosage regimen were made. The next follow-up evaluation might be planned to occur in 90 days to reevaluate the continued success of the entire care plan.

Improved   Measurable progress is being realized in achieving the patient's goals of therapy. Goals have not been completely achieved at this time; however, no changes in drug therapy will be implemented at this time because more time will be required to observe the full benefit from this drug regimen.

> **Example**   Consider a 55-year-old male patient whose depressive signs and symptoms such as loss of energy and disturbances in sleep and eating patterns have improved following an initial 3 weeks of drug therapy with 100 mg daily of the antidepressant drug sertraline (Zoloft).

Although his depressed mood and ability to concentrate have still not fully responded, no changes in his dosage regimen will be instituted at this time. In this case, an additional follow-up evaluation would be scheduled for 4 weeks.

Partial improvement   The evaluation indicates that some positive progress is being made in achieving the patient's goals of therapy, but adjustments in drug therapy are necessary at this time in order to fully meet all of the goals of therapy by the next scheduled follow-up evaluation.

Example   A 47-year-old female patient whose arthritic pain has been somewhat relieved following 2 weeks of therapy with ketoprofen (Orudis) 12.5 mg four times daily, desires additional relief from her discomfort. The practitioner's evaluation indicates that greater effectiveness might be realized by increasing the total daily dosage of ketoprofen to 75 mg taken as 25 mg three times daily. The next follow-up evaluation is scheduled to occur in two more weeks to determine if this adjustment in the dosage regimen of the nonsteroidal anti-inflammatory medication produces continued and/or additional relief for the patient without intolerable stomach irritation, headache, or fluid retention.

Unimproved   The practitioner's clinical evaluation is that, to date, little or no positive progress has been made in achieving the patient's goals of therapy, but further improvement is still anticipated given more time. Therefore, the patient's care plan will not be altered at this time. Thus, the unimproved status evaluation is dependent on the timing of the follow-up evaluation.

Example   An adult male patient who is allergic to penicillin is started on erythromycin 250 mg orally four times a day for the treatment of a localized soft tissue infection following a work-related injury to the right forearm. Twenty-four hours after initiating erythromycin therapy the patient experiences some nausea from the antibiotic, and the injured area on the arm is still inflamed and slightly swollen. The practitioner reassures the patient about the nausea and provides him with a suggestion as to how to minimize this undesirable side effect commonly associated with erythromycin, and documents an evaluation of the current effectiveness of therapy. The practitioner reports that although the arm is unimproved at this early stage in therapy, no dosage changes are indicated, and that 3–5 days would be an appropriate time to make another evaluation of the potential effectiveness of the erythromycin therapy.

Worsened   The practitioner's evaluation describes a decline in the health of the patient despite an adequate therapeutic trial using the best possible drug therapy for this individual. Because the goals of therapy are not being achieved, changes in the patient's drug therapies are necessary at this time. The drug dosage may need to be increased and/or additive or synergistic drug therapies might need to be added. A future follow-up evaluation should be planned to examine the status of the patient's condition once the changes in the care plan have been instituted.

> **Example**   A 17-year-old athlete whose elbow stiffness and muscle pain have progressively become more bothersome over the past 4 days despite the use of acetaminophen 325 mg three times each day and ice packs. This worsening condition might call for increasing the aceta-minophen dosage and/or adding a topical analgesic such as capsicum. Two days after increasing the acetaminophen dosage to 1000 mg three times a day and adding topical capsicum, the practitioner would follow-up again to determine the effectiveness in reducing the pain and stiffness in this varsity athlete.

Failure   The practitioner's evaluation indicates that the present care plan and associated drug therapies have been given at adequate dosages and for an adequate amount of time, yet they have failed to help the patient achieve the goals of therapy. Therefore, the present therapy should be discontinued and alternate pharmacotherapy initiated. In these situations, the desired outcomes have not been realized and the initial treatment is considered to have failed.

> **Example**   A 37-year-old female patient whose symptoms of seasonal allergic rhinitis have not improved with 2 weeks of chlorpheniramine therapy at 24 mg per day. Therefore, it will be discontinued, and new drug therapy initiated such as loratadine (Claritin) 10 mg daily. The next follow-up evaluation is planned in 5 days to examine the effectiveness of loratadine in controlling the patient's symptoms of rhinitis.

Expired   The fact that the patient dies while receiving drug therapy is documented in the pharmaceutical care record. Any important observations about contributing factors, especially if they are drug-related, should be noted.

Using this standard pharmacotherapy outcome status terminology is a powerful tool in analyzing and improving your ability to care for patients, maintain a viable practice, and communicate effectively with other practitioners. The term *initial* is used to describe the status of the patient at the time drug therapy is first initiated and goals of therapy are being established. This represents the beginning of therapy and allows the practitioner to determine the length of time required to achieve the observed clinical outcomes. Carefully documented follow-up evaluations can provide important summary data to address vital questions such as "How long does it take for your patients with hypertension to become stable on their new antihypertensive drug therapies?" or "Which of my patients receiving antidepressants are unimproved, or only partially improved, after 60–90 days of therapy?" Outcome data supporting the positive contributions of pharmaceutical care require person-to-person follow-up evaluations and systematic, explicit clinical decisions and documentation of patient outcomes over time.

A summary of the outcome status terminology is given in Table 9-4.

Table 9-4   Summary of outcomes status terminology

Pharmacotherapy outcome status	Definition (progress toward goal and action required)
Resolved	Goals of therapy have been achieved. Drug therapy has been completed or can now be discontinued. Usually associated with therapy for an acute disorder.
Stable	Goals of therapy have been achieved. The same drug therapy will be continued. Usually associated with therapy for chronic disorders.
Improved	Adequate progress is being made toward achieving the goals of therapy at this point in time. The same drug therapy will be continued.
Partially improved	Some measurable progress is being made toward achieving the desired goals of therapy, but adjustments in drug therapy are required. Usually dosage changes or the addition of additive or synergistic therapies is required.
Unimproved	No measurable progress in achieving goals of therapy can be demonstrated at this time. It is judged that more time is needed to produce adequate response. No changes will be made. The same drug therapy will be continued at this time.
Worsened	There has been a decline in health status while receiving the current drug regimen. Some adjustments in drug product selection and/or drug dosage are required.
Failure	The goals of therapy have not been achieved despite adequate dosages and adequate duration of therapy. Discontinuation of the present medication and initiation of new drug therapy is required.
Expired	Patient died while receiving drug therapy.

Other Outcomes Associated with Drug Therapy

In addition to clinical outcomes, drug therapies can also have a dramatic economic influence on patients and their families. Some drug products can represent a substantial economic burden; however, in general, drug therapies are among the most cost-effective forms of treatment available within modern medicine.

Economic outcomes are described in terms of cost-to-response data, cost avoidance, or savings amounts. Treatment failures are probably the most expensive problem associated with drug therapies. The high negative costs associated with treatment failures or inadequate dosages result from the fact that all of the costs of the health care system are incurred, but none of the benefits are realized.

> **Example** A 52-year-old business woman who is suffering with weakness, fatigue, cold intolerance, muscle cramps, and other signs and symptoms of hypothyroidism seeks care. This patient must recognize the need for care, and then commit the time away from work and consume the other resources necessary to seek care. The patient's physician must spend time assessing the patient's complaints, history, physical examination, review of systems, and obtain relevant laboratory tests to rule out other causes of these symptoms. To establish the diagnosis of hypothyroidism, appropriate thyroid function tests need to be analyzed. Once the diagnosis of hypothyroidism has been established, treatment is initiated. Levothyroxine (synthetically derived thyroid hormone—Synthroid) 100 μg per day therapy is started. If after 2 months, this drug therapy fails to improve her condition because the dosage of levothyroxine is not sufficient to create the desired euthyroid state for this patient, then she must repeat the entire care process. She must recognize she needs additional care, and commit the time and resources to seek care. A physician must conduct an examination and collect additional laboratory tests and determine the cause of her poor clinical presentation and abnormal laboratory results. All these additional expenses are incurred because of a drug therapy problem of *dosage too low*. For the lack of a few additional micrograms of levothyroxine, hundreds and thousands of dollars in health care resources had to be consumed. In addition to the expenses, the patient also had to continue to suffer the negative manifestations of a disease that is manageable.

Drug therapies can also influence humanistic outcomes. These are described as patient satisfaction with treatment, addressing concerns, allaying fears, as well as improving quality of life. Addressing these successfully can have a significant impact on future outcomes.

Patient Outcome Versus Practitioner Output

Dictionaries define *outcome* as the final result, or consequence. As applied to pharmaceutical care, outcomes refer to that which is a direct consequence of the collaborative efforts of practitioners and patients. This is particularly important when the physical and psychosocial aspects of the patient's medication experience are examined.

Much has been spoken and written about outcome evaluations and the positive outcomes that will result from various practitioners providing pharmaceutical care. However, much of this discourse is somewhat hollow. In fact, much of what is described as outcomes of drug therapy, or outcomes of providing pharmaceutical care, has little to do with patient outcomes at all. Much of this energy is misdirected toward counting and measuring *outputs* of practitioner activities. These practitioner outputs often include actions such as doses changed, number of prescriptions substituted with a formulary approved generic product, or percentage of time that prescribers agree with the recommendation of the pharmacist. These outputs may or may not have any measurable influence on the health and welfare of the patient. In fact, some of these activities may adversely affect the patient. Outcomes are the result of outputs.

Patient outcomes do not include whether or not the prescriber followed the pharmacist's recommendation to change a dose. Patient outcomes do not include successfully substituting a less expensive drug product for another. It is also important to note that patient outcomes do not include implementing a protocol for a group of patients with a particular disorder, and outcomes do not include counseling patients on how to properly administer medications. Each of these well-meaning and frequently useful interventions may or may not have a positive impact on any given patient. To determine positive and/or negative clinical outcomes, the effectiveness and safety of the patient's drug therapies must be evaluated and documented.

There are no shortcuts to positive patient outcomes. Patient outcomes resulting from drug therapy and associated pharmaceutical care cannot be determined from a distance. Outcomes cannot be measured from the boardroom, they cannot be measured from the hallway, and they cannot be generated by a computer program. If one is truly concerned with the impact that drug therapy and pharmaceutical care have on patients, there is no other method available to determine clinical outcomes than by personally contacting each and every patient at appropriately planned intervals and eliciting information describing the effectiveness and safety of pharmacotherapy. Only through the direct clinical approach can the impact of drug therapies be fully understood.

To fully accept responsibility for patient outcomes associated with drug therapy, the practitioner must be prepared to recognize not only the positive outcomes that can be anticipated, but also the negative. It is important to keep in mind that even the most carefully designed care plans and associated drug therapies cannot be expected to always result in positive outcomes. The performance of an appropriately scheduled, comprehensive, and continuous follow-up evaluation of effectiveness and safety is an essential responsibility within the practice of pharmaceutical care.

Having command of clinical outcomes vocabulary becomes noticeably important when one considers the complexity of patients encountered in practice. Some patients for example, have acute or self-limiting conditions that might be expected to be totally resolved by appropriate drug therapy. Patients with acute bacterial infections represent common examples in which one might establish a realistic goal to *resolve* the infection within a certain timeframe (10–14 days). However, the vast majority of patients suffer from chronic disorders such as hypertension, depression, hyperlipidemia, asthma, and/or arthritis for which patient's goals of therapy do not include the complete resolution, but rather include interim (surrogate) goals such as reducing blood pressure or blood glucose or improving the condition by reducing signs and symptoms, correcting abnormal test results, and/or improving the patient's endurance or ability to ambulate.

EVALUATION FOR NEW DRUG THERAPY PROBLEMS

Another purpose of follow-up evaluations is to identify new medical conditions that require treatment with drug therapy or determine if any new drug therapy problems have developed. This assessment requires the application of the same skills used throughout the assessment step of the pharmaceutical care process. The practitioner must assess the appropriateness of the indication, effectiveness, safety, and compliance of all of the patient's pharmacotherapies using the Pharmacotherapy Workup (refer to Chapter 6).

A negative patient outcome at the follow-up evaluation is considered a new drug therapy problem and must be prioritized as such and resolved as expeditiously as possible. In pharmaceutical care practice, negative patient outcomes are resolved in the same way that other patient-specific drug-related needs are addressed.

> **Example** If your patient's major depressive disorder has not improved after the recommended 12 weeks of antidepressant therapy, then your patient's therapy has not resulted in a positive clinical outcome. If the clinical decision is that the outcome at this point would be considered a failure, then you would describe this new drug therapy problem as "the patient is receiving ineffective drug therapy for depression." You are now responsible to institute whatever interventions are needed in order to improve the patient's medication experience. Despite your best efforts, corrective action is required. You will need to discontinue the failed drug therapy and identify a new pharmacotherapeutic approach to manage this patient's depressive illness.

SCHEDULE FOR CONTINUOUS FOLLOW-UP EVALUATIONS

The last activity of a well-conducted evaluation is to establish the schedule and plan for continuous follow-up evaluations. The therapeutic relationship serves as the basis for providing continuous care and constantly improving the management of the patient's medications. Providing continuous care is an active process and requires a commitment to keep in contact with each patient throughout the entire course of therapy.

DOCUMENTING THE FOLLOW-UP EVALUATION

Documentation of the follow-up evaluation is required. The main objective when documenting your findings from a follow-up evaluation is to establish the association or connections between the patient's indication, pharmacotherapy, and actual outcomes. Figure 9-4 will help to recall the relationship between the three steps of the patient care process.

It is essential that when you conduct a follow-up evaluation, you record the patient outcomes and your clinical evaluation of the patient's status while receiving drug therapy.

The Therapeutic Relationship

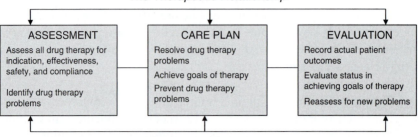

ASSESSMENT	CARE PLAN	EVALUATION
Assess all drug therapy for indication, effectiveness, safety, and compliance Identify drug therapy problems	Resolve drug therapy problems Achieve goals of therapy Prevent drug therapy problems	Record actual patient outcomes Evaluate status in achieving goals of therapy Reassess for new problems

Continuous Follow-up

Figure 9-4   Relationships between assessment, care plans, and follow-up evaluation in the patient care process.

The outcome status is recorded using the standard pharmacotherapy outcome terminology of resolved, stable, improved, partially improved, unimproved, worsened, or failure. These terms represent your clinical judgment. Supporting evidence for your judgment can include improvements in clinical and/or laboratory values. These are balanced or compared to evidence (or lack of evidence) of adverse drug effects documented as undesirable changes in clinical and/or laboratory values caused by drug therapy.

Recommended changes in drug therapy are documented at the follow-up evaluation, and the care plan is modified to reflect the new therapy. Changes in product, dose, interval, duration, and/or instructions need to be clearly and completely understood by your patient. Lastly, you will record the schedule for the next follow-up evaluation.

You should place your signature on the evaluation record. This step, in essence, completes a circle of care, at least up to this time. Furthermore, patients, other practitioners, and payers must be able to link the care provided with a specific practitioner, not just the clinic, pharmacy, hospital, or the health plan. Care represents a people process, so new practitioners should establish the clinical habit of signing all work.

Figure 9-5 is an example of a follow-up evaluation documentation form.

Pharmacotherapy Workup© **NOTES**	**EVALUATION**

Medical Condition: _____

	Outcome Parameter	Pretreatment Baseline (Date)	First Follow-up (Date)	Second Follow-up (Date)
EFFECTIVENESS	Sign/symptom			
	Sign/symptom			
	Lab value			
	Lab value			
SAFETY	Sign/symptoms			
	Signs/symptoms			
	Lab value			
	Lab value			
	Other			
STATUS	STATUS **Initial:** goals being established, initiate new therapy **Resolved:** goals achieved, therapy completed **Stable:** goals achieved, continue same therapy **Improved:** adequate progress being made, continue same therapy **Partial Improvement:** progress being made, adjustments in therapy required **Unimproved:** no progress yet, continue same therapy **Worsened:** decline in health, adjust therapy **Failure:** goals not achieved, discontinue current therapy and replace with different therapy			
	New Drug Therapy Problems Identified		__none at this time __documented	__none at this time __documented

Date	Schedule for next follow-up	Comments

Signature_____ Date_____

Figure 9-5 Follow-up evaluation documentation form (© 2003 The Peters Institute of Pharmaceutical Care).

SUMMARY

The follow-up evaluation supports and maintains a positive therapeutic relationship. It is the only method available to determine patient outcomes. Outcomes are what the patient experiences as a result of specific drug therapies and related drug information, advice, and other pharmaceutical care interventions. Follow-up evaluations are the critical points at which the effectiveness and safety of the patient's care plan and associated drug therapies are determined and balanced against one another, and where decisions concerning further adjustments in drug therapy are made.

There are several important activities and skills required of the pharmaceutical care practitioner in order to conduct an appropriate follow-up evaluation. During the follow-up evaluation, patient outcomes are observed and recorded, progress in meeting goals of therapy is appraised, effectiveness and safety of drug therapies are evaluated, and an assessment is made to determine whether new problems have developed since the last encounter. The connections the practitioner establishes throughout each follow-up evaluation include the patient's medical condition, the medication(s) used to manage that condition, the clinical outcome as at the time of the evaluation, the practitioner's clinical judgment as to the outcome status, and any changes in drug therapies that are necessary to improve the patient's medication experience.

Practitioners must be willing to engage in critical, reflective reviews of all of their clinical decisions. The follow-up evaluation provides an ideal situation in which to grow as a practitioner. Pharmacotherapy is a classic example of a biological system in which one introduces an exogenous chemical influence (drug) into a complex biological system (patient), and the result (outcome) is neither consistent nor predictable. Pharmaceutical care practice requires practitioners and patients to make decisions in areas of uncertainty. In practice, patient outcomes are not always predictable and not always positive. The best practitioner is on a constant quest to improve. This means that each practitioner can learn from every follow-up evaluation by recognizing failures or mistakes and work diligently toward improvement (see Chapter 12 for a discussion of the reflective practitioner).

EXERCISES

9-1 The follow-up evaluation is said to be the most informative of the three steps in the patient care process. Why is this?

9-2 Describe all of the patient's responsibilities at the follow-up evaluation.

9-3 Describe the information you will have to consider during a follow-up evaluation to evaluate the effectiveness of your patient's pharmacotherapy.

9-4 Give at least two reasons why it is essential to determine the actual dosage of medication your patient is taking as part of the follow-up evaluation.

REFERENCES

1. Ernst, F.R., Grizzle, A.J., Drug-related morbidity and mortality: updating the cost-of-illness model. *J Am Pharm Assoc* 2001; 41(2):192–199.
2. Johnson, J., Bootman, JL, Drug-related morbidity and mortality: A cost-of-illness model. *Arch Intern Med* 1995; 155(18):1949–1956.
3. Johnson, J.A., Bootman, J.L., Drug-related morbidity and mortality and the economic impact of pharmaceutical care. *Am J Health Syst Pharm* 1997; 54(5):554–8.
4. Cipolle, R., Strand, L.M., Morley, P.C., *Pharmaceutical Care Practice*. New York: McGraw Hill; 1998.

CHAPTER TEN

ETHICAL CONSIDERATIONS IN PRACTICE

Key Concepts

1. *Pharmaceutical care involves applied ethics in that it consists of the practical application of moral standards to specific ends.*

2. *Pharmaceutical care practitioners should not only be clinically competent, but must also adhere to the law, professional codes of conduct, and ethical standards.*

3. *The pharmaceutical care practitioner must learn to recognize when his/her personal values (political views, religious beliefs, or social expectations) interfere with professional responsibilities and mandated behaviors.*

4 *As a general rule, clinical problems should be identified and resolved first, followed by legal issues, and if an ethical dilemma remains it can then be resolved systematically and comprehensively.*

5 *The process for resolving ethical issues in practice is to (a) recognize when a patient encounter raises an important ethical problem, and gather the relevant facts involved; (b) work with the patient to describe the problem that has to be resolved; (c) determine what each of you consider to be an acceptable resolution to the case; (d) generate reasonable alternatives to resolve the ethical dilemma, and consider each option in relation to the fundamental ethical principles and the patient's position; (e) select the resolution that you and the patient will implement; (f) critically examine the decision that has been made, and justify it; (g) do the right thing—implement it.*

INTRODUCTION

Ethics is the study of the rightness or wrongness of human conduct. In any situation involving two or more individuals, values may come into conflict and ethical issues may develop. This is especially true in the case of health care where pain and suffering are involved, and limited resources exist. Patient care involves applied ethics in that it consists of the practical application of moral standards to specific ends. In the case of pharmaceutical care, one of these ends is to benefit patients through the appropriate utilization of pharmaceuticals, using the essential knowledge that should always accompany such clinical intervention. The practitioner should not only be clinically competent, but should also adhere to the law, professionally determined codes of conduct, and ethical standards.

Pharmaceutical care is dependent upon human interactions. These interactions include patients, family members, pharmaceutical care practitioners, other clinicians, support personnel, managers, and administrators. These individuals are likely to have different values, beliefs, and preferences. Whenever two people with different value systems interact, there is the potential for an ethical problem to develop. Because ethical problems are common in practice it is important that practitioners know how to identify and resolve them when they arise.

Identifying and addressing ethical problems would be easier if they were not so often confused with clinical and legal issues. These three issues—clinical, legal, and ethical—can be so closely associated that they appear to be the same problem. It will be helpful if the three issues can be separated, when possible, because a successful resolution to each issue is arrived at slightly differently. Each situation requires different knowledge for its recognition and a somewhat different process for its resolution.

Although each patient situation is unique, as a general rule, *clinical* problems should be identified and resolved first, followed by *legal* issues, and if an *ethical* problem remains, it can then be resolved effectively. Thinking in this order will make the identification and resolution of the ethical problem more manageable. The first nine chapters of this book focused on clinical issues; let us now discuss issues of the law and ethics.

ISSUES OF THE LAW

Pharmacy law consists of rules, regulations, and actions that are promulgated by governments and are binding on its constituents. Law and ethics, while in most cases clearly demarcated, often overlap and sometimes appear contradictory.[1]

> **Example** Should a pharmacist, based on her clinical judgment at the time of an emergency, provide a patient with a life-saving drug not authorized by a physician's prescription, when technically she is breaking the law, but is arguably acting ethically?

Legal issues often have explicit statutes that provide a solution. In pharmacy, there are many laws that govern what practitioners may and may not do with prescription drug products. Here again, professional standards require practitioners to both know and follow the law. In those relatively few situations where the law is not clear regarding what can and cannot be done, practitioners should always follow the professional and ethical mandate to do no harm and when it is possible, to do good for the patient.

> **Example** Is it ethical to knowingly dose a patient with an amount of drug that is so small it has little or no chance of successfully treating the medical problem? If the pharmacist's clinical judgment is that the patient's drug therapy problem is that the dosage is too low, then it is legally necessary to obtain the consent of the prescriber in order to increase the dose.

Being an active *moral agent* can conflict with the law and often does. It should go without saying that practitioners have a duty to know the law and act accordingly. The law prescribes codes of conduct that are usually reasonable, clear, and direct. Thus, we divide actions into two classes: *legal* and *illegal*. Ethical analysis requires critical examination of actions and their consequences and are not so easily differentiated as appropriate and inappropriate.[1]

PROFESSIONAL CODES OF CONDUCT

The standards for professional behavior (described in Chapter 3) as well as the code of ethics for a profession provide even more guidance for the practitioner. However, no code of ethics can contain all the necessary detail to address all issues that arise on a daily basis. Rather, it is to be seen as a somewhat sweeping statement on the overall ethical mandate of a profession. In this sense, it makes a public statement concerning a collective commitment to certain values, principles, and duties.

A code of ethics is a public pledge to meet certain responsibilities and perform duties for those who do not share the knowledge, expertise, or professional mandate. It is also a public pledge to adhere to the standards and ideals of conduct and to enforce them through mechanisms that will punish those who violate the essentials of the pledge.

CODE OF ETHICS FOR PHARMACISTS*

Preamble Pharmacists are health professionals who assist individuals in making the best use of medications. This Code, prepared and supported by pharmacists, is intended to state publicly the principles that form the fundamental basis of the roles and responsibilities of pharmacists. These principles, based on moral obligations and virtues, are established to guide pharmacists in relationships with patients, health professionals, and society.

   I. *A pharmacist respects the covenantal relationship between the patient and pharmacist* Considering the patient-pharmacist relationship as a covenant means that a pharmacist has moral obligations in response to the gift of trust received from society. In return for this gift, a pharmacist promises to help individuals achieve optimum benefit from their medications, to be committed to their welfare, and to maintain their trust.

   II. *A pharmacist promotes the good of every patient in a caring, compassionate, and confidential manner* A pharmacist places concern for the well being of the patient at the center of professional practice. In doing so, a pharmacist considers needs stated by the patient as well as those defined by health science. A pharmacist is dedicated to protecting the

* Adopted by the membership of the American Pharmacists Association October 27, 1994.

dignity of the patient. With a caring attitude and a compassionate spirit, a pharmacist focuses on serving the patient in a private and confidential manner.

III. *A pharmacist respects the autonomy and dignity of each patient* A pharmacist promotes the right of self-determination and recognizes individual self-worth by encouraging patients to participate in decisions about their health. A pharmacist communicates with patients in terms that are understandable. In all cases, a pharmacist respects personal and cultural differences among patients.

IV. *A pharmacist acts with honesty and integrity in professional relationships* A pharmacist has a duty to tell the truth and to act with conviction of conscience. A pharmacist avoids discriminatory practices, behavior or work conditions that impair professional judgment, and actions that compromise dedication to the best interests of patients.

V. *A pharmacist maintains professional competence* A pharmacist has a duty to maintain knowledge and abilities as new medications, devices, and technologies become available and as health information advances.

VI. *A pharmacist respects the values and abilities of colleagues and other health professionals* When appropriate, a pharmacist asks for the consultation of colleagues or other health professionals or refers the patient. A pharmacist acknowledges that colleagues and other health professionals may differ in the beliefs and values they apply to the care of the patient.

VII. *A pharmacist serves individual, community, and societal needs* The primary obligation of a pharmacist is to individual patients. However, the obligations of a pharmacist may at times extend beyond the individual to the community and society. In these situations, the pharmacist recognizes the responsibilities that accompany these obligations and acts accordingly.

VIII. *A pharmacist seeks justice in the distribution of health resources* When health resources are allocated, a pharmacist is fair and equitable, balancing the needs of patients and society.

Practitioners must understand the serious nature of a professional standard. To do otherwise can bring about acts or utterances that, while perhaps not illegal, can profoundly impact the life of an errant clinician and prove harmful to the patient. Conduct that contravenes the content of the code can have consequences that are equal to, or greater than, some legally binding expectations of performance. Therefore, it is important to study the standards for professional behavior and the standards of care (refer to the Appendix) with the intent to apply them in the case of each patient and prevent as many ethical problems from occurring as possible.

COMMON ETHICAL CONSIDERATIONS IN PHARMACEUTICAL CARE PRACTICE

Now the focus turns to actual ethical problems that are routinely experienced in the practice of pharmaceutical care. Experience with over 20,000 patients was reviewed, and a number of situations were identified that occurred commonly enough to warrant comment here.

The most common situations that involved ethical issues could be grouped into two different types: (1) those which consist of privacy and confidentiality, conflict of interest, respect for patient autonomy, duty to warn, and value conflicts and which occur daily during the patient/practitioner interaction and (2) those which involve the allocation of resources, rationing, justice, and competency, are more episodic and patient-specific, and occur in the institutional context. Competency refers not only to the practitioner's grasp of pharmaceutical knowledge, but also adherence to standards and to their protection. The phrase *clinically competent* should refer to a practitioner who is pharmaceutically, legally, culturally, and ethically informed and has a commitment to draw upon appropriate available knowledge bases when meeting a patient's needs and resolving problems (Table 10-1).

Patient Confidentiality and Privacy Issues

Pharmaceutical care practitioners deal with patient-specific information that is personal and sensitive, therefore patient confidentiality and privacy must be maintained at all times. This includes all written documents and records, as well as all verbal discussions, which must be held in the strictest of confidence. Patients trust practitioners not to disclose any personal information

Table 10-1 Common ethical dilemmas in pharmaceutical care practice

Patient-practitioner interaction	Institutional context
Patient confidentiality and privacy issues	Allocation of resources and rationing
Conflicts of interest	Personal competency, colleague
Respect for patient autonomy	competency
Duty to warn	Protection of standards
Patient/practitioner conflicts in values	

about them to any person who is not directly involved in their care. This includes the prohibition of practitioners from discussing individual patient cases with friends, family members, or any other clinicians or lay individual without the express permission of the patient.

> **Example** It would be considered unethical to discuss or disclose personal health-related information about your patient with one of your friends or family members who is not a health care provider and who is not involved in the care of that patient.

Conflicts of Interest

Practitioners are expected to always try to *do good* for patients. The patient is the focus of the practitioner's actions. Doing good for the patient may or may not benefit the practitioner. Beneficence on the part of a health care practitioner means that all the work, decisions, and actions taken are intended to benefit someone else. Keeping the patient's best interest in mind sometimes requires that a practitioner set his/her own interest aside. Conflicts of interest are not acceptable in patient care environments.

> **Definition** Conflict of interest (for an individual): An individual has a conflict of interest when a personal, financial, or political interest exists that undermines his or her ability to meet or fulfill primary professional, ethical, or legal obligations.[2]

Conflicts of interest can best be identified and dealt with when specific practitioner's roles and relationships—and their ethical underpinnings— are clearly defined, understood, and universally accepted. Within the context of pharmaceutical care, we have argued that the practitioner's primary obligation is to patients and their well being. Meeting patient's needs comes first, and their best interests are to be sought, upheld, and protected at all times.

> **Example** There is a potential for a conflict of interest if the practitioner is in a position to personally benefit from the selection and use of a particular drug product unless that product is unique and no acceptable alternatives exist. In either case, the practitioner needs to disclose his/her personal interest in that product to the patient.

Self-interest and the interests of employers or institutions, should not be placed before those of the suffering. Practitioners must critically examine all patient care decisions to expose any conflict of interest issues that may harm the patient. Personal bias and financial or political interests that affect judgment, reasoning, motivation, or behavior should be suppressed by practitioners who *put the patient first.*[2]

Patient Autonomy

Patients expect practitioners to respect their autonomy. Practitioners must avoid being coercive. All of the information about drug therapies that practitioners share with patients must be accurate and true. Practitioners often need to be persuasive when helping patients decide, but patients must be allowed to make and participate in their own decisions. Patient autonomy is best maintained by negotiating a mutually acceptable care plan.

> **Example**   It would be considered a breech of your patient's autonomy to provide misleading drug information or withhold information in order to *convince* your patient to use the pharmacotherapy you are recommending. Practitioners need to assist and allow patients to be the final decision maker when it comes to their own health.

Practitioners can find themselves feeling strongly that a patient *needs* some specific form of pharmacotherapy. Health care practitioners often disguise paternalism as behaving in the best interest of the patient. It is difficult to act on someone's behalf if he/she does not want you to do so. However, some would ague that when patients are ill they lose some of their autonomy, and by treating them (acting in their best interest) you have helped them regain some autonomy. In patients who are critically ill, it is often the responsibility of the practitioner to make decisions that are deemed to be in the best interest of the patient.

Duty to Warn

Drugs can save lives, improve health, and prevent illness. However, they can also cause harm. Some of the harm caused by drug therapies is unpredictable, but many of the harmful effects of medications can be expected and are therefore predictable. Practitioners who treat patients with medications have a duty to warn patients of the known risks associated with drug therapies. Pharmaceutical care practitioners are the most knowledgeable clinicians in areas such as pharmacology, toxicology, and pharmacotherapeutics. Patients have the right to expect the pharmaceutical care practitioner to provide appropriate warnings of any harmful actions that the drug regimens may cause. Joined with the duty to warn is the obligation to follow-up to determine if patients experienced harmful effects from drug therapy.

> **Example** It would be considered a failure of your duty to warn not to inform your patient of the potential harmful effects that drinking alcohol can have while taking a course of metronidazole to treat an infection.

Conflicts in Value Systems

Patients and practitioners often come from different backgrounds, religions, educational systems, and cultures. The practitioner must examine his/her own value system. It is important to understand that each patient can have a different set of values and that in some cases, the patient's way of acting or deciding will be very different from the practitioner's. These conflicts in values should be managed on a daily, and sometimes moment-to-moment, basis. Understanding the patient's perspective can be enlightening and empowering in deciding how to manage potential ethical dilemmas. It is your professional responsibility not to put yourself in practice situations where you can anticipate that your personal value system will conflict with your practice obligations.

> **Example** Practitioners who hold personal beliefs that all forms of contraception are wrong have the obligation to see that patients requiring contraceptive pharmacotherapy have access to those products and associated drug information.

Allocation of Resources

How decisions are made to allocate resources can generate ethical dilemmas. Resource allocation impacts many patients. Allocation of resources most often involves financial considerations. These decisions are made on a population basis by health care planners and managers. These guidelines are carried out on a patient-by-patient basis by practitioners. It is the responsibility of individual practitioners to advocate on the patient's behalf to secure the resources necessary to provide the appropriate level of care. Resource-based dilemmas can often place the practitioner at odds with health care managers, administrators, or payers. It is the practitioner's duty to argue and support the clinical merits of the case.

> **Example** Practitioners can find themselves in an ethical dilemma if management requires that they provide care for too many patients without adequate resources.

Competency

Health care practitioners practice within a community of other clinicians; therefore it is incumbent upon each practitioner to make certain that his/her colleagues are competent in their own practices. Health care practitioners review and evaluate one another. Allowing a practitioner who is not competent to provide care to patients can create a serious ethical dilemma. Similarly, each practitioner has the duty to maintain his/her own competency in the knowledge and skills necessary to provide appropriate safe care. In order to be considered competent, a practitioner must recognize the limits of his or her knowledge and inform patients and colleagues.

> **Example**   If a practitioner does not maintain an acceptable level of knowledge about the safety and efficacy of the drug products he/she recommends to patients, it would be considered a case of clinical and ethical incompetency.

IDENTIFYING ETHICAL PROBLEMS

Identifying an ethical problem is not always an easy task. Identifying *right* and *wrong* for oneself is perhaps easier than performing the same evaluation for someone else. At least we like to think that we know right from wrong, and we frequently appeal to faith-based reason, or claims of conscience, in order to arrive at the particulars of both our judgment and its justification.

In a clinical context, where patient-centeredness, patient choice, and autonomy are highly valued and rigorously guarded, identifying ethical issues is, in essence, a central part of communication. Through discussion the practitioner can gather information from the patient thereby establishing some measure of specificity concerning the patient's desires, values, expectations, beliefs, and needs (patient's medication experience). Thus, within the context of communication—the social matrix of pharmaceutical care—we find the beginnings of ethical analysis. Problem identification, at clinical, legal, and ethical levels of involvement, is where we begin to explore the possibility of ethical issues that will influence decisions and recommendations.

Elsewhere we have noted the importance of practitioners engaging in both the introspective and interactive dimensions of values clarification (see Chapters 3 and 12). Knowing oneself well cannot be underestimated as it relates to knowing others and understanding values conflict. As we move from "self" to "other", we must be aware of our cultural and ethical *baggage* so as not to presume that our baggage is the same as our patients' or colleagues'. Interventions based on such an unexplored life frequently have a deleterious affect on those we strive to help no matter how well-intentioned our motives.

Assuming that all practitioners, both neophyte and experienced, will over time increase their levels of self-awareness—something that only they can do—their next step is to improve their understanding of the patient. Familiarity with social, economic, political, cultural, and ethical dimensions of life can be developed. To put it another way, such understanding must be developed if competency, as referred to earlier, is to be maximized and applied.

Socio-cultural understanding, along with that of ethical understanding and clinical knowledge, are to be seen as prerequisites to the provision of patient care. Patients exist in a socio-cultural context with all its complexities and nuances. This is where patients' ethical and cultural baggage emerges, this is where they live and die. Attention to such dimensions of illness, patient experience, and personal biography, results in more integrated patient-specific caring practices and shows appropriate respect for persons in context, rather than as abstract organ systems or disease states. The lived experiences of the patient consist of a complex web of affiliations, memories, and stories, all of which are defining characteristics of personhood. Moreover, these personal characteristics shape attitudes, expectations, hopes, and fears. To know the patient is the first step to achieving any success at authentic caring. This discussion helps to emphasize the importance of taking the time to understand each patient's medication experience.

Following is a number of guidelines that take the form of questions which should routinely be asked whenever differences between the practitioner and patient occur and must be resolved. These inquiries include the following:

1. Is this a situation in which I am allowing my personal values (political views, religious beliefs, social norms) to interfere with my professional responsibilities?
2. Is this a situation that involves a clinical problem and therefore requires me to use my expertise and clinical judgment?
3. Is this a situation that involves a legal decision and therefore following the law is the solution?
4. Finally, is this an ethical problem that requires a systematic problem-solving process to address it successfully (see the Workup of an Ethical Problem described below)?

Ethical problems emerge within the context of two or more individuals acting autonomously, but with shared goals and objectives. In this sense, the practitioner requires some direction. Establishing an instructional method for the systematic analysis of ethical concerns is a highly useful objective. Such needs can be met through a procedure that may be termed an *ethics work-up.*[2]

WORKUP OF AN ETHICAL PROBLEM

Just as practitioners have a structure to identify, resolve, and prevent drug therapy problems, they also have a useful method to address ethical problems encountered in patient care. The following can be used to guide practitioners through the careful thought process involved in identifying, resolving, and preventing common ethical problems. It is adapted from the work of Philip Hebert described in his book *Doing Right.*[3]

First, and foremost, the Work-up of an Ethical Problem is an attempt to formalize the decision-making process. This permits the practitioner to structure dialogue and analysis in a framework that provides greater clarity of issues. It also serves to critically examine issues relevant to the understanding of shared, yet different, principles and positions. Central to this enterprise are the patient's perspectives and needs. Essentially, the Work-up of an Ethical Problem is a practical framework used to *map* the most important elements that emerge during the practitioner's deliberations and guide action in therapeutic interventions.[3] However, the practitioner should be aware that the decision-making procedure presented here is not to be seen as a "moral algorithm" that will "churn out right answers."[3] Remember, ethical decision-making is not an exact science; all too often decisions are made in less than ideal circumstances with less certainty than anything destined to produce complete peace of mind for all concerned. Hebert is correct in his conclusion that:

> Unfortunately, we have to make do with such decisions. While we may arrive at solutions for a case, our feelings and uncertainties may remain unresolved. In hard cases ethical principles may not determine the right outcome, but they do provide assurance that we have done the best we could, especially if applied in a trustworthy way.[3]

Hebert has produced a very useful Workup of an Ethical Problem that provides a framework for decision-making.[3] His procedure consists of seven steps. While every case may not require practitioners to work through the entire procedure, it is useful to address each step "when one wishes to ensure that one's decision is backed up by careful reflection."[3] For a discussion of the fundamental ethical principles involved in the Workup of an Ethical Problem, refer to Chapter 3.

WORKUP OF AN ETHICAL PROBLEM*

1. *Recognize when a patient encounter raises an important ethical problem, and gather the relevant facts* (What are the clinical facts? What are the legal facts? What are the ethical facts?)

2. *Work with the patient to describe the problem that has to be resolved* (What is the ethical dilemma? What ethical principles are involved?)

3. *Determine what each of you (practitioner and patient) consider to be an acceptable resolution to the problem*

4. *Generate reasonable alternatives to resolve the ethical problem, and consider each option in relation to the fundamental ethical principles and the patient's preferences* (What are the possible strategies to address the problem? What are the practical possibilities?)

Autonomy:	What does the patient want?
Paternalism:	How am I affecting the patient?
Beneficence:	What good can be done for the patient?
Nonmaleficence:	Is harm to the patient being avoided?
Justice:	Is the patient receiving what is fair?
Veracity:	Is the patient being told the truth?
Confidentiality:	Is the patient's privacy being protected?

5. *Select the resolution that you and the patient will implement* (What should be done? What is the final decision that you plan to implement?)

6. *Critically examine the decision that has been made, and justify it* (What makes this the best choice? What would make you change your mind?)

7. *Do the right thing—implement it* (How am I going to accomplish this? What is the best strategy to implement the solution? How will I know if my actions were appropriate or not? Follow-up with the patient.)

Step 1: Recognize when a patient encounter raises an important ethical problem, and gather the relevant facts In this step, the practitioner recognizes value conflicts and can identify an ethical problem. The practitioner should be committed to increasing his/her ethical consciousness through reflection, reading, discussion, and any other means. Gather as much information as possible, examine it, and discuss it with the patient. Always remember that the patient's perspectives and preferences are of paramount importance. In essence, the practitioner begins any encounter prepared to ask questions concerning the possibility and/or probability of ethical problems.

This is not a retrospective exercise in which one acts and then examines the action taken for any ethical issues. Inform the patient that ethical issues are a significant part of any therapeutic intervention. Involving the patient at the outset is more useful than bringing an ethical problem

---

* Adapted from Hebert.[3]

back to this individual for a somewhat belated *ethics autopsy*. For lack of a better expression *ethics surprises* tend to alienate patients and rarely play a positive role in determining therapeutic outcomes. At all times, work with the patient, overtly address ethical issues, and make their discussion an integral part of problem identification and resolution.

Step 2: Work with the patient to describe the problem that has to be resolved   The second step requires that the central problem be stated. Once stated the problem can be discussed and the essentials that require resolution pursued. Are the practitioner and the patient *on the same page*? Clarification is fundamental!

Step 3: Determine what each of you (practitioner and patient) consider to be an acceptable resolution to the problem   In this step the practitioner asks, "What would a solution look like?" Solutions may be simple, or they could be complex. What does the practitioner think is reasonable? The patient? Do both agree? What desired outcome can be agreed upon by both parties? Are the views expressed divergent? What is reasonable? What is considered unreasonable or unacceptable? Are there any irreconcilable differences?

Step 4: Generate reasonable alternatives to resolve the ethical problem, and consider each option in relation to the fundamental ethical principles and the patient's preferences   The practitioner focuses on possible options as they relate to autonomy, beneficence, and justice. Hebert considers this step to be difficult. While the patient's preferences "come first, it is important to keep in mind that preferences will depend on such things as the availability of resources, or access to options that are viable."[3] Of course if the patient's preferences are illegal, or may harm others, the practitioner can reject them. Also, should the patient prefer a course of action that is burdensome to others, then the practitioner has a responsibility to draw attention to this and ask if this is the right thing to do. It should be emphasized that when deciding upon an appropriate course of action among options, discussion is essential. The "unstated", silent or silenced voice, creates problems, and rarely if ever solves them. Communication skills are of primary importance and should be seen as central to both the ethical and clinical decision-making procedure.

Step 5: Select the resolution that you and the patient will implement   This is the moment when the practitioner decides on a resolution to the specific problem. Here, a decision must be made, and the practitioner should conclude that this is a justifiable resolution and the best of all possible options. When any disagreement arises as a consequence of this decision the practitioner should be in a position to articulate why this is the best course of action and why he or she finds the alternatives unacceptable.

Step 6: Critically examine the decision that has been made, and justify it This step requires the practitioner to critically reflect on the course of action that is recommended. Hebert asserts the importance of making a decision that "you can live with." Do you feel comfortable with the decision? Additionally, "will you be able to sleep soundly given your decision?"[3] The role of emotions in decision-making is important.

Hebert asserts the following:

> Do not be pushed by abstract ethical principles to do something that your conscience or emotions tell you is wrong.... Emotions can be a helpful corrective to reason.[4] Until you get a better feel for ethics, it would be unwise to do something that you instinctively feel is wrong.

The issue of conscience surfaces on many occasions most notably on issues that are highly controversial or emotionally charged, and when it is seemingly impossible to arrive at any position of consensus. Matters of religious conviction such as contraception/abortion, euthanasia, and stem cell research, come to mind as good examples of beliefs and actions (or non-actions) that give rise to a considerably emotionally charged debate as well as personal angst. Societies do not function in a state of equilibrium; rather they exhibit considerable evidence that conflicts of religious, ideological, political, and moral nature do exist and are frequently dysfunctional in that they often render individuals paralyzed with indecision. This is a more realistic expectation of daily life than the utopian notion that reasonable individuals can always arrive at harmony. Decisions are made in a dynamic socio-cultural context, and they involve more than individual choices isolated in time and space/place from prevailing tensions between people and institutions and all their normative rules and expectations. Always consider context and social tensions as these relate to individual choices. To do otherwise limits our understanding of the patient as a social being with values, preferences, needs, and expectations.

Step 7: Do the right thing—implement it The seventh and final step in the process urges the practitioner to do *the right thing*. Of course, arriving at the right thing is a collaborative exercise. Given the general tenets of pharmaceutical care practice, such a partnership is essential to work toward determining what is right and appropriate, ethically and clinically, for the patient.

Throughout this procedure it is clearly the case that the practitioner is constantly engaging in critical reflection on all dimensions and details of the questions asked and the answers received. Critical thinking, along with meaningful discussion, and a willingness to modify or change positions is a vital part of this important work-up.

Listening—hearing the patient, is to be seen as an indispensable part of the Pharmacotherapy Workup and the Workup of an Ethical Problem. Well-defined, clearly stated, ethical decisions are an integral part of any therapeutic relationship. This is as much to do with building trust as it is with professional responsibilities. Indeed, trust is largely based on ethical commitment to a purpose shared by all those concerned. Keeping this in mind at all times helps clinicians to do *the right thing*.

SUMMARY

In sum, ethics is inescapable! With this in mind, the pharmaceutical care practitioner must be cognizant of ethical considerations at all times and make every attempt to incorporate the principles of ethical behavior into all clinical decisions and judgments. To do otherwise is wrong for the patient and becomes problematic for the practitioner. Unethical conduct is rarely ignored, and never excused.

EXERCISES

10-1 Use the Workup of an Ethical Problem to work through the following scenario:

Mr. Z., age 63, has had two heart attacks in the past. He now has a prescription for a medication to prevent recurrences of heart attacks that must be taken regularly to be effective. He tells you that he does not think he will bother to take the new medication because he does not believe another heart attack will harm him. How would you approach his care?

10-2 Select a colleague with work experience. Between the two of you, identify a real-life situation involving an ethical problem. Apply the Workup of an Ethical Problem to work through the dilemma.

10-3 Select a colleague with practice experience. Describe one example of an ethical dilemma that contains each of the following common ethical considerations in practice:

   (a) Patient confidentiality

   (b) Conflicts of interest

   (c) Patient autonomy

   (d) Duty to warn

   (e) Conflicts in value systems

   (f) Allocation of resources

   (g) Competency

10-4 Each practitioner must create a set of guidelines that he/she will use to identify when an ethical dilemma is occurring. Describe your guidelines, and explain why each one is on your list.

REFERENCES

1. Fremgen, B.F. *Medical Law and Ethics*. Upper Saddle River, New Jersey: Prentice-Hall; 2002, p. 4.
2. Shamoo, A.E., Resnik, D.B. *Responsible Conduct of Research*. New York: Oxford University Press; 2003.
3. Hebert, P.C. *Doing Right: A Practical Guide to Ethics for Medical Trainees and Physicians*. Toronto: Oxford University Press; 1996, Chapter 1.
4. Callahan, S. The role of emotion in ethical design in Hastings Center Report, 1988, vol. 18, pp. 9–14, in: Hebert, P.C., *Doing Right*. Toronto: Oxford University Press; 1996.

ELEVEN

ACQUIRING THE KNOWLEDGE
YOU NEED TO PRACTICE

Key Concepts

1. *The expertise of the pharmaceutical care practitioner is focused in the disciplines of pharmacology, pharmacotherapy, and pharmaceutical care practice.*

2. *The knowledge you will need to provide pharmaceutical care can be categorized into three types: knowledge about the patient, knowledge about diseases, and knowledge about drug therapies.*

3. *The scope of knowledge about patients can be grouped into personal, social, and physiological information.*

4. *The scope of knowledge about diseases can be grouped into characteristics of the disease, intent of treatment, and goals of therapy.*

5. *The scope of knowledge about drug therapies can be grouped into characteristics of the drug, actions of the drug in the patient, and the outcomes of drug therapy.*

6 *The knowledge you need can most effectively and efficiently be learned within the structure of the Pharmacotherapy Workup and then applied in the patient care process.*

7 *The most useful approach to learning this knowledge is to begin with those patient characteristics, diseases, and drug therapies that are most commonly seen in practice.*

BECOMING FAMILIAR WITH WHAT YOU NEED TO KNOW

The contribution of a pharmaceutical care practitioner is measured by his/her ability to apply a unique body of knowledge to resolving drug therapy problems for patients. This unique knowledge focuses on pharmacology and pharmacotherapy and is applied in pharmaceutical care practice to resolve drug therapy problems and improve the medication experience.

However, the mere accumulation of knowledge is not sufficient; the key is applying this knowledge in order to help patients. Caring for patients and resolving drug therapy problems requires that you integrate patient, disease, and drug knowledge and then apply it to the specific patient. There are often other practitioners such as physicians or nurses, who will know more than you do about patients and diseases, but no other patient care provider will know more about drug therapy. Therefore, "learn your pharmacology; learn your pharmacology; learn your pharmacology."

Learning all that is required may seem like an enormous task, but there are three basic concepts that can get you started:

1. The knowledge you must learn, integrate, and use in practice can be classified into three broad categories: knowledge about *patients*, knowledge about *diseases*, and knowledge about *drugs*. All three categories of knowledge are equally important, however your unique expertise will lie in drug therapies. Because you will be using this knowledge to make patient-specific decisions, you will always think about and apply it in a specific order: understand the patient; understand the patient's disease, illness, or medical condition; and understand the drug therapy used to treat the medical condition.
2. Although it will be necessary to gain knowledge in a number of different sciences, the foundation of your knowledge will be how drugs work (pharmacology), how drugs are used to treat and prevent diseases

(pharmacotherapy), and how we apply this knowledge to help patients (pharmaceutical care practice).

3. It will be prudent to begin your learning with those patients, diseases, and drug therapies that are most commonly encountered in practice.[1] Do not try to learn everything immediately; start with the drug therapy problems that patients experience most frequently. Data from over 20,000 patients are now available, and a learning agenda can be created based on the medical conditions and drug therapies most frequently encountered in practice (these will be presented throughout this chapter). Build your expertise based upon what your patients need to know, and learn from your patients.

These three general concepts can serve as a place to begin the process of learning what is required to become a practitioner. The most efficient way to learn this knowledge is to understand how it is applied in practice. Therefore, the practice of pharmaceutical care generally—and the Pharmacotherapy Workup specifically—is the framework in which to learn the patient, disease, and drug knowledge you will need to practice. An organizing theme used throughout this book is that the more comprehensively you understand pharmaceutical care practice, the easier it will be to learn all of the new information needed about patients, diseases, and drugs to become a successful practitioner. The practice process will provide you with the appropriate questions to ask, and the challenge is to have or find the appropriate answers.

As you might imagine, becoming a competent practitioner is quite an extensive process, however, it is not a difficult one. You can become qualified through your formal educational process within pharmacy and experiential training in practice. At this time, the formal educational process is only beginning to teach the practice of pharmaceutical care in a way that can be helpful. There are still few experiential training sites that provide and teach pharmaceutical care. Therefore, the more active role you play in your learning process, the more quickly and extensively you will learn.

Your success will depend on your ability to take control of your learning agenda, your commitment to learning the pharmaceutical care process, and your dedication to provide pharmaceutical care.

UNDERSTANDING THE IMPORTANT RELATIONSHIPS: PATIENT-DISEASE-DRUG THERAPY

Schools and colleges of pharmacy have continuously expanded the amount of knowledge pharmacy students require for graduation. However, acquiring knowledge is only a portion of what is necessary to practice pharmaceutical care. First, you must determine that you are acquiring the appropriate knowledge, and second, you must do this in a manner that allows you to apply it for the specific purpose of identifying, resolving, and preventing drug therapy problems.

Traditionally, patient, disease, and drug information have been taught as though they can be learned in isolation. Pharmacology is often taught as drug actions on cells or organ systems. Disease knowledge is often presented as though there is a single, predictable course for every patient. Similarly, patient characteristics are studied as though they are static and independent of disease and drug. In clinical practice, it quickly becomes evident that for a specific patient, the status of his/her medical condition and the impact of drug therapy all influence how the patient will respond to drug therapy decisions, advice, and instructions. Therefore, the integration of patient, disease, and drug therapy knowledge must occur from the beginning of the learning process and then continue throughout your career.

KNOWLEDGE YOU NEED ABOUT THE PATIENT

The patient is central to pharmaceutical care practice. You must know your patient. You must discover your patient's wants, needs, and concerns and understand how he/she will respond to your advice.

Table 11-1 describes the patient information required to understand patients in general and each patient individually.[2] This table also describes the environmental factors that can influence your patient's drug-related needs including living conditions, employment, and cultural background. Finally, the physiological information required for pharmaceutical care includes a patient's signs and symptoms, allergies, and risk factors for illness, toxicity, or treatment failures. This table will be helpful to you on two different levels. First, it describes the scope and organization of information about a specific patient that you will need to care for him/her (refer to the assessment step of the patient care process described in Chapter 6). Second, it describes how to organize the knowledge you learn about patients, as you acquire it. For example, content from a medical sociology course and content from a laboratory medicine course all *fits* into this organizational framework. You should use this table as a map of knowledge you will need about patients to practice pharmaceutical care.

This organizational framework is presented for the purpose of visualizing the scope of knowledge necessary to become an effective pharmaceutical care practitioner. Understanding the scope and finding a *place* for

Table 11-1   Patient information needed for practice

	Dimensions		
Timeframe	Personal	Environmental	Physiological

Present	Health concerns
	Expectations of
	  treatment outcomes
	Understanding of
	  disease and drug
	  therapies
		Living situation
		Who lives with the
		  patient
		Who cares for the
		  patient
			Indications for
			  drug therapy
			Diagnosis,
			  conditions
			Signs and
			  symptoms
			Medications

History of
present
condition
	Change in mood
	  or behavior
	Change in habits
	Change in mental
	  outlook
		Change in living
		  situation
		Change in physical
		  environment
			Change in signs
			  and symptoms
			Change in
			  physical
			  condition
			Change in
			  medications

Background	Personality traits
	Coping mechanisms
		Socioeconomic
		  status
		Cultural influences
		Job/employment
		Insurance
		  benefits
		Personal
		  relationships
			Risk factors
			Allergies/alerts
			Family history
			Hereditary
			  factors
			Cultural traits

newly acquired knowledge will facilitate its recollection in practice when it is needed.

KNOWLEDGE YOU NEED ABOUT THE PATIENT'S MEDICAL CONDITIONS

The practitioner must also have a standard set of knowledge related to commonly encountered diseases in order to provide pharmaceutical care. In pharmaceutical care practice, one of the first decisions the practitioner must make is whether the indication for the drug is clinically appropriate. You must know the primary indication for each drug your patient is taking, and your patient should understand this as well.

The indication and its presentation (clinical signs and symptoms) also serve as parameters that are used to establish goals of therapy. That is, reducing or eliminating the presenting signs and symptoms often becomes the goal of therapy. The status of these signs and symptoms will be evaluated at follow-up and thus serve to determine the effectiveness of the drug therapy. The indication dictates the goals of therapy, and achieving the goals of therapy determines the outcomes of drug therapy.

The association between the presenting signs and symptoms (documented in the assessment), the goals of therapy (agreed upon and documented in the care plan), and the patient outcomes (documented at each follow-up evaluation) serves as the core set of data used by the pharmaceutical care practitioner to make clinical decisions at every encounter.

An organizational structure illustrating the scope of knowledge regarding medical conditions used by pharmaceutical care practitioners is shown in Fig. 11-1. The structure illustrates how you will apply knowledge about the patient's diseases in practice.

Table 11-2 displays the knowledge you will need about each medical condition you encounter. It should be emphasized that you do not need to know all the information described in this table for all medical conditions, but learn to use this table to help find the necessary information when you encounter a medical condition with which you are unfamiliar.

It is almost overwhelming to think that you will need to understand all of this information about all the diseases experienced by patients in practice. Therefore, it will be helpful to approach this challenge with a manageable goal. The most logical method is to begin with common medical problems, and learn them one at a time. This is achievable because pharmaceutical care has been provided to enough patients so the most common medical problems are well known and represent a relatively manageable number of medical conditions.

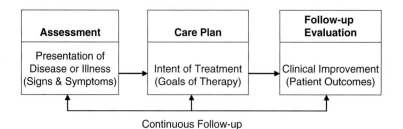

Figure 11-1   Application of knowledge regarding medical conditions.

Table 11-2   Disease information for pharmaceutical care practice

	Dimensions

Characteristics of the disease	Definition of the disease:
	    Presentation of the disease
	    Structural abnormalities—disturbances of the normal
	      anatomic and/or biochemical conformation of the body
	    Functional abnormalities— disturbances in the normal
	      performances and actions of cells, tissues, and/or organs
	    Results including clinical presentation, signs, symptoms, and
	      laboratory abnormalities
	Epidemiology:
	    Frequency and distribution of causes
	    Incidence—rate at which a disease occurs (number/time)
	    Prevalence—total number of cases in existence at a given time
	Cause/etiology:
	    What brings about the condition or produces the effect?
	Natural course:
	    Onset
	    Severity/intensity
	    Prognosis

Intent of treatment	Specify:
	    Pharmacotherapy
	    Nondrug therapy
	For the following purposes:
	    Curative
	    Preventive
	    Palliative
	    Diagnostic

Goals of therapy	Clinical (physiological):
	    Resolution of signs and symptoms, laboratory abnormalities
	Improvement in:
	    Physiological activities
	    Quality of life
	Behavioral (psychological)
	    Patient satisfaction
	    Compliance
	Economic (cost savings)
	    Avoid unnecessary clinic or office visits
	    Reduce drug costs
	    Reduce employee sick days
	    Prevent emergency department visits
	    Prevent admission to long-term care facility
	    Prevent hospitalizations

Common Conditions are Common

In a generalist practice such as pharmaceutical care, the practitioner encounters numerous patients with common medical conditions, who are treated with commonly used medications. Therefore, the learning curve of a generalist practitioner can be steep. It is important to realize that being reflective and learning the most you can from every patient encounter accelerates learning (see Chapter 12 for a detailed description of reflective practitioner skills).

The more efficient you are at dealing with the most common problems, the more time and effort you can spend meeting the less common drug-related needs of your patients. This process of rapidly recognizing and dealing with common patient needs and constantly expanding your ability to deal with more complex patient needs is the foundation of becoming a competent practitioner.

The results generated from over 59,000 pharmaceutical care encounters from numerous community-based practices provide an informative description of the common medical conditions encountered. Table 11-3 lists the 20 most commonly encountered clinical indications managed with drug therapy in pharmaceutical care practice.

In the text, *20 Common Problems in Primary Care*,[1] Barry D. Weiss described, the results of the National Ambulatory Medical Care Survey (NAMCS) which revealed that the most frequent medical indications resulting in a primary care clinic visit included disorders requiring treatment, prevention, and risk assessment. Table 11-4 lists these *Top 20*. Weiss noted in the preface that: "If the primary care practitioners develop

Table 11-3 Top 20 indications for drug therapy in pharmaceutical care practices[a]

1. Hypertension	11. Asthma
2. Hyperlipidemia	12. Arthritis pain
3. Osteoporosis prevention	13. Bronchitis
4. Diabetes	14. Sinusitis
5. Vitamin/dietary supplements	15. Menopausal symptoms
6. Allergic rhinitis	16. Otitis media
7. Depression	17. Anxiety
8. Esophagitis	18. Insomnia
9. Pain—general	19. Headache pain
10. Hypothyroidism	20. Cardiac dysrhythmias

[a]Data generated from 20,761 patients receiving pharmaceutical care from independent pharmaceutical care practitioners. The database is described in Chapter 2.

Table 11-4 Common problems treated in primary care

Cough	Sore throat and nasal congestion
Back pain	Sprains and strains
Depression	Anxiety
Osteoarthritis	Headache
Abdominal pain: dyspepsia	Chest pain
Urinary tract infection	Preventive health examinations
Birth control	Hypertension
Earache	Obesity
Cigarette smoking	Diabetes mellitus type II
Dermatitis-eczema	Hidden problems of:
	Domestic violence
	The problem drinker
	Low literacy

a firm mastery of these problems, those individuals will be able to diagnose and treat most of the conditions for which patients present for care...."[1]

Compare Tables 11-3 and 11-4. The results of these practices reaffirm the concept that this is a generalist practice in that the medical conditions seen by pharmaceutical care practitioners in the community are similar to the most common medical conditions resulting in visits to primary care medical practitioners. Of possibly greater interest to the student practitioner are the following facts:

1. *What you need to learn is known.* A limited number of medical conditions and illnesses represent a large portion of the information that you will need to understand in order to become a successful practitioner.[1,3–6]
2. *The data you will need are available.* Much is known about virtually all of these common medical conditions, so you can easily find information concerning etiology, presenting signs and symptoms, diagnostic criteria, effectiveness of various treatments, and recommended follow-up procedures.[4–6]
3. *You will have numerous, effective solutions available for your patients.* There are several very efficacious drug therapies available to treat and/or prevent these common medical conditions giving you numerous therapeutic alternatives (prescription, nonprescription, herbal remedies, dietary supplements) from which to select in order to meet the individual needs of your patients.[3–9]

The most useful advice to the new practitioner is to acquire knowledge when you discover you need it (take control of your learning process), and practice providing pharmaceutical care at every opportunity you have.

KNOWLEDGE YOU NEED ABOUT THE PATIENT'S DRUG THERAPIES

There are well defined, standard categories of drug-related information that a practitioner must be able to integrate and apply in order to meet his or her patient's drug-related needs. In practice, having command of drug-related information in a format that can be applied to individual patients with unique clinical conditions is essential. Patients, other practitioners, and colleagues expect the pharmaceutical care practitioner to possess a level of understanding of pharmacotherapy and the ability to apply clinical pharmacological principles that is the highest among all patient care providers. Your colleagues will expect you to have a command of in-depth and expansive pharmacotherapeutic knowledge in order to identify, resolve, and prevent drug therapy problems regardless of patient, disease, or drug products involved (Table 11-5).

As described throughout this text, the rational, well-reasoned, problem-solving approach, which is at the core of pharmaceutical care practice, is nothing less and nothing more than a structured method to assess the drug-related needs of individual patients through the application of accepted clinical pharmacological principles. The pharmaceutical care practitioner repeatedly cycles through problem solving in the areas of indication, effectiveness, safety, and compliance.

Most clinical pharmacology knowledge is developed and reported in the following four areas:

1. **Indication**—therapeutic uses or intent for the drug or drug products due to the known pharmacological actions of the active ingredient(s).
2. **Efficacy**—desired pharmacological action resulting in the somewhat predictable benefit of a medication in a patient population with a specific disease or illness.
3. **Safety**—side effects, toxicology, and other undesirable pharmacological actions that the drug is known to exhibit at the doses used to treat patients.
4. **Compliance**—onset and duration of action (pharmacokinetic and pharmacodynamic characteristics) of the drug product and their influence on the instructions for use by patients.

Efficacy is used to describe benefits to a population, while *effectiveness* describes benefits to individuals.

Table 11-5   Pharmacotherapeutic knowledge needed for pharmaceutical care practice

	Dimensions
Characteristics of the drug	Description of the drug
	Efficacy for an indication
	Dosage regimen for the drug
	Dose (initial and maintenance)
	Dosing interval
	Frequency
	Duration
	Pharmacology (action of the drug)
	Mechanism of action
	Sites of action
	Toxicology
	Contraindications
	Adverse effects
	Precautions
Activity of the drug in the patient	Pharmaceutical process
	Bioavailability
	Physicochemical properties
	Formulations and dosage forms
	Methods of drug administrations
	Pharmacokinetic process
	Absorption
	Distribution
	Metabolism
	Elimination
	Pharmacodynamic process
	Impact of a drug on cell, tissue, or organ
	Time course of the effects
The outcomes of drug therapy	Therapeutic process
	Effectiveness: The therapeutic effect— expected beneficial pharmacological effects of the drug on the course of the patient's disease or illness
	Improvement in signs, symptoms, and/or laboratory findings
	Safety: Detrimental pharmacological effects of the drug on the patient
	Undesirable or harmful effects and adverse drug reactions

Example "The efficacy of this new drug has been well-established in clinical trials of patients with major depression. This new selective serotonin reuptake inhibitor (SSRI) product has been demonstrated to be efficacious in 60–75% of patients with hypertension."

The term effectiveness is used to describe the positive result a drug has on an individual patient.

Example "My patient's aspirin therapy has been very effective at reducing the pain and swelling in her right elbow. However, her atorvastatin (Lipitor) was not effective at reducing her cholesterol."

Practitioners train themselves to make decisions based on the series of questions described below. These questions serve as the basis for every assessment of each patient's drug therapy regardless of the patient, disease, or drug therapy involved. The information you gather during this process will become the database and clinical experience you will use to form your own drug-related knowledge base.

Questions that shape your pharmacotherapeutic knowledge

1. Are all of my patient's medications appropriately indicated at this time? (Indication)
2. Are all of the patient's clinical indications for drug therapy being appropriately treated or prevented with medications at this time? (Indication)
3. Are the drug product(s) that my patient is taking producing or likely to produce the desired outcomes for each medical condition? (Effectiveness)
4. Are the dosage regimen(s) that my patient is taking producing or likely to produce the desired outcomes for each medical condition? (Effectiveness)
5. Are any of the drug products causing or likely to cause my patient to experience an adverse reaction? (Safety)
6. Are any of the dosage regimens causing or likely to produce toxic side effects? (Safety)
7. Are the instructions for all drug therapy regimens understood and can my patient incorporate them into his/her daily life as recommended? (Compliance)

This is a good time to point out the relationships between the practice of pharmaceutical care and the principles of the discipline of clinical pharmacology. The need for pharmaceutical care practice is not new. Over 25 years ago, Goodman and Gilman described the need for the clinical application of pharmacological principles primarily to avoid therapeutic failures and unnecessary adverse effects. They called for the *rational use of drugs* and stated that the practitioner

> ...is advised to examine each therapeutic effort in a systematic manner, questions similar to the following; Is there a valid indication for this drug? Is it the agent of choice? Are its effects modified by the patient's illness or concurrent medications? Is the dosage schedule appropriate? Is ancillary medication indicated? What is the therapeutic objective and what evidence of efficacy and potential adverse effects should be monitored? Is the patient adequately informed and instructed about the medication and can his/her compliance be expected?[9]

In this concise description of a rational process for thinking about a patient's drug-related needs, these pharmacologists established the scientific framework for what has eventually become the practice of pharmaceutical care. This framework is a well-reasoned thought process based on established clinical pharmacological principles, beginning with a critical assessment of whether the patient has a valid *indication* for each drug he/she is taking. The practitioner must then work with the patient to establish measurable goals of therapy, evaluate *effectiveness* of therapy as well as the *safety* of those therapies, finally working with the patient to ensure the best understanding and *compliance* possible.

It is noteworthy that the rational thought process which is at the foundation of the Pharmacotherapy Workup and pharmaceutical care practice has its roots in the discipline of clinical pharmacology. The role of the clinical pharmacologist was to narrow the gap between the quantity of available scientific information on drugs and their safe and effective use in practice. Pharmaceutical care practice is intended to accomplish this same goal one patient at a time.

> **Note**   One could describe pharmaceutical care as the practical application of well reasoned, clinical pharmacology principles in the primary care setting in order to ensure effective and safe drug therapy for every patient.

The drug knowledge required to provide pharmaceutical care goes well beyond pharmacology and includes a thorough understanding of pharmaceutical, pharmacokinetic, and pharmacodynamic processes (refer to Table 11-5). Pharmaceutical processes describe how a drug gets into the patient. The application of pharmacokinetic principles to predict and control drug concentrations at the drug's site of action is also important. Pharmacodynamic processes describe the intensity and the timeframe of the effects that the drug has on the patient.

Clearly, the practitioner's clinical judgment is most influenced by the therapeutic processes (refer to Table 11-5). These include most notably how to determine if the desired therapeutic outcome did in fact occur (effectiveness) and if the patient experienced any detrimental effects from drug therapy (safety). Effectiveness and safety are the two primary processes that practitioners must assess and evaluate continuously in each patient, for every disorder, at every patient-practitioner encounter.

Learning the process of identifying, resolving, and preventing drug therapy problems, rather than simply finding *answers* to questions is what will make the pharmaceutical care practitioner useful to patients well into the future.[10]

Common Drugs are Common

There are thousands of drug products available to treat and prevent diseases. The Food and Drug Administration approves a new drug product for use in the United States approximately every 10 days.[11] Learning all that is required about them can seem like a formidable task for the student practitioner. There is much to be learned. Learning the characteristics listed in Table 11-5 for classes of drugs can be helpful, but sometimes confusing. We have tricyclic antidepressants which are grouped based on their chemical structure but used in practice for numerous indications other than depression (enuresis). Antihistamines are grouped based on their mechanism of action. There are histamine H_1-receptor antagonists. We also have a category of relatively nonsedating antihistamines grouped because of a lower incidence of a side effect. H_2-blockers act at another histamine site of action but are not generally referred to as antihistamines.

Nonsteroidal anti-inflammatory drugs (NSAIDs) are grouped based on a chemical structure that they do not possess. Grouping of drug products by similarities in chemical structure, mechanism of action, or selected indication does not yield mutually exclusive categories and therefore can cause some confusion for the early learner. It is important to understand all of a drug's actions on your patients, not just the intended or marketed actions.

There is an efficient way to begin or to expand your pharmacotherapy learning process. Create a personal learning agenda that begins with the drug products you will encounter most frequently. The most common prescription and nonprescription products selected for use by practitioners and patients are listed in Tables 11-6 and 11-7.

The most efficient learning method is to begin caring for patients, under supervision. Care for as many patients as possible. The best practitioners in any field are the busiest practitioners. Busy practitioners must be effective

Table 11-6 The twenty most frequently dispensed[a] prescription products in the United States for 2002 (based on volume of prescriptions)

1. Lipitor (atorvastatin)	11. Celebrex (celecoxib)
2. Synthroid (levothyroxine)	12. Amoxicillin
3. Premarin (conjugated estrogens)	13. Levoxyl (levothyroxine)
4. Norvasc (amlodipine)	14. Zithromax (azithromycin)
5. HYCD/APAP (hydrocodone, acetaminophen)	15. Toprol-XL (metoprolol)
6. Zoloft (sertraline)	16. Zyrtec (cetirizine)
7. Zocor (simvastatin)	17. Furosemide
8. Paxil (paroxetine)	18. Atenolol
9. Prevacid (lansoprazole)	19. Prilosec (omeprazole)
10. Albuterol	20. Allegra (fexofenadine)

[a]Listed items represent approximately 19% of the total U.S. prescription market share for 2002. There were 3.34 billion prescriptions dispensed in the United States in 2002.

and efficient at providing care. The best way to become effective and efficient is to learn first how to care for patients with common problems.

Building upon this base of core clinical knowledge will allow you to eventually help patients with more complex and/or less commonly encountered problems. This is the method used by all successful patient care practitioners to establish and continually expand their clinical expertise.

SUMMARY

The pharmaceutical care practitioner will need patient, disease, and drug knowledge in every case, and much of this information is known and available to you. The key point to learn early in the developmental stages of becoming a successful practitioner is that you must have command of all three categories of information in every clinical situation. The patient-specific information, the disease-related information, and the drug knowledge are always related and must be considered as a whole. Separating any one of these three linked elements removes it from its true context and distorts or diminishes the value of the other two. Knowing the patient and the drug but not the indication makes it virtually impossible for the practitioner to add any value to the patient's drug-related needs. Knowing the drug therapy and the disease but not having adequate information about your patient makes it difficult for you to offer him/her any individualized service, information, or drug therapy. Only by collecting, critiquing, integrating, assessing, and

Table 11-7 Most frequently used nonprescription products in the United States[12–15]

1. Multivitamins 　Centrum 　Centrum Silver 　One-A-Day 　Flintstones	9. Laxatives (liquid) 　Metamucil 　Citrucel 　Fleet 　Perdiem
2. Analgesics (internal) 　Tylenol 　Advil 　Aleve 　Bayer	10. Laxatives (tablets) 　Ex-Lax 　Dulcolax 　Fibercon 　Senokot
3. Cold/allergy/sinus 　Benadryl 　Alka-Seltzer Plus 　Theraflu 　Sudafed	11. Foot care products 　Dr. Scholl's 　Lotrimin AF 　Lamisil AT 　Tinactin
4. Cold/allergy/sinus liquids 　Vicks Nyquil 　Tylenol Cold 　Dimetapp 　Triaminic	12. Acne treatment 　Neutrogena Acne Wash 　Clean & Clear 　Clearasil 　Oxy Balance
5. Cough syrup 　Robitussin DM 　Delsym 　Vicks Formula 44 　Diabetic Tussin	13. Adult incontinence products 　Depend 　Depend Poise 　Serenity 　Sure Care Slip On
6. Antacids (tablets) 　Tums Extra 　Rolaids 　Pepcid AC 　Zantac 75	14. Topical anti-itch treatments 　Cortizone 10 　Benadryl 　Cortaid 　Aveeno
7. Eye and lens care products 　Renu Multiplus 　Opti-Free Express 　Visine 　Aosept	15. Herbal supplements 　Nature's Resource 　Sundown 　Estroven 　PharmAssure
8. Weight control/nutrition 　Ultra Slim Fast 　Ensure 　Pedia Sure 　Boost	

applying information about your patient, the diseases or illnesses requiring pharmacotherapy, and all of your patient's drug therapies can you provide a meaningful, effective, and comprehensive service.

EXERCISES

11-1 Each practitioner needs to constantly construct a learning agenda for him/herself. Begin constructing yours by listing the five types of patient characteristics you want to learn more about, the five medical conditions you want to better understand, and the five different drug therapies you plan to study.

11-2 Refer to each of the tables of knowledge contained in the chapter (Tables 11-1, 11-2, and 11-5). Select a colleague. Consider the different types of knowledge described in each table. Each of you decide which three pieces of knowledge you think are most important about each (the patient, diseases, and drug therapy) and explain why they are more important than the rest. Discuss the similarities and differences between your two lists.

11-3 With the list created in exercise 2 above, select a patient type, a disease, and a drug therapy with which you are unfamiliar. Now identify appropriate references and learn the three most important pieces of knowledge about each one.

11-4 This book puts forth the argument that it is more efficient to learn all this knowledge after the practice of pharmaceutical care is understood. Many academics argue that you need the knowledge first and then you can learn the practice at the end of the educational experience. Take a position and describe your reasoning.

REFERENCES

1. Weiss, B.D. *20 Common Problems in Primary Care*, 1st ed. New York: McGraw-Hill; 1999.
2. Norman, D.D. *Perceptions of the Elderly Regarding the Medicating Experience: A Discourse Analysis of the Interpretation of Medication Usage (Ph.D. thesis)*. Minneapolis, MN: University of Minnesota; 1995.
3. Cipolle, R., Strand, L.M., Morley, P.C., *Pharmaceutical Care Practice*. New York: McGraw Hill; 1998.
4. Dipiro, J.T., et al. *Pharmacotherapy—A Pathophysiologic Approach*, 5th ed. New York: McGraw-Hill; 2002.
5. Koda-Kimble, M.A., Young, L.Y., *Applied Therapeutics: The Clinical Use of Drugs.* 7th ed. Baltimore, MD: Lippincott Williams & Wilkins; 2001, p. 24.

6. Gray, J. *Therapeutic Choices*, 4th ed. Canadian Pharmacists Association; Ottawa, Ontario, Canada; 2003.

7. Vaczek, D. *Top 200 Drugs of 2002*. www.pharmacytimes.com; 2002.

8. *Drug Facts and Comparisons*, St. Louis, MO: Wolters Kluwer Health, Inc, 8th ed. 2004.

9. Gilman, A.G., Hardman, J.G., Limbird, L.E. *Goodman & Gilman's The Pharmacological Basis of Therapeutics*, 10th ed. New York: McGraw-Hill; 2001.

10. Schwinghammer, T.L., et al., *Pharmacotherapy Casebook: A Patient-Focused Approach*, 5th ed. New York: McGraw-Hill; 2002.

11. Peterson, M. *New Medicines Seldom Contain Anything New, Study Finds*. New York: The New York Times; 2002.

12. Pinto, D. (ed), Over-the-counter drugs: Market analysis: Business holds promise, peril for drug chains. *Chain Drug Rev* 2001; 23(9):21.

13. Pinto, D. (ed), Over-the-counter drugs: Category stuck in the doldrums. *Chain Drug Rev* 2001; 23(9):29.

14. FDA approval rate reflects growth of biotech. *Chain Drug Rev* 2003; 25(4):RX11. Pinto, D. ed.

15. Pinto, D. (ed), CDR/IRI H&BA Report: The Data Shows "Who is Winning, Who's Losing, What Had an Impact." *Chain Drug Rev* 2002; 24(11):185–282.

CHAPTER TWELVE

ACQUIRING THE CLINICAL SKILLS YOU NEED TO PRACTICE

Key Concepts

1. *The clinical skills required to practice pharmaceutical care include obtaining information from the patient, applying knowledge to individual patients, communicating with patients and colleagues, and being reflective in practice.*

2. *Obtaining information from patients requires observational, interview, and physical assessment skills.*

3 *Applying knowledge to individual patients allows you to generate hypotheses, solve problems, and make rational and logical decisions about the patient's pharmacotherapy.*

4 *Documenting the care provided in practice reflects commitment to the patient, adherence to practice standards, and the desire to learn from clinical experience.*

5 *Reflective skills allow you to convert clinical experience into clinical knowledge.*

INTRODUCTION

The practice of pharmaceutical care requires the mastery of a number of clinical skills. The four sets of skills that are used on a continuous basis are gathering information, evaluating and applying information, communicating information, and learning from your experience. Because the information practitioners need and use can be complex, and is often technical, special skills are required to master this unique body of knowledge.

The first skill set requires that practitioners learn to retrieve, gather, and assemble patient, disease, and drug information from patients. You will need observational, interview, and physical assessment skills to accomplish this. Frequently, the patient will present with a medical condition that is unfamiliar, a drug therapy that is new, or a unique set of circumstances that require you to gather information from books, the literature, colleagues, or the internet. Retrieving information in an effective manner will improve your ability to care for patients.

The second set of clinical skills are those required to apply the knowledge you have accumulated to the patient for whom you are caring. This will allow you to generate hypotheses, solve problems, and make rational and logical decisions about the patient's pharmacotherapy. These skills rely on the practitioner's inquiry, discovery, and creativity abilities.

The third skill set includes the ability to communicate what the practitioner knows and the decisions he/she has made. A practitioner's communication skills often determine the level of success he/she has in practice. Both written and verbal communication skills are important and communication with patients as well as with other practitioners is required to be successful. Written communication, in the form of documentation in the pharmaceutical care patient chart and medical record, is also a skill that must be mastered.

The fourth category is the skills required to be reflective in practice, so that you can learn from each patient care experience. Reflective skills allow you to convert clinical experience into clinical knowledge. This skill set allows the practitioner to reflect on a patient encounter to determine what went well and why, what did not go as expected and why, and what must be changed in the future. These skills help you to learn on a daily basis from both the patient and colleagues. Reflective skills are powerful as they allow practitioners to learn from both successful and unsuccessful experiences. Although these skills are discussed frequently in the nursing and medical literature, pharmacy programs have not uniformly developed these skills in their practitioners. The basic skill of being reflective in practice will have a significant impact on how quickly you become a competent pharmaceutical care practitioner.

Clinical skills are like any other skill set. To master them requires training, practice, and reflection. The student practitioner can work to develop these skill sets in stages. Although all are required to provide pharmaceutical care for a patient, it is useful to focus on one set at a time while you are developing your clinical skills.

For the new practitioner there is no substitute for practice. The more patients you see and provide direct care for, the more proficient you will become. New practitioners should avail themselves of every possible opportunity to provide pharmaceutical care to patients. Internalizing the clinical skills and decision-making processes necessary to perform at a level dictated by the standards of practice requires considerable time and a variety of patient cases for a new practitioner to.

OBTAINING CLINICAL INFORMATION FROM THE PATIENT

Eliciting relevant information from your patient is not only the first goal you will have to accomplish, but it is one of the most important when providing care. The quality of the information you elicit will determine the quality of the care you can provide. This skill set integrates observational, interview, and physical assessment skills.

Observational Skills

The first skill to learn is gathering information from observation. Although the amount of physical effort involved in this skill is small, the amount of insight and sensitivity required to optimize the information you elicit through observation can be substantial. Observational skills require you to collect information with your eyes and your powers of deduction. Table 12-1 describes the information you can often elicit with these skills, and the table includes suggestions as to how you might document this information in the pharmaceutical care chart.

Improving your observational skills first requires you to become conscious of the variables that will have an impact on your care plan. If you teach yourself to be aware of these items you can save yourself and your patient a significant amount of time and effort. Becoming sensitive to nonverbal clues will help you throughout the Pharmacotherapy Workup.

Table 12-1   Information obtained from observational skills

Patient variable	Examples of values to document
Age	Approximate age in years or decades for older patients *Example*: A gentleman who appears to be in his 80s.
Height, weight	Approximate height and weight *Example*: Normal weight, slightly obese, very obese
Gender	Male, female
Overall health status	Assessment of physical/mental health *Example*: Excellent, good, poor
Physical grooming and personal hygiene	*Example*: Neat, clean, unkempt, disheveled
Posture and general ability to ambulate	Level of physical activity No difficulty ambulating Difficulty ambulating *Example*: Good posture, poor posture
Ability to communicate	Language ability, use of hearing aid
Outward signs of illness	Normal or pallid skin tone Energetic, lethargic *Example*: Well nourished, malnourished
Apprehension, fear, agitation	Example: Anxious, distressed, preoccupied
Willingness and ability to participate	Cooperative, uncooperative *Example*: Good historian, quiet

Respect the power of keen observational skills. You can collect this information in the first moments of your assessment. Simply make mental notes of the data you collect before you begin your assessment interview so that it does not get lost or overlooked. You will want to record this information in writing as soon as it is appropriate.

After you have taught yourself to be effective at observation, then you are ready to develop your listening skills.

Interview Skills

You will gain most of your information from your patient during the assessment. The assessment consists of primarily patient-specific information collected using the process described in Chapter 6. The assessment interview is a purposeful conversation which differs from casual or friend-to-friend conversations. An effective assessment interview requires that the practitioner become skilled at using open-ended inquiries to elicit patient responses and then explore the topic more extensively through pointed questioning.

Learning these assessment interview skills requires practicing to be an active listener. Active listening means taking the time and energy to hear and understand what your patient has just told you. As a student, you will want to practice listening to patients' stories about their medication experiences and the impact that drug therapies have had on their lives.

Students tend to ask the patient a question and then immediately start to think of what the next question should be. Experienced practitioners approach the assessment interview much differently. Skilled practitioners listen very carefully to the patient's response, and after fully hearing and understanding what was said, formulate the next logical question. The next question in an effective assessment interview should be related to the patient's response to the previous question. Therefore, you will not know what the next best question should be until you have understood what your patient is telling you. Listen, then listen more, and then listen even more. If all you hear is your voice, change your approach.

Take your time to formulate questions. If it requires a few moments, that is not a problem. The time you take to formulate your next question may seem like an uncomfortable lull to you, but the pause usually does not bother patients.

Students often feel nervous and hurried when conducting their first few assessment interviews. Remain calm, and proceed in a relaxed manner. Let your patient know about how long you anticipate the assessment will take, and let him/her do most of the talking. Establish and maintain good eye contact and be conscious of your posture and body position. Sit up straight in the chair or stand without leaning, and avoid nervous repetitive movements.

Listen with an open mind   When you first begin to develop your assessment skills, you may not feel you are adequately prepared to deal with some of the issues that patients present to you. Some practitioners may feel that the sexual, psychiatric, or interpersonal problems the patient discusses may be beyond their scope to manage in an assessment interview. However, this information may have a direct impact on the course of action your patient is willing to pursue, and it may impact the outcome of therapy, so it is important that you obtain the relevant information.

> **Example**   The topic of sexual activity is often thought of as a *private matter*, and is too often avoided. Interviewing a patient about sexuality and sexual problems can be a complex and difficult dimension of the Pharmacotherapy Workup. In a world in which human immunodeficiency virus (HIV), acquired immunodeficiency syndrome (AIDS), and numerous other sexually transmitted diseases (STDs) cause significant morbidity and mortality, practitioners must understand these conditions and develop the ability to obtain appropriate information during an assessment. Drug therapy is an essential form of treatment and prevention of many sexually transmitted illnesses. Practitioners need to inform the patient of the need to ask some questions about his/her sexual life. Questions of how their illness has affected their sexual life can be helpful in evaluating the effectiveness of drug therapy. Similarly, inquiring as to how the patient feels that his/her drug therapy has impacted sexual activity can identify adverse drug reactions that require adjustment in pharmacotherapy.[1]

Listen with empathy   Demonstrating empathy for your patient's emotional situation can be comforting for him/her. Being empathetic—having the ability to imagine yourself in your patient's position—will positively impact the relationship you establish with the patient. The challenge of learning empathic skills lies in learning the primary approaches of reflecting and legitimating and then integrating an interpersonal style that feels genuine to you and is likely to be perceived as genuine by the patient.

Reflecting refers to the practitioner describing the emotional experience of the patient.

Example   "I can see that you are upset by this."

Legitimating confirms that the emotion is understood and accepted.

Example   "I can understand why that would make you upset."

Your patients will want to know that you intend to be supportive of their needs. Skillfully explaining that they can depend on your assistance is reassuring. This can be accomplished by explaining: "I would like to work together with you to develop the best possible treatment plan once we have agreed on what goals we will try to achieve."[1]

It is not necessary to wait until the end of an assessment interview to summarize. By summarizing what you have heard and your interpretation of that information, you can get immediate feedback as to whether you and your patient have the same understanding. Summarizing is also an effective method of regaining control of the conversation and redirecting it as you feel is necessary.

Did you miss anything important? This question perplexes new practitioners during their first few assessment interviews. The best method to be confident that you did not omit an important area is to give your patient ample opportunity to respond to: "Is there anything else you feel I should know?" After you share your summary of the assessment with the patient, make certain that the patient has ample opportunity to add information that may not have been mentioned. This technique helps the patient feel that you have done your best to understand his/her needs or problems.

Becoming efficient at collecting patient information   You must first become *effective* at conducting a comprehensive assessment of a patient's drug-related needs before you attempt to become *efficient*. Efficiency is effectiveness over time, and therefore an ineffective approach to patient assessment will never result in an efficient process. As a student practitioner, take your time, and learn how to get it right. Most patients appreciate someone spending sufficient time to fully hear their story.

Collect only the information you will use   During the assessment process, you should only gather information that you will use to make your clinical judgments and decisions. It is often difficult for students to know what information will be necessary and/or useful. As you become more experienced in patient assessment, you will find that you can select the most useful and important questions within each assessment. You will feel more confident that you have a clinically sound idea of your patient's drug-related needs and can identify his/her drug therapy problems. Experts use surprisingly few pieces of key data to make their initial clinical judgments, and then proceed to gather more facts in order to verify or refute their initial decisions.[1,2]

There are no shortcuts to collecting patient, disease, and drug information and knowing specifically what information is needed and when. You will not find effective recipes for care. Patient care does not provide a list of necessary ingredients (information) and a formula (knowledge) of how to combine them. The best way to learn what information you need to gather in order to make clinical decisions is to gather it, then decide if it was actually helpful to you when you made the decision. If so, you have learned how that particular information can be applied to make patient-specific clinical decisions about drug therapies. If you find that the information you gathered did not help, then you will have learned from that as well.

Physical Assessment Skills

Pharmaceutical care practitioners primarily use physical assessment skills to evaluate the effectiveness and safety of their patient's medications. The physical assessment skills used within the diagnostic process far exceed those required for the pharmaceutical care process. However, physical assessment skills are essential to determine if your patient is experiencing positive or negative effects from their drug therapy.

The follow-up evaluation in the pharmaceutical care process calls for the collection of clinical and/or laboratory parameters necessary to determine if the patient's drug therapies are being effective and/or causing any harm. Drug effectiveness is often determined based on the improvement of clinical signs and symptoms. The practitioner uses physical assessment skills to detect side effects caused by medications.

There are a number of basic physical assessment skills that students need to acquire and understand in order to provide pharmaceutical care. The specific techniques are beyond the scope of this text, but are described in detail in textbooks used by medical, nursing, pharmacy, and other students of the health sciences.[3] As an example, the core set of physical assessment skills would include measuring the patient's vital signs.

Vital signs   Measurement of vital signs includes the patient's blood pressure, heart rate, respiratory rate, and temperature. These basic clinical parameters are essential to determine the effectiveness and safety of a great majority of medications commonly used today. A sphygmomanometer is commonly used to measure your patient's blood pressure, a thermometer is required to determine temperature, and a functional timepiece is helpful to accurately measure a pulse rate, but no other equipment or expense is involved in obtaining a patient's vital signs.

Hypertension is among the most common indications for the use of prescription medications. The effectiveness of antihypertensive drug therapy and much of the evaluation of its safety are based on the measurement of blood pressure. This is a skill that every pharmaceutical care practitioner will use throughout his/her career.

Temperature is the hallmark sign of most infectious processes. Antibiotic drug therapies are evaluated based on the improvement of signs, symptoms, and laboratory parameters. The patient's temperature often serves as the primary clinical indicator of effectiveness. Numerous techniques and innovative technologies are available to obtain the patient's temperature and familiarity with their application is a useful clinical skill.

The patient's pulse or heart rate can be greatly influenced by drug therapies. Most cardiovascular agents increase or decrease the pulse when used at pharmacologically active dosages. Drugs that slow the heart rate can put patients at risk of becoming dizzy or losing consciousness due to lack of blood supply to vital organs including the brain.

> **Example**   The pulse rate is one of the common parameters used to evaluate the safety of digoxin dosing in patients with heart failure or cardiac dysrhythmias, and beta-blockers such as atenolol and metoprolol used to manage patients with angina pectoris or hypertension.

Improving the patient's breathing symptoms is frequently a goal of drug therapy. The respiratory status of the patient includes the rate, rhythm, depth, and effort of breathing, all of which can be observed and easily counted. Respiratory rates are often essential in determining the effectiveness of drug therapy to manage asthma, pneumonia, bronchitis, congestive heart failure, chronic obstructive pulmonary disease (COPD), and cystic fibrosis.

Retrieving Information

No matter how good you become as a practitioner, you will always have to retrieve information from books and the literature. Pharmacotherapy changes continually, and it is virtually impossible to remember everything you need to know to practice pharmaceutical care. Your ability to retrieve necessary information at the right time is an important skill.

As students begin to develop their clinical skills, subscribing to one important guideline can be helpful: *Look it up now.* If you come across information you need to retrieve from a book or other source, find the answer immediately. Retention of newly acquired knowledge is easier and more efficient when that new knowledge is placed in a clinically appropriate context, that is, the care of a patient. If you stop and put forth the effort to retrieve these data when you need to apply them to identify or resolve a patient problem, you will retain that new knowledge.

Students and experienced practitioners tend to use different sources as references because they generally have different needs. Students, especially early in their studies, are best served by texts containing full descriptions of pharmacological actions, disease processes, and pharmacotherapeutic approaches. References with this level of detail and comprehensive explanations are useful to provide new practitioners with the necessary overall understanding of the topic. Following is a list of these types of references.

References for new practitioners

- *The Pharmacological Basis of Therapeutics,* Goodman and Gilman[4]
- *Pharmacotherapy: A Pathophysiological Approach*[5]
- *Handbook of Nonprescription Drugs*[6]
- *Applied Therapeutics: The Clinical Use of Drugs*[7]
- *Principles of Internal Medicine*[8]
- *American Hospital Formulary Service Drug Information*[9]
- *Natural Medicines Comprehensive Database*[10]

Busy practitioners already have a general and often thorough understanding of the topic, but they need a small piece of data to support a specific decision that has to be made. Therefore, while students need comprehensive pharmacology, pathophysiology, and pharmacotherapy textbooks at their disposal, experienced practitioners tend to make better use of reference handbooks from which they can quickly retrieve a single piece of data needed to complete the clinical decision-making process. Following is a list of these types of references.

Useful reference handbooks

- *Facts and Comparisons*[11]
- *Handbook of Clinical Drug Data*[12]
- *Drug Information Handbook*[13]
- *Therapeutic Choices*[14]

- *Griffith's 5-minute Clinical Consult*[15]
- *Geriatric Dosage Handbook*[16]
- *Pediatric Dosage Handbook*[17]
- *Laboratory Test Handbook*[18]
- *Tyler's Honest Herbal: A Sensible Guide to the Use of Herbs and Related Remedies*[19]
- *The Top 100 Drug Interactions: A Guide to Patient Management.*[20]

There are many texts in these areas, and the selection of an appropriate one can be confusing. New practitioners must be certain that the books they use to establish their reference library will be the most useful. It is useful for students to choose an example topic and examine that section in a book before it is purchased. Did it answer the questions? Can the topic be understood? How the text is indexed is especially important because you will often need to refer to the index to identify and learn new material quickly and effectively.

Some references deal only with products licensed for use in one country; some contain information on products only available without a prescription. Other references focus on herbal and natural products. Students may need several references just to learn about all of the medications that patients take. In order to look up information for a patient taking an herbal product, two prescription medications, and a commonly used nonprescription drug product, a student may use three separate texts. Efficiently using these references requires an understanding of how each reference organizes and presents information. Some references list drug information alphabetically by generic names, some organize the drug information by therapeutic class, and some organize information by the primary pharmacological actions of the drug.

The use and retrieval of primary literature sources is a skill that every practitioner must possess in order to continue learning. Because it often requires 1–3 years to bring a new reference book to publication, professional journals are considered the best source for contemporary information, controversial topics, alternative approaches, and comparison studies. Contemporary topics such as severe acute respiratory syndrome (SARS) or HIV are best researched using the primary literature. Also, individual case reports and unusual or rare events are most frequently published in primary sources and can be helpful to verify whether your patient's outcome has been reported in other patient cases. Searching for information from the primary literature has become extremely efficient through the Internet. Many professional journals make the full text of articles available on their websites.

Obtaining information from the Internet can be the most efficient method to obtain access to the current literature and information. Remember, however that it is important to verify that you are using only reputable sources. In general, the information explosion that has occurred in pharmacotherapy knowledge over the past few decades is well served by the capacity and timeliness of the internet. For example, many of the major pharmaceutical firms provide open access to the current understanding of the pharmacology, efficacy, and safety of their products. Additionally, information about new products that are still in the developmental process can be researched via the Internet. There are many sites on the World Wide Web that provide useful information about diseases or drug therapies. A common advantage of these sites is that the explanations and descriptions are written with terms that can be understood by patients. For examples, visit www.medicinenet.com, www.webmd.com, www.diabetes.org, and www.americanheart.org.

COMMUNICATION SKILLS

This text is not intended to teach you to master the basic skills involved in human communication. There are a number of other useful texts for that purpose.[1,2,21,22]

We begin with the assumption that students who have been successful at securing a position in a professional education program have a basic command of the skills required to communicate verbally and in writing. Therefore, this is not intended to be a basic or theoretical discussion of communication skills. Instead, we want to present the unique aspects of communicating with patients and other health care professionals about drug therapy issues in pharmaceutical care practice.

Patient-focused Communication

Communication with patients brings together many of the dimensions of pharmaceutical care practice. At the center of communication is the relationship between the patient and the practitioner. The nature and ethical framework of the relationship that is required to practice pharmaceutical care dictates the specific guidelines for the communication that occurs between patient and practitioner (see Chapter 10 for a discussion of the ethical dimensions of pharmaceutical care and Chapter 4 for a discussion of the therapeutic relationship).

Ruesch captures this in his definition of therapeutic communication: "Therapeutic communication can be defined as a skill that helps people to overcome temporary stress, to get along with other people, to adjust to the unalterable, and to overcome psychological blocks which stand in the way of self-realization."[23]

The key to building a therapeutic relationship as well as successfully communicating with patients is to create an environment for the patient that has the right conditions for fostering good communication. Empathy, positive regard, and congruence define these conditions. Empathy is the process of communicating to patients the feeling of being understood; it is putting yourself in the patient's situation. Positive regard is the process of communicating support to the patient in a caring and nonjudgmental way; it is communication that is genuine, unthreatening, and unconditional. Communicating congruence involves the honest expression of the practitioner's own thoughts and feelings; it requires that the caring professional will respond honestly to the patient and attempt to be genuine in his or her relationship with the patient.

As a pharmaceutical care practitioner you have three primary objectives or reasons to communicate with the patient: (1) to elicit necessary information from the patient to make your decisions; (2) to negotiate the terms of the goals of therapy and the patient's role in achieving them; and (3) to educate the patient about the drug therapy he/she is receiving and/or taking. A significant amount of space in this text has been devoted to explaining the assessment interview skills required to practice pharmaceutical care (see Chapter 6 for a detailed discussion of the assessment process). We will not repeat this information but focus on the skills required to educate patients about their drug therapy.

Educating the patient about drug therapy is most beneficial if you first understand the patient. You will be most effective if you establish with the patient:

1. what your patient *wants* to know;[24]
2. what the patient *already knows*;
3. the best way to recognize this difference is to
   - determine the preferred language of the patient;
   - determine the level of comprehension best suited to the patient—this will determine the vocabulary/terms that are familiar to the patient; and
   - identify any cultural or religious issues that are relevant to communicating with the patient.

The following material should be conveyed to all patients, unless you have identified a patient-specific reason for not sharing this information. This is considered to be the basic information about the patient's medication that will help him or her to actively engage in the care plan and be compliant with his or her medications. You will want to explain the following to the patient:

1. The reason the patient is taking each medication. (Indication)
   - Explain how the medication works
   - Use pictures and diagrams whenever possible
   - Provide patients with information and labeling to take home with them that ties the reason for taking the medication to the drug product, to the directions for administration to the goals of therapy, and to a timeframe for meeting the goals.
2. The specific instructions of how to take the medication explained in a manner the patient can understand.
   - Use the same terms from one encounter to the next
   - Use phrases that are familiar to the patient so they are not misunderstood (twice a day, dissolved in water, with food)
   - Start from your patient's point of reference (when do they eat, what time do they go to bed)
3. A description of how the patient will know that the medication is working well. (Effectiveness)
   - Describe how the patient's symptoms will change and when to expect these improvements
   - Create an understandable system for complicated terms (clinical parameters or laboratory values)
   - Include specific values that will serve as endpoints
   - Communicate how confident you are that the patient's pharmacotherapy will be effective
4. Explain the undesirable effects that might be expected. (Safety)
   - Be specific about when adverse reactions are most likely to occur.
5. Be clear about what the patient should do if a dose of the medication is missed or if he/she takes an extra dose of the medication. (Compliance)
6. Inform the patient of when and how you intend to follow-up to evaluate effectiveness and safety of the medication.
   - Provide the patient with clear instructions of what to do if any problems arise with the medication.
7. Provide the patient with a way to contact you if the medication is not working within the timeframe you discussed.

Care must be taken when communicating this much information. Be sure to speak slowly as much information about medications may be new to the patient. It may also be the case that the practitioner's first language is not the patient's first language. Be sure to evaluate the extent of understanding by him/her when you are finished communicating this information. Provide the patient with written information whenever possible to reinforce the major points made during the discussion.

Written correspondence with patients   It can be reinforcing to correspond with the patient in writing. Written correspondence might be used to provide him/her with literature about the medication being taken or a reminder about an appointment. This activity can be important in achieving the desired goals of therapy for a patient. It is worth remembering that written correspondence of all types is a reflection on you as a professional and a practitioner. You will always want to proofread this correspondence well. When communicating with a patient in writing, be sure to print the material in a size that the patient can easily read.

Everything we discussed for optimizing verbal communication with your patient applies to written communication. Before communicating with your patient in writing, be sure you have determined how much information your patient wants and what the patient already knows. Your purpose for communicating is always the same, to fill the gap between what the patient wants to know and already knows in a way that a particular patient can best understand. It is not helpful to give the patient more information than is needed or wanted.

Practitioner-focused Communication

Practitioners use a specific practice vocabulary, and it should be employed when communicating with health care providers, whether verbally or in writing. We have emphasized the use of the glossary in this book for this very reason (see Appendix). You should not create new definitions for practice terms or use practice terms differently than intended. All practitioners have an obligation to learn and to use standardized terms so that communication is facilitated at all times.

Your purpose for communicating with colleagues usually involves patient care. You may be asking for help with the care of a patient or providing help to a colleague who is caring for a patient. You may be sharing the care of a patient with a coworker or sharing your knowledge more generally with colleagues and students in the practice setting. All of these clinical situations require effective communication.

It is important that you be precise when discussing a patient's care because confusion can precipitate costly errors on your part. Be concise when you talk with colleagues because neither you nor your colleague has time to waste. You must be complete because anything not mentioned is assumed to be normal, and this could lead to significant misunderstanding.

Going back to "fill in" information for a colleague can be very time consuming.

The Pharmacotherapy Patient Case Presentation Format, which is presented in Chapter 13, presents the standard format for how pharmaceutical care practitioners present patient cases for the purpose of seeking help or provide help to colleagues. It is the format that should be used for discussing a patient case with a colleague, whether verbally or in writing.

Written correspondence with other practitioners   Corresponding with health care providers in writing requires the same attention described for verbal communication with practitioners.

You will be communicating with practitioners in writing most frequently about the care of a specific patient. Identify for your colleague the patient to whom you are referring early in your correspondence. You often will be providing recommendations for specific changes in a patient's drug therapy or initiation of drug therapy. There are a few rules that might be helpful. Always try to provide the patient care provider with two different options from which to choose. However, make sure both options are acceptable to you before presenting them as alternatives. Make clear which of the options you recommend and why you believe this to be the better of the two. When you explain your rationale always compare and contrast effectiveness and safety evidence. You may want to explain to the practitioner under which conditions the second option is better.

Make your written correspondence to other patient care providers precise, concise, and complete so the practitioner does not have questions at the conclusion. If the practitioner has to contact you with questions or is confused by your correspondence, you have created more work, not less. Your purpose should always be to facilitate the care of a patient, not interfere with it.

Only provide information that is necessary for the practitioner to make a decision or to be informed. Reading written correspondence takes time, as does responding to written correspondence. Therefore, whenever possible, provide the practitioner with a quick and easy way to respond. Perhaps checking off or initialing an approval box and returning it is a good alternative.

DOCUMENTATION IN PRACTICE

Another form of written communication that must be mastered by the pharmaceutical care practitioner is the documentation of the care you provide in the pharmaceutical care patient chart.

Documentation is mandatory. The patient chart is the means by which practitioners communicate in a universal language. The pharmaceutical care practitioner must contribute in the same manner as other patient care providers. However, the practice of pharmaceutical care is relatively new, so a clear expectation of where the care is to be recorded in the patient chart might be different in each practice setting. Regardless of where the documentation is located, the most important point is that the care of a patient is always appropriately documented.

> **Definition** Documentation refers to all the patient-specific information, the clinical decisions, and the patient outcomes that are recorded for use in practice. This includes everything written down in long-hand, or entered into a computer program that becomes data and is used to facilitate the care of the patient.

It is not an overstatement to suggest that if you are not documenting the care you provide in a comprehensive manner, then you do not have a practice.

The Pharmaceutical Care Patient Chart

The patient chart is a record of the information collected by practitioners, the decisions made, the actions taken, and the outcomes that result, at the time these events occur. Patient charts are created one patient at a time. The output of this type of documentation is a database describing the patient, drug, and disease information, decisions related to drug choice, dose determinations, modalities of administration, parameters for patient monitoring, and patient outcomes in terms of efficacy, length of treatment, incidence of side effects, toxicity, and other drug-related behaviors.

There are two primary options for the structure of the pharmaceutical care patient chart. This information can become a section in the patient's medical chart, or you can create a separate pharmaceutical care patient chart. In either case, there must be a standard, clearly identifiable pharmaceutical care record for the patient. A progress note may be the way you communicate with a physician in the medical chart, but this will not adequately serve as a pharmaceutical care record.

The pharmaceutical care patient chart must be easily and quickly retrievable at all times. How this is implemented is institution specific because each institution has its own policy governing medical records. Most pharmaceutical care practices establish a separate pharmaceutical care patient chart therefore, this is the context in which documentation will be discussed.

Guidelines for Documenting Pharmaceutical Care

The standards for documentation are described throughout the patient care process (see Chapters 6–9), however, a few general suggestions as to how to improve your skills are discussed here.

Although it takes time to document well, the benefits of a complete and timely patient care record far outweigh the effort. Documentation of patient care is not optional in our health care system. It is mandatory. Patient care cannot be provided, ethically, without a written record of what occurred.

Be timely Learn to document a patient's care as soon as possible after providing the care. This is only logical in that critical information can be forgotten or confused with the passing of time. Also, other people may need to use the information you have about a patient for the patient's benefit, making it necessary to have the information available as soon as possible.

Practitioners themselves usually document the care they provide, however if resources are available, it is possible to dictate the information to be included in the patient chart or to have technical support complete the documentation. Whichever approach is taken, make documentation a priority. The quality of your care depends upon information being available where and when you need it.

Be precise The care of your patient will depend upon details about laboratory values, clinical signs and symptoms, descriptions of your patient's preferences, and much more. It is important that you report exact values, specific impressions, and clear descriptions. Do not guess, do not estimate, and do not be inconclusive about your judgments. Other practitioners may have to make decisions based on what you record—be precise.

Be concise It is important to be short, the point, and not waste words. It takes time to read written or computerized material. Therefore, chose your words carefully, and make each word communicate something specific and unique. This will take practice.

Be complete Costly mistakes are caused by missing information in documentation recording .patient information. When information is missing, practitioners assume that information is either normal or not relevant and both assumptions could be costly to your patient. Suggestions of what to document and how to document it are made in each of the chapters describing the patient care process (see Chapters 6–9).

Reasons to Document Care in Practice

There are a number of reasons to create a pharmaceutical care patient chart in practice. These include to (1) meet the documentation standards that exist for all patient care practitioners; (2) be effective and efficient at caring for patients; (3) limit legal liability; (4) communicate with the patient and the patient's other care providers; (5) obtain reimbursement; (6) present patient cases for learning purposes and to have clinical experience on which to reflect and convert to clinical knowledge; and (7) manage a practice.

Meeting the documentation standard for patient care Patient care practitioners are expected to record the information they use to make decisions about a patient's care, the decisions that were made, and the results of those decisions. Pharmaceutical care is a new practice that will be expected to meet these same practice expectations. All patient care providers have an ethical obligation to be accountable for the decisions they make and the actions they take as well as the results they produce. This is impossible without appropriate documentation. The patient chart is the means by which practitioners communicate with one another about a patient's care. Most, if not all, patient care involves collaborative efforts by multiple patient care providers. Documentation is necessary for this to occur efficiently and effectively. It will be impossible for the practice of pharmaceutical care to be recognized, legitimized, and accepted without proper documentation of the care that is provided on a patient-specific basis by the practitioner.

Being effective and efficient at patient care An important reason for creating the pharmaceutical care patient chart is to provide high quality care to the patient. Documenting patient care information, as well as clinical decisions and outcomes, is a responsibility of each pharmaceutical care practitioner. Documentation is essential because the patient's conditions, needs, and outcomes are constantly changing. The amount of information required to provide pharmaceutical care is so voluminous as to necessitate the recording of the relevant information. No one can remember all the clinically relevant information about an individual.

As the practitioner sees patients repeatedly, and the practice grows, good care will depend on accurate and complete patient records. Records must report decisions made, on a continuous basis, and reflect input from multiple practitioners. Each patient care decision made is based on accumulated results and data derived from all of the previous decisions and outcomes. Therefore, patient care documentation must be a chronological record that can be constantly updated and evaluated to improve patient care.

Also, it will seldom be the case that a practitioner works entirely alone. Technicians, support personnel, and other pharmaceutical care practitioners will all require access to the written patient record. Therefore, it must be complete, consistent with other patient care providers, easily retrievable, and up to date.

Legal purposes   An obvious reason for documentation today, and the one that comes to mind first, is legal liability. All activities performed for another individual must be documented. If, in the future, legal action is brought against the practitioner, appropriate documentation must be available. Comprehensive documentation certainly provides the practitioner with an advantage and can minimize liability. However, even more important, the more comprehensive the documentation, the better it is for the patient because good care depends upon complete and accurate information.

Now, let us concern ourselves with other patient-centered reasons for documenting the pharmaceutical care provided to patients.

Communication purposes   Providing pharmaceutical care is a collaborative effort between the practitioner and the patient as well as the patient's other health care providers. Therefore, there will be numerous occasions for the pharmaceutical care practitioner to communicate with one or all of these individuals. This requires a record of the patient's care.

It may be necessary to generate correspondence to the patient or the patient's care providers, to elicit information about a drug product from a pharmaceutical manufacturer, or to provide information to a clinic or a hospital. All of this requires complete and up-to-date information about the patient and the patient's care.

Reimbursement purposes   The pharmaceutical care patient chart is the physical evidence that care was provided, and this is necessary if you are requesting reimbursement for your services. No third party payer will reimburse a patient care provider unless there is evidence of the specific service provided and a mechanism for auditing the quality of the service. Payers work on the assumption that *if the service was not documented, then it was not done*. Payers usually require specific information be provided to them for the purpose of being reimbursed for a service. There are many different approaches to this, and they are discussed in the First Edition of this text.[25] Whichever approach to reimbursement is used by the practitioner, it will require the generation of a patient care chart.

Patient case presentations and reflection in practice   Practitioners communicate with each other through the recorded patient chart, previously discussed. They also communicate frequently through the presentation of patient cases for the purpose of getting advice, asking questions, sharing responsibilities, or teaching the student (refer to Chapter 13 for a description of the Pharmacotherapy Patient Case Presentation Format). Therefore, information about a patient's case should be quickly and easily accessible to the practitioner. Documentation is necessary for this to occur. The pharmaceutical care patient chart must be accessible, well organized, and consistently kept up to date so that information can be extracted and presented in a timely manner. Sometimes this is a matter of extreme importance for the patient's welfare.

A well-documented patient record is necessary for this to occur. It is necessary to refer back to previous experiences, to recall what decisions you made, and to determine what occurred when certain drug therapies were used.

Managing a pharmaceutical care practice   Although the management of a practice may not be your focus at this time, it will become necessary for you to understand the basic requirements of managing a patient care practice in the not too distant future. Managing a successful practice requires frequent monitoring of practice functions. Workload measurement, performance appraisal, appointment scheduling, billing, and revenue generation, to name just a few, are all functions that require documentation of practice on a daily basis. Without the necessary records, a financially viable practice cannot be maintained.

Most data used to generate management reports come from the patient chart. Therefore, if information is omitted, it is not possible to demonstrate the cost effectiveness of the service, set appointment schedules, or to establish a reimbursement fee.

Paper and Electronic Documentation

Two approaches to documentation are a written paper format and a computerized software program. As early as 1995, pharmaceutical care practitioners stated that is was impossible to imagine providing care without the aid of a computerized software program. This is even more the case today.

The vast amount of patient information that is necessary, the myriad of functions required of those data, and the convenience that is now available from computerized software makes this avenue mandatory. However paper systems may be functional in those situations where students are learning to provide pharmaceutical care. An argument can be made that the initial learning activities could occur without the interference of technology, although even that could be debated. Nevertheless, we present both options here with the understanding that good care requires the management of patient data at a level that requires computerization.

The paper chart   The documentation format that has been developed to support the learning of pharmaceutical care practice can be found in the Appendix. The use of this format for documentation is described in the context of the practice in Chapters 6 through 9. Although there are many different *forms* available today, those presented here were developed specifically to support the practice of pharmaceutical care and are the result of 25 years of experience in providing care to over 20,000 patients.

Advantages of the paper chart   When a student is learning to practice pharmaceutical care, it may be advantageous if he/she does not have to be burdened with learning the nuances of a computerized documentation system at the same time. It is also difficult to use the computer to document a process that is not yet well understood by the student. Therefore, paper may be more efficient during the learning process.

The majority of patient charts in institutions are still paper documents. Although there is obviously a trend to computerize health care functions, the patient chart has been one of the slowest to convert completely to a computerized document. Therefore, this may be an argument for creating a paper chart for pharmaceutical care practice. However, it is certain that in the near future, patient charts will be computerized as well.

Limitations of the paper chart   The paper chart can be time consuming to maintain. Manually recording all the information involved in patient care can be a major undertaking. In addition, the retrieval of information that has been entered manually can be time consuming, often confusing, and sometimes impossible. When information is entered in different locations on the form, handwriting is difficult to interpret, or key elements are omitted, the value of a paper system is compromised. At times care is difficult if more than one practitioner needs the patient chart because its physical location limits its access.

It is very time consuming to conduct research, sort data, evaluate your practice, or make changes when all the patient data is recorded on paper. Reviewing patient charts is time consuming, and it is difficult to translate hand-written text into data.

The use of a computerized program   Few would argue that a computerized documentation system is much more effective and efficient than a paper system. Although it can be cumbersome to learn a new computer system or program, in the long term, the benefits have been shown to far outweigh the costs.

Advantages of the computerized documentation system   Even if you intend to use the data for a number of different purposes, as long as your program can manage relational databases, it is only necessary to enter most information once. The computer program allows you to query, analyze, and generate reports from the data—all the functions that are necessary to become a competent practitioner.

The data entered into the computer is more standardized than freehand documentation. The program requires certain data for all patients, asks for responses in structured formats, and can establish a standard of care for patients that is consistent and comprehensive.

The patient record can be accessed, if necessary, by multiple practitioners in multiple sites. The information can usually be entered from multiple locations so the practitioner is not limited to the physical location of the paper patient chart.

The computerization of patient data is absolutely necessary if there is any intention to conduct research in practice or to justify the establishment of a new practice. Any task that requires easy, quick access to time-bound data will require electronic capabilities.

Limitations of the computer system   Initially, computer documentation systems can be more expensive than paper systems. Practitioners need to take the time to learn the computer software system well so it becomes an asset for the practitioner and not a time-consuming burden. Some practitioners may not be comfortable with technology to the point they can efficiently enter information and extract data as necessary for patient care.

The use of SOAP notes to document pharmaceutical care practice   The question is frequently asked as to why Subjective-Objective-Assessment-Plan (SOAP) notes are not included in the documentation system developed for pharmaceutical care practice. This question results from the use of SOAP notes in other approaches to pharmacist activities and their somewhat extensive use in the practices of nursing and medicine. There are a number of reasons why they are not encouraged in pharmaceutical care practice:

1. There is no common understanding of what S—subjective, and O—objective refers to in the acronym. This often leads to confusion and inconsistency in the information contained in these two sections.
2. Because SOAP notes are written in long-hand and there is no standardization, they can ramble, be difficult to read, and not contribute unique information to the care of the patient.
3. The common practice is to SOAP the medical problem. There is no reason for one more practitioner to SOAP the same medical problem being managed by physicians and nurses. In pharmaceutical care, there is no reason to SOAP the medical problem. The only item that would be rational to SOAP is the drug therapy problem, but the system described in Chapters 6 through 9 deals with drug therapy problems in a much more direct manner and requires more extensive management than what a SOAP note allows.
4. The data in SOAP notes cannot be consolidated and retrieved because they are written in long-hand. Therefore, they cannot be evaluated, summarized, or reported in any standardized format.

The experience of medicine and nursing with this approach suggests that SOAP notes are not as effective or as efficient as they were originally envisioned to be. Even Weed, the creator of the SOAP note suggests that the concept should be rethought.[26] Subjective has become a pejorative term implying that what patients tell us is *all in the mind*, while the data that we clinicians capture is often biased and anything but *objective*.[27,28] Therefore, we suggest using the documentation system described in Chapters 6 through 9 and presented in the Appendix for the practice of pharmaceutical care.

LEARNING TO BE REFLECTIVE IN PRACTICE

Self-improvement must be a goal of all patient care providers. Drug knowledge is constantly expanding, and health care is too complex to know everything all the time, obligating practitioners to establish an active learning routine. There are two important skills you will have to develop to become actively engaged in the self-improvement process: (1) learn how to be reflective in practice to learn the most you can from every patient experience and (2) become proficient at presenting patient cases so you can learn from your colleagues. We will focus on how to become reflective in the remainder of this chapter and discuss how to present patient cases in Chapter 13.

Each interaction with a patient is an opportunity to gain more knowledge. To turn this experience into the most valuable learning situation that is possible, new practitioners need to develop a few reflective skills. These reflective skills take only a few moments, but can dramatically enhance learning, knowledge, and confidence.[29]

Note   Always take a moment and recollect your thoughts and feelings about the encounter you just had with the patient.

As the term implies, reflecting upon what just occurred between you and your patient simply requires a few moments immediately after each patient encounter to critically examine a few key ideas:

- How do you feel about the last patient encounter?
- What went well during the patient visit and why?
- What did not go as well as you would have liked and why not?
- What would you do differently?
- What did you learn from this experience?

Critical reflection is the hallmark of adult learning. Kitchener and King claim it is the seventh stage of learning that only develops in a person's late 20s and early 30s.[30] This would help to explain why students in the professional program do not demonstrate this skill without prompting and are slow to internalize the process to make it part of their routine learning agenda.

These skills can be developed when they are taught, expected, modeled, and reinforced. However, because faculty and mentors must be reflective themselves to teach these skills, there is not as much teaching of reflective skills as is necessary. Therefore, you need to make these skills a learning agenda item in your own active learning process.

Many different strategies have been suggested to develop the skills required in reflection. One of the most useful is the strategy described by the acronym LEARN. These steps can be implemented by you in any practice setting for all types of patients. This strategy combined with the work of Atkins and Murphy helps to create a comprehensive understanding of the skills required to promote reflection in practice. The results are described in Table 12-2 next to each of the skills required to promote reflection.[31]

Table 12-2 Skills to promote reflective learning

Skill	Definition	Strategy to promote reflection
Self-awareness	An honest examination of feelings. How did this experience affect me? How is this experience important to me?	Look back at an experience or event that happened in your practice recently. Review it in your mind as if you were watching a video.
Description	Accurate recall of experiences in detail. What happened including thoughts and feelings?	Elaborate and describe, verbally or in writing, what happened during the event. How did you feel, and how do you think others felt? What were the outcomes? Were you surprised by what happened during the event, or did it turn out as you expected?
Critical analysis	Examining all aspects of the experience including: Challenging assumptions; identifying current knowledge; seeking alternatives. What sense can I make of this experience? What are the significant aspects of this experience? How is this like other experiences?	Analyze the outcomes. Review why the event turned out the way it did. Why did you feel or react the way you did, and why did others feel/react the way they did? If the event or outcomes were not what you expected, consider how you could improve on them next time. This is an opportunity to question your beliefs and assumptions, and ask yourself what the experience reveals about what you value. It is also a great time to ask for feedback from others.
Synthesis	Integration of new and current knowledge to creatively solve problems and predict consequences. How will I apply this to another experience? What will I change or complement in my practice?	Revise your approach based on your review of the event and decide how, or if, you will change your approach. This might involve asking others for ideas for dealing with the situation next time or how to work on a learning need. With your new learning, you may decide to try a new approach, learn more about the subject, or decide that you handled the situation very well.

(Continued)

Table 12-2 (*Continued*) Skills required to promote reflection

Skill	Definition	Strategy to promote reflection
Evaluation	Making value judgments using criteria and standards. How has this experience changed my values, my beliefs? How do I think about others?	New trial. Put your new approach into action. This may require anticipating or creating a situation in which you can then try out your new approach.

This skill is so important that you will want to look for opportunities to develop it whenever possible.[32–35] Selected strategies for stimulating reflection include reading journals, constructing professional portfolios, conducting small group discussions, and performing self-assessments.[36] The reflective process needs to be applied to each patient you care for, from your very first to the very last. Self-improvement needs to be the goal of all patient care practitioners.[36]

SUMMARY

The practice of pharmaceutical care requires the development of a number of clinical skills. These skills include obtaining necessary information from patients, books, available literature and the internet; communicating with patients and practitioners; documenting care in practice and being reflective in practice. None of these skills is complicated, but all of them require time, discipline, and practice to perfect.

EXERCISES

12-1 Select a patient for whom you will provide pharmaceutical care. Seek permission from the patient and schedule a 30–45 minute encounter. Provide care as described in previous chapters. Pay particular attention to the information you elicit from the patient before you ask any questions. Record this information as quickly and completely as is feasible. Reflect on this *observational* information after the patient encounter is completed.

12-2 Practice taking vital signs, including blood pressure and pulse, of at least five different colleagues.

12-3 Obtain permission to review the medical charts of three patients. Complete an assessment documentation form (see Chapter 6) using each chart. Determine the availability and completeness of immunization history, drug allergies, current medical conditions and medications, and past drug therapies.

12-4 Retrieve the following information from the appropriate references:

(a) What are the common presenting signs and symptoms of allergic rhinitis?

(b) What are the most common side effects of St. John's Wort?

(c) What is the evidence that etanercept (Enbrel) is efficacious in the treatment of rheumatoid arthritis?

(d) What is the mechanism of action of losartan thought to be in the treatment of hypertension?

REFERENCES

1. Cole, S.A., Bird, J. *The Medical Interview: The Three-Function Approach.* St. Louis, MO: Mosby Inc.; 2000, pp. 127–128.
2. Lipkin, M.J., Putman, S.M., Lazare, A. *The Medical Interview: Clinical Care, Education, and Research.* New York: Springer; 1995, p. 10.
3. Bickley, L.S., Szilagyi, P.G. *Bates' Guide to Physical Examination and History Taking,* 8th ed. Baltimore, MD: Lippincott Williams and Wilkins; 2003.
4. Gilman, A.G., Hardman, J.G., Limbird, L.E., *Goodman & Gilman's The Pharmacological Basis of Therapeutics,* 10th ed. New York: McGraw-Hill; 2001.
5. Dipiro, J.T., et al. *Pharmacotherapy—A Pathophysiologic Approach,* 5th ed. New York: McGraw-Hill; 2002.
6. Berardi, R.R., DeSimone, E.M., Newton, G.D., Oszko, M.A., Popovich, N.G., Rollins, C.J., Shimp, L.A., Tietze, K.J. *Handbook of Nonprescription Drugs: An Interactive Approach to Self-Care,* 13th ed. Washington, DC: American Pharmaceutical Association; 2002.
7. Koda-Kimble, M.A., Young, L.Y. *Applied Therapeutics: The Clinical Use of Drugs.* Baltimore, MD: Lippincott Williams & Wilkins; 2001, p. 24.
8. Braunwald, E., Fauci, A.S., Kasper, D.L., Hauser, S.L., Longo, D.L., Jameson, J.L., *Harrison's Principles of Internal Medicine,* 15th ed. New York: McGraw-Hill; 2001.
9. McEvoy, G.K. (ed), ASHP, *American Society of Health-Systems Pharmacists. AHFS Drug Information.* Bethesda, MD: American Society of Health-Systems Pharmacists; 2002.
10. Jellin, J.M., Batz, F., Hitchens, K., *Pharmacist's Letter/Prescriber's Letter. Natural Medicines: Comprehensive Database.* Stockton, CA: Therapeutic Research Faculty; 1999.

11. *Drug Facts and Comparisons*. Pocket version, 8th ed. St. Louis, MO: Wolters Kluwer Health; 2004.

12. Anderson, P.O., Knoben, J.E., Troutman, W.G. *Handbook of Clinical Drug Data*, 10th ed. New York: McGraw-Hill; 2002.

13. Lacy, C.F., Armstrong, L.L., Goldman, M.P., Lance, L.L. *Lexi-Comp's: Drug Information Handbook—APhA*, 11th ed. Hudson, OH: Lexi-Comp Inc.; 2003.

14. Gray, J. *Therapeutic Choices*. Canadian Pharmacists Association; 2000. 4th ed. Toronto, Ontario, Canada; 2003.

15. Dambro, M.R. *Griffith's 5-Minute Clinical Consult*, 11th ed. Philadelphia, PA: Lippincott Williams & Wilkins; 2003.

16. Semla, T.P., Beizer, J.L., Higbee, M.D. *Geriatric Dosage Handbook*, 2nd ed. Cleveland, OH: Lexi-Comp Inc.; 1995.

17. Taketomo, C.K., Hodding, J.H., Kraus, D.M. *Pediatric Dosage Handbook*, 3rd ed. Cleveland, OH: Lexi-Comp Inc.; 1996.

18. Jacobs, D.S., DeMott, W.R., Oxley, D.K. *Laboratory Test Handbook*, 2nd ed. Cleveland, OH: Lexi-Comp Inc.; 2002.

19. Foster, S., Tyler, V.E. *Tyler's Honest Herbal: A Sensible Guide to the Use of Herbs and Related Remedies*, 4th ed. New York: The Haworth Press; 1999.

20. Hansten, P.D., Horn, J.R. *The Top 100 Drug Interactions: A Guide to Patient Management*. Edmonds, WA: H&H Publications; 2003.

21. Coulehan, J.L., Block, M.R. *The Medical Interview: Mastering Skills for Clinical Practice*. Philadelphia, PA: F.A. Davis Company; 2001, p. 156.

22. Isetts, B.J., Brown, L.B., Patient Assessment and Consultation, in: Berardi, R.R., DeSimone, E.M., Newton, G.D., Oszko, M.A., Popovich, N.G., Rollins, C.J., Shimp, L.A., Tietze, K.J. (eds), *Handbook of Nonprescription Drugs: An Interactive Approach to Self-Care*, 14th ed. Washington, DC: American Pharmaceutical Association; 2004, in press.

23. Ruesch, J. *Therapeutic Communication*. New York: W.W. Norton & Company Inc.; 1961, p. 7.

24. Ziegler, D.K., Mosier, M.C., Buenaver, M., Okuyemi, K. How much information about adverse effects of medication do patients want from physicians? *Arch Intern Med* 2001; 161:706–713.

25. Cipolle, R., Strand, L.M., Morley, P.C. *Pharmaceutical Care Practice*. New York: McGraw Hill; 1998.

26. Weed, L.L. *Medical Records, Medical Education, and Patient Care*. Case Western Reserve, Cleveland, OH: University Press; 1971, p. 18.

27. Wyatt, J.C. Clinical data systems. Part 1. Data and medical records. *The Lancet* 1994, 344(8936):1543–1547.

28. Weed, L.L. New connections between medical knowledge and patient care. *Br Med J* 1997; 315(7102): 231–235.

29. Isetts, B.J. Evaluation of pharmacy students' abilities to provide pharmaceutical care. *Am J Pharm Educ* 1999; 63:11–20.

30. Kitchener, K.S., King, P.M. The reflective judgement model: transforming assumptions about knowing. *Fostering Critical Reflection in Adulthood*. San Francisco: Jossey-Bass; 1990.

31. Atkins, S., Murphy, K. Reflection: a review of the literature. *J Adv Nursing* 1993; 18:1188–1192.

32. James, C.R., Clarke, B.A. Reflective practice in nursing: issues and implications for nurse education. *Nurse Educ Today* 1994; 14:82–90.

33. Jarvis, P. Reflective practice and nursing. *Nurse Educ Today* 1992; 12:174–181.

34. Reed, J., Koliba, C. *Facilitating Reflection: A Manual for Leaders and Educators*. Accessed August 26, 2003, www.uvm.edu/~dewey/reflection manual/.

35. Schon, D.A. *The Reflective Practitioner: How Professionals Think in Action*. Basic Books Inc. USA; 1983.

36. Rideout, E. *Transforming Nursing Education through Problem-based Learning*. Mississauga, CA: Jones and Bartlett Publishers; 2001.

THIRTEEN

THE PHARMACOTHERAPY PATIENT CASE PRESENTATION

Key Concepts

[1] *Practitioners present patient cases to seek help from colleagues, provide help to colleagues, and share information about unique patient cases.*

[2] *The specific format ensures that complete and accurate information is communicated by the practitioner and understood by the audience (often other practitioners).*

[3] *The structure of the presentation follows the Pharmacotherapy Workup and the patient care process of (1) practitioner's assessment of the patient's drug-related needs; (2) identification of drug therapy problems; (3) care plan development; and (4) follow-up evaluation.*

[4] *Guidelines for presenting a patient case are as follows:*
  - *Prepare*
  - *Describe your purpose for presenting the case*
  - *Describe the associations between the patient, his/her diseases, and the drug therapy being taken/administered*
  - *Include evidence of effectiveness and safety of the drug therapies*
  - *Practice, practice, practice*

[5] *Common problems include using inappropriate terminology, not following a structured organization, including too little or too much information, and not being clear and concise in your speaking.*

[6] *Written patient case presentations follow the same format as verbal presentations.*

PURPOSE OF THE PATIENT CASE PRESENTATION

A practitioner is judged by peers according to how well he/she cares for patients. Interestingly, practitioners usually do not directly observe their colleagues as they provide care, yet all practitioners develop opinions regarding who is skilled and who is not. Have you ever considered how practitioners develop these opinions? Opinions are formed when practitioners present patient cases.

Patient cases are presented to colleagues on a daily basis, for three primary reasons. First, one practitioner needs another to assume responsibility for a patient when leaving a shift, taking a vacation, or sharing responsibilities. Second, a practitioner needs advice from a colleague concerning the care of a patient. Third, and most frequently in the case of student practitioners, to present patient cases to a mentor/practitioner when learning to care for patients. You will be expected to present numerous patient cases, so it is important to learn the skills to do this properly as early in your career as possible.

NEED FOR A SPECIFIC FORMAT

All patient care providers present patient cases to their colleagues including physicians, nurses, dentists, and veterinarians. The specific format for the case presentation is dictated by each practitioner's primary function. The physician presents patient information for the purpose of arriving at a diagnosis of the medical problem. The nurse focuses on presenting nursing care problems and the dentist on dental problems. Therefore, the case presentation for each practitioner is slightly different from the others. This is also true for the pharmaceutical care practitioner. The case presentation format in pharmaceutical care practice is structured to present patient information for the purpose of identifying, resolving, and preventing drug therapy problems. Therefore, sharing information about a patient requires skill and proficiency, but it starts with knowing your role and responsibilities.

The case presentation is a specific speaking format that allows efficient transfer of information that can be technical and complex.[1,2] The Pharmacotherapy Case Presentation Format is such a structure. A case presentation should consist of selected and processed data from the Pharmacotherapy Workup and must be delivered in a lucid, precise manner. The oral presentation of a patient's case is usually an abbreviated effort. It includes all of the important positive findings and a few pertinent negative findings; however, information that you may have gathered, but did not use to make decisions or provide care for the patient are not included in your presentation.

All pharmacotherapy case presentations begin with a brief description of the patient. They contain the same core information, including medical conditions, drug therapy problems, associated drug therapies, and resulting outcomes. All case presentations end by summarizing the information you feel is most relevant to your understanding of how to optimize the patient's medication experience.

You will always use the same order for the presentation because both the presenter and the practitioners listening to the case follow the same structure. The listeners are prepared to listen a certain way. They expect you to describe the patient's case using a specific format. The best way to organize your case presentation is the same way you conduct the work, according to the Pharmacotherapy Workup. Table 13-1 describes the major

Table 13-1 Pharmacotherapy Patient Case Presentation Format

Assessment

Brief description of the patient (age, gender, appearance)

Primary reason for the patient encounter or visit

Additional patient background/demographics

The medication experience as reported by the patient (wants, expectations, concerns, understanding, preferences, attitudes, and beliefs that determine the patient's medication taking behavior)

Comprehensive medication history (allergies, alerts, social drug use, and immunization status)

Current medication record: description of all medical conditions being managed with pharmacotherapy with the following associations made:

Indication–Drug product–Dosage regimen–Result to date

Relevant past medical history: outcomes of past medication use

Review of systems

Identification of drug therapy problems: description of the drug therapy problem, medications involved, and causal relationships

Prioritization of multiple drug therapy problems

Summary of the assessment

The Care Plan (for each indication)

Goals of therapy

Clinical and laboratory parameters used to define the goals of therapy

   Observable, measurable value and timeline for each

How you plan to resolve the patient's drug therapy problems

   Therapeutic alternative approaches considered

   Rationale for your product and dosage selections

How you plan to achieve the goals of therapy

Nonpharmacologic interventions

Prevention of drug therapy problems

Schedule for follow-up evaluation

Follow-up Evaluation

Clinical and/or laboratory evidence of effectiveness of drug therapies for each indication

Clinical and/or laboratory evidence of safety of every drug regimen

Evidence of compliance

Evaluation of outcome status

Changes required in drug therapies

Schedule for future evaluations

Summary of Case

sections of the Pharmacotherapy Patient Case Presentation Format presentation in detail.

Colleagues will expect you to have done your work in order to present your patient's case. It will be unfair to present a patient for whom a comprehensive Pharmacotherapy Workup has not been completed. Therefore, if there are any aspects of the workup you have not completed, this must be made known during the case presentation.

During a case presentation your decisions are described and your rationale is explained. Drug therapy problems are a good example. During the presentation of your patient's case, you will need to describe which drug therapy problem your patient has and how you decided to resolve it. Case presentations are not like novels or mystery stories for your listeners to try to solve. You have already completed the assessment, identified drug therapy problems, constructed care plans, and may have evaluated your patient's outcomes. The case presentation tells the story of what you found, what you did, and what happened.

Some case presentations are designed for the purpose of obtaining assistance from a colleague. You might need help in determining what your patient's drug therapy problem is or what might be the best approach to achieving the goals of therapy. In either situation, your presentation should inform your colleague what help you need.

> **Example** "I have not been able to determine why my patient is not responding to her drug therapy. I would appreciate your opinion about what the drug therapy problem might be in this case."

Listening to the presentation of a patient case, one can tell if the presenter knows his or her patient's drug therapy problems and can properly process and organize data. Even the most complicated case should be presented in a minimum amount of time. The story becomes lengthy when the student is not confident of his or her skill in identifying the clinically relevant information. The more thought and organization that goes into it, the shorter the presentation becomes. When the story rambles on and on, it often means that the presenter cannot organize the clues or his/her thoughts, make decisions or solve the patient's problems.

YOUR FIRST CASE PRESENTATION

Case presentations employ a unique format, contain new vocabulary, and often involve patients, diseases, and drug therapies that are new to the student. Therefore the first time a student is asked to present a patient case to a group of colleagues or faculty can be quite intimidating. To become proficient at case presentation skills, start with the fundamentals. Do not feel as though you need to master all of these new skills and all of the new information during your first attempt.

Your first few attempts need not display the student's pharmacotherapeutic prowess, but rather these initial presentations are best used to practice organization, communication, and decision-making skills. To get started, focus on a few key steps of the process. These include: a brief description of your patient; the primary reason for the encounter; and your patient's active medical conditions with associated drug therapies. Be clear about the drug therapy problem(s) you decide your patient has. For each care plan, describe the goals of therapy, the changes you recommend in your patient's drug therapy, and your plan and schedule for the next follow-up evaluation.

Note that all of these fundamental items inform your audience of who your patient is, what illnesses are presently being managed with medications, what you are attempting to achieve, and when you will know if your plan is working. Note that the drug therapies and interventions you recommend are only one portion of your case presentation. Although these *answers* may seem important, learning the case presentation structure is the focus of your first presentations.

It is useful to present your first few cases as though you are asking a colleague for advice in determining the nature of your patient's drug therapy problem.

> **Example** "I would like your help in identifying my patient's drug therapy problem. G.W. is a 57-year-old…" This presentation can continue through the first three fundamental steps and end with "what do you think my patient's drug therapy problem might be?"

The primary purpose is to practice clearly describing the patient, by organizing the patient's information about medical conditions and/or illnesses being managed with drug therapies, and their effectiveness up to now. This can be a considerable amount of information to have gathered, analyzed, researched, and organized within your Pharmacotherapy Workup. Presenting this much of a patient's case for the first few times lets you become comfortable with the structured format of a pharmacotherapy case presentation.

Future case presentations can focus on determining a clinically appropriate care plan and follow-up evaluation schedule. The focus of these case presentations is planning the timing for the parameters to determine the effectiveness and safety of all of the patient's drug therapies.

Any advice you intend to request from a colleague, instructor, mentor, or practitioner concerning one of your patients must be asked for within the Pharmacotherapy Case Presentation Format. For instance, if you are asking your colleague whether an unusual side effect can be caused by a certain drug your patient is taking, you will ask it in the context of your patient's case.

> **Example** "Dr. Johnson, I would like to know if you have ever heard about or seen a patient who has had this side effect from a medication. My patient is a 59-year-old male taxicab driver who weighs about 150 lb and has presented with a new complaint of swelling and edema of both ankles and feet which he thinks started shortly after he began taking a new drug treatment for his back pain..."

In order to become comfortable, competent, and confident at making case presentations, you need to practice. However, repetition alone is not sufficient. Repeating mistakes and bad habits can slow your development as a competent practitioner. As a student practitioner, you need to take full advantage of every opportunity to obtain feedback on your ability to make case presentations. There are numerous methods to obtain the necessary help in developing your case presentation skills.[3] Students, instructors, and/or mentors can listen to your presentations and provide constructive feedback. Student colleagues can help one another by providing honest feedback. Videotaping yourself while making case presentations can be especially instructive in the areas of nonverbal communication skills as well as revealing speech habits that you may not be aware that you use.

ASSESSMENT OF THE PATIENT'S DRUG-RELATED NEEDS

Brief Description of the Patient

All case presentations begin with a brief description of the patient. This provides your colleagues with a mental picture of this individual. Practitioners need to *see* the patient to care for him or her. This should be simple, straightforward, and include how the patient appeared to you (physically, emotionally, and health-wise). Your introduction of the patient should include age, gender, and physical description (height, weight, and ethnic origin if it is germane to the care this patient). Be sensitive to the words you use and how you say them. Patient names and other patient identifiers (address, telephone numbers) are seldom appropriate in a case presentation as you are responsible to always maintain patient confidentiality.[4] An exception to this is if you are formally transferring or referring a patient to another practitioner. In these situations you will give the patient's full name to your colleague. Your goal is to provide your audience with a mental picture of a person they may not have met.

> **Example**   M.J. is a 23-year-old female who is 5 ft 3 in tall and weighs 132 lb.

> Mr. W. is a 71-year-old Caucasian male who is approximately 6 ft tall and of average weight.

> B.L. is a 55-year-old, 6 ft 3 in 220 lb male construction worker who appears very uncomfortable due to his recent work-related injury to his right hand.

Reason for the Patient Encounter

The next item discussed is the description of the patient's reason for the encounter with the practitioner. Your description should focus on the patient's initial request or the precipitating event.

It is most helpful to use the patient's own words when describing his/her initial request for care. Therefore, your description may include direct quotations from the patient describing his or her perceptions of need. This might include items the patient does not understand, expressed concerns, or expectations that are unrealistic. Using the patient's own words avoids adding your own bias or interpretation onto the patient's description of his/her primary concern.[5]

When presenting a description of the patient's original reason for the encounter, be certain to describe how that *chief complaint* directed your assessment interview. You may also need to include the patient's presenting signs, symptoms, or illness behavior and a description of the patient's general health.

> **Example**   M.J. presented to our pharmaceutical care clinic with a cough that has "kept me awake for the past two nights."

> Mr. W. was referred to me by Dr. Samuelson for assessment and continued follow-up of his anticoagulant therapy. Mr. W. explained that he has "been taking these pills for over 6 years, and I don't know why they keep taking blood samples."

B.L. asked us to contact his primary care physician and obtain "a new drug that will work" to relieve the pain and inflammation in his injured right hand.

The patient background summarizes the context in which the patient lives. The intent is to provide your colleagues with a more complete image of your patient as an individual. In order to fully understand your patient's drug-related needs, you may need to describe his/her employment, family support, and socioeconomic status. Lifestyle, living conditions, occupation, and family (or other care-givers affected by the person's illness) can all impact the patient's medication taking beliefs, behaviors, and outcomes. A patient's functional capacity (physical, emotional, and social) should also be included here.

The last portion of the background will include a description of any special needs the patient has. Language barriers, physical limitations (hearing or sight, walking restrictions), or diverse cultural backgrounds (beliefs, religion, traditions) should all be noted if they impact the drug therapy decisions that will be made. It is important to be respectful of individual differences and sensitive when describing patient characteristics that represent beliefs or lifestyles that differ from your own.

Example   M.J. has a history of animal allergies and has recently begun taking care of her partner's three cats.

Mr. W. lives alone in a gated retirement community. He uses a cane to assist with walking and requires large print books and newspapers to read due to his failing eyesight.

B.L. recently moved from Mexico and speaks very little English. His oldest daughter accompanied him to help as an interpreter.

Medication Experience Reported by the Patient

The patient's medication experience includes a summary of the relevant events in a patient's lifetime that involve drug therapy. This summary will include the patient's attitudes, beliefs, and preferences about drug therapy that have been shaped by the patient's experiences, traditions, religion, and culture. This information is most useful when it, too, is presented in the patient's own words. The focus of this portion of your presentation is to describe how your patient makes decisions about using medications.

The patient's medication experience is important because it forms the context in which to understand the remaining information in the case. This information helps you to understand the *whole* person and will be necessary as you try to identify common ground on which to develop the care plan.

> **Example**   M.J. explained that this type of cough has occurred "at least three or four times in the past, whenever my partner brings her cats to my apartment. I think it is because of the cats, but I really like animals."
>
> Mr. W. has been meticulously observant of all his appointments to have his INR measured and his warfarin dosage adjusted. He keeps a record of all his past INR results in his wallet.
>
> B.L. asked his daughter to ask why he had to see a physician, just to get some more pain medication. In his hometown in Mexico, that was not required. He could purchase most medications his family needed at any pharmacy.

Now that your audience has a fairly complete description of the patient as a person, the reason for the encounter, and an understanding of the medication experience, it is necessary to focus on the patient's medication history and current medication record. A comprehensive description of your patient's medications involves several important areas. These include allergies, alerts, immunization records, and social drug use that may impact your decisions about medications as well as all of your patient's current medical conditions or illnesses and pharmacotherapies used to manage them at this time.

Comprehensive Medication History

Allergies and alerts/social drug use/immunization record   To describe a complete medication history and to include all the information necessary to prevent drug therapy problems, it is necessary to describe any allergies (and associated allergens) or adverse reactions to previously taken drug therapy. In your case presentation, it is important to clearly differentiate drug allergies from adverse drug reactions that your patient may have experienced in the past. To do this, you will want to include the nature of the reaction, the timing of the reaction relative to the specific drug therapy, and the consequences of the episode. Describing how the episode was treated is often useful. It is also important to describe your interpretation of future risk to the patient should he/she be exposed to the drug.

Smoking, alcohol, and recreational drug use can all influence your patient's risk for certain diseases and drug therapy outcomes. Therefore, a clear and honest description of this information is necessary, as well as a determination of the consequences it can have on this patient's care. It should be emphasized that patient confidence and consent should be assured as they relate to reporting recreational drug use. Your responsibility is to emphasize the association between sensitive information and the drug therapy decisions being made that you choose to share with your colleagues.

Prevention is one of the primary responsibilities in pharmaceutical care. Therefore, the patient's immunization history is an essential aspect of the Pharmacotherapy Workup and case presentation. This is especially true in vulnerable populations such as children, immunocompromised patients, and the elderly. The degree to which your patient's immunization status is current is an important part of every pharmacotherapy case presentation. Plans to provide necessary immunizations can also be included. Up-to-date information should be reported, and when it is not available, it should be sought.

> **Example** M.J. reports no drug allergies, but is allergic to animal dander and some forms of nuts which manifest as severe itching and rash that respond to benadryl (diphenhydramine) and cool compresses. She has never used tobacco and drinks 1 or 2 alcoholic beverages only on social occasions.
>
> Mr. W. indicated he was allergic to codeine. He reported that he had to go to the emergency department because he developed angioedema shortly after he took his first dose of Tylenol with codeine for a dental procedure in 1998. He quit smoking cigarettes after his wife died in 1991. He reports no use of alcohol of any type.
>
> B.L. reports no history of any drug or food allergies. He describes his alcohol use as *two beers after work* and does not smoke cigarettes or cigars.

Current Medication Record: Indication–Drug Product–Dosage Regimen–Outcome

An essential portion of every pharmacotherapy case presentation is the patient's current medication record. Pharmaceutical practitioners add substantial and useful information to every patient's case by gathering and analyzing patient, disease, and drug data and creating new information in the format of indication–drug therapy–outcome.

The pharmacotherapy case presentation format calls for a specific approach to describing your patient's current drug regimens. This format uses a comprehensive method to describe each drug the patient is taking. First the indication is described, then the specific drug product, then the dosage regimen the patient is taking and how long he/she has been taking it at that dosage, and finally the response the patient has exhibited or described that has resulted from that drug therapy.

Recall that the framework for your Pharmacotherapy Workup asked you to assess the relationships between indication, drug product, dosage regimen, and outcome. This same unique framework is applied to the method you use to describe your patient's medication usage.

> **Example**   M.J. is presently treating tendonitis of the right elbow with ibuprofen 600 mg taken three times each day for the past 5 days. She is satisfied with the relief of both the pain and stiffness and has not experienced any gastrointestinal side effects.

> Mr. W. is presently taking warfarin 2.5 mg orally each morning for prevention of a stroke or myocardial infarction secondary to his long-standing atrial fibrillation. His most recent INR was 2.2 last month and he has not experienced any bleeding therefore no dosage adjustments were made at that time.

> B.L. has been taking aspirin, 325 mg two times each day, for the past 3 days with no relief of his pain or inflammation of the right hand.

The medication record is organized by therapeutic indication. When your patient is taking several medications for one indication, all of them are described together.

> **Example**   Mr. W. is presently taking warfarin 2.5 mg orally each morning for prevention of a stroke or myocardial infarction secondary to his long-standing atrial fibrillation. His INR last month was 2.2, and no dosage adjustments were made at that time. His heart rate and rhythm have been successfully controlled for the past three years with digoxin 0.25 mg orally every day, furosemide 20 mg each morning, and oral potassium supplement of 20 meq daily. A review of systems revealed that Mr. W. has not experienced any adverse reactions from his drug therapies.

The medication record is complete when you describe the patient's overall understanding of the medications he/she is taking and the patient's ability and willingness to comply with instructions.

Past Medical History and Associated Drug Therapies

Next you may need to describe the pertinent portions of the patient's past medical history. Keep in mind that this is a pharmacotherapy case presentation and not the presentation of a patient's complete medical workup. Therefore, present only the information and experience you used to make current drug therapy decisions. Past medical history is used most often to describe those experiences in the patient's past that suggest a risk factor or contraindication to drug therapy. These situations may include: serious illnesses, hospitalizations, surgical procedures, accidents and injuries, pregnancies, deliveries, and complications to any medical treatments.

> **Example** M.J. was diagnosed with exercise-induced asthma at 7 years of age but has not needed any drug therapy or other medical care for that condition for the past 8 years.
>
> Mr. W. had dental surgery last April at which time his warfarin was discontinued for 7 days and then restarted without incident.

Providing any evidence of success or failure of past attempts at treating or preventing an illness can be a very informative portion of your case presentation. If you discover that a specific form of drug therapy had failed to produce the desired response in your patient in the past, then explaining that finding can clarify why you have chosen certain other forms of pharmacotherapy. Similarly, if you know that a drug product or a dosage regimen was effective at treating the same problem your patient has at this time, then that information becomes essential to include in your pharmacotherapy case presentation.

> **Example** M.J. is presently treating tendonitis of the right elbow with ibuprofen 600 mg taken three times each day for the past 5 days. She is satisfied with the relief of both the pain and stiffness. The week prior, she attempted to treat her tendonitis by taking 200 mg twice daily but felt no relief.
>
> M.J. also reported that she attempted to treat a similar cough with dextromethorphan last spring, but "that medication did not help much and it upset my stomach."
>
> In 1999, Mr. W. was instructed to take 2.5 mg of warfarin every other day, alternating with 5 mg, but he could not seem to keep track of his dosing schedule. He was seen in clinic on two occasions that year with

bleeding from the nose. He reported that his INR was "way too high because I was taking too much medicine."

Review of Systems

There are several situations in which you will need to present positive or negative findings from the review of systems:

- To establish the relationship of the finding to the drug therapy the patient is taking. This is either evidence of the presence or absence of a side effect or adverse drug reaction.
  "The review of systems revealed that the patient was not nauseous or agitated and has not experienced headache or dizziness and showed no other side effects from her fluoxetine."
- To identify additional drug therapy needs of the patient that were not discovered during your assessment interview.
  "The review of systems revealed that the patient has experienced excessive bruising over the past 3–4 months thought to be related to..."
- To present your interpretation of any abnormal or unexpected findings.
  "The review of systems revealed that the patient experienced a feeling of fullness in the abdomen, which subsided when she started her ranitidine therapy.

The report of the review of systems represents a systematic review of physical findings, descriptions, and experiences offered by the patient and laboratory values not already associated with a specific medical condition (and reported earlier). The review of systems must be presented in a concise and useful manner. Only the important positive and pertinent negative findings and laboratory tests should be reported.

> **Example** The review of systems was unremarkable except for his report of intermittent nausea over the past 2 weeks which the patient feels is a result of his new diet.

Always make the association between the finding and drug therapy for the listener. If you have a series of values to report, presentation of the data in a flow sheet or graph is preferable.

Summary of the Assessment

The summary of the assessment should include a brief review of your clinical judgment regarding the patient, his/her active medical conditions, associated drug therapies, and any drug therapy problems identified. Your summary should report your judgment as to whether you think that all of your patient's drug therapy is appropriately indicated, the most effective available, as safe as possible, and whether the patient is taking it as intended. This summary informs your colleagues where you are in the course of the case presentation.

> **Example**   "The summary of my assessment of M.J. is that she is a healthy 23-year-old female who is bothered by coughing in the evening, which is disrupting her sleep and is felt to be a manifestation of her allergies to cat dander. We will need to provide drug therapy to control these symptoms as she will be in contact with cats for the next 2 weeks."

The summary need only be a few sentences as you are only including the most important data that were used to make your clinical decisions.

DRUG THERAPY PROBLEM IDENTIFICATION

Problem–Drug Therapy–Cause and Effect

If drug therapy problems have been identified, they must be stated clearly during your presentation of the patient's case. There is a specific format used to describe a patient's drug therapy problems. This format has three parts that must be described together: (a) the medical condition associated with the drug therapy problem, (b) the drug therapy involved, and (c) the relationship (cause and effect) between the medical problem and the drug therapy. It must be clearly stated so your colleagues can understand your clinical decision.

> **Example**   "The patient's ibuprofen dosage of 200 mg twice a day was too low to provide effective relief of her tendonitis."
>
> "The patient requires potassium supplements to prevent diuretic-induced hypokalemia."
>
> "The patient has developed orthostatic hypotension due to the excessive dosage increase of her enalapril."
>
> "The patient prefers not to take his cefuroxime suspension for pharyngitis because of the poor taste."

Remember this represents one of the most important clinical decisions you make. The identification of the patient's drug therapy problems is to the pharmacotherapy case presentation what the diagnosis is to the medical case presentation. The drug therapy problems should be prioritized based on the patient's needs, and those being addressed currently should be differentiated from those to be addressed in the future.

In addition, if your patient has any risk factors for specific drug therapy problems that need to be prevented at this time, this should also be stated here.

THE CARE PLAN

Identifying your patient's drug-related needs, as well as resolving and preventing drug therapy problems, requires an organized care planning process. Therefore, presenting the care plans you have constructed for your patient also requires organization. The care plan should be organized and prioritized by active medical conditions being managed with drug therapy. The problems should be presented in order of risk, severity, and importance to the patient.

The care plan is complete when you can describe how to manage the medical condition with drug therapies and other nondrug interventions. For each medical condition, you will need to present your plan to resolve any drug therapy problems associated with that medical condition, a clear description of the goals of therapy, and the interventions you intend to make to achieve the goals of therapy and prevent any drug therapy problems from occurring in the patient.

> **Example** "Our goal is to eliminate the orthostatic hypotension by holding her enalapril for 1 day and then reducing the daily dosage regimen of enalapril to 10 mg twice each day, beginning on Tuesday."

When describing the goals, be certain to include the timeframe in which you expect to achieve each goal.

> **Example** "The goal of therapy is to reduce and then maintain her blood pressure at a systolic of 120–130 mmHg and a diastolic of 70–80 mmHg within the next 4 weeks."

Generally, therapeutic alternatives to resolve drug therapy problems are only presented if controversial, if you are still uncertain about your decision, or if your mentor needs to know that you have considered all of the reasonable therapeutic choices. When presenting the therapeutic alternatives considered and the drug therapy selected, be sure to explain the rationale for your choice. When describing pharmacotherapy rationale always explain both the efficacy and safety considerations for each alternative. What is the comparative efficacy, and what is the comparative safety of the multiple products you considered? Additional considerations (cost and convenience) can be described here too, but efficacy and safety are always the required minimum.

Interventions are complete if they include who is responsible for the activity: you, the patient, or another practitioner. The final information you will present in your care plan section of the presentation is the schedule for follow-up meetings with the patient. This plan should also include the parameters you intend to use to evaluate the effectiveness of your plan and the parameters you plan to use to evaluate the safety of your patient's drug therapies.

> **Example** "The patient will take her own blood pressure every morning and record it on her medication diary. She will also record any feelings of dizziness or lightheadedness. I will evaluate these records at the next appointment on August 23. I will evaluate renal function using blood urea nitrogen, serum creatinine, and potassium determinations at that visit. I will also inquire to determine if she has developed a cough from her enalapril therapy."

FOLLOW-UP EVALUATION

Some case presentations focus on a single, recent follow-up evaluation.[1] In these situations, your presentation generally follows the above outline with respect to briefly describing the patient, the main conditions, and the drug therapies involved. For presentations of the follow-up evaluation, your focus is on the evidence of success or failure of past care plans and interventions.

The presentation of a follow-up evaluation generally has three sections. First, you must briefly review the patient and what you were trying to achieve at previous visits. This generally focuses on resolution of drug therapy problems and achieving goals of therapy. Second, you will describe what happened to the patient (patient outcome) since the last visit. You will need to compare the patient's outcomes to what was intended (goals of therapy). This comparison is based on clinical and/or laboratory findings used as evidence of effectiveness and safety of drug therapies and patient compliance. Third, you present your clinical judgment (evaluation) of the patient's progress toward achieving the goals of therapy as of the date of the follow-up presentation being described. It is most useful to be consistent in your use of outcome terminology. The terms to describe pharmacotherapy outcome status include resolved, stable, improved, partially improved, worsened, and failure. It is important to be clear in your use of these outcome status categories (see Chapter 9).

Finally, report any new drug therapy problems the patient may have developed since the previous evaluation.

> **Example**   "As you will recall, we had reduced this patient's dosage of enalapril 4 weeks ago due to episodes of orthostatic hypotension. I think we have successfully resolved that drug therapy problem. Today, she reports one episode of slight dizziness that diminished within 2 minutes. She has no other complaints including no cough associated with her drug therapy. Her renal function tests have not changed over the past month and all remain within normal limits. Her blood pressure readings over the past month have steadily declined to a daily range of 124–130 over 75–80 mmHg, which are within the planned goal of 120–130 over 70–80 mmHg. My evaluation at this visit is that her blood pressure control has improved, and no changes should be made in her drug regimen at this time. She has no new problems to report at this time. I plan to reevaluate her hypertension pharmacotherapy in 3 months."

SUMMARY OF THE CASE

The case presentation ends with a brief summary of the most cogent points. Be sure to summarize the drug-related needs of the patient, the resolution and prevention of drug therapy problems, as well as evidence of effectiveness and safety of the patient's pharmacotherapy.

COMMON PROBLEMS IN THE CASE PRESENTATION

Because case presentations are indicative of a student's capacity to process data and solve clinical problems, some common errors should be mentioned. Items frequently omitted from student case presentations include the primary reason the patient sought care, the original reason for admission to the hospital or clinic, the nonprescription medications being used as self-care and their indications, evidence of the patient's ability to understand and adhere to the medication instructions, and evidence that the drug therapy is being effective. Such deficiencies invariably lead to confusion and questions that interrupt the case presentation.

The terminology used in patient case presentations will communicate your preparedness, your experience, and your standard of care. Be sure to use appropriate practice vocabulary and be precise in the words you choose. It is also important to be as concise as possible because you are either seeking help or providing it, and the listener's time is valuable.

The objective of the patient case presentation format is to make the presentation of the case efficient. This depends on your organization of the patient information, your clinical decisions, and the patient responses. Be complete, but do not include any information that is not directly relevant to the objective for presenting the case. Remember that omitted information is the source of the most confusion in case presentations.

The strength of the case presentation format is its simplicity. Be sure not to negate this by being confusing, long-winded, or making the case appear complex when it is not. These are the most common problems encountered by new practitioners.

WRITTEN CASE SUMMARIES

Written case presentations are very similar in format to the verbal presentations described in this chapter. The outline and contents are the same, but a few differences exist.

A written case presentation, often referred to as a *write up*, should include headings or subheadings for major sections (description of patient, current medication record, drug therapy problems) to help the reader locate information.[2] It is necessary to use quotations when using the patient's own words. Write-ups often include tables to summarize multiple drug therapies and/or laboratory results.

Your write-up may become part of the patient's permanent record, so attend to the accuracy and concise nature of the words you include. Always sign your work and indicate how others can contact you if they have questions.

EXAMPLE OF A PHARMACOTHERAPY CASE PRESENTATION

The following is an example of a Pharmacotherapy Case Presentation.

Brief description of the patient M.J. is a 23-year-old female who is 5 ft 3 in tall and weighs 132 lb.

Primary reason for the encounter   She presented to our pharmaceutical care clinic concerned about a cough that she explained has "kept me awake for the past two nights."

Additional patient background   M.J. has a history of animal allergies including cat dander and has recently been taking care of her partner's three cats. She feels the cough is related to the cats, but would like to continue to care for the cats until her partner returns in 2 weeks.

Medication experience   She has not attempted to treat this episode of the cough, but she did attempt to treat a similar cough last spring using dextromethorphan. M.J. described that she prefers not to take dextromethorphan again, as it caused her to "feel nauseated and it did not help much".

Comprehensive medication history   She reports no drug allergies and does not use tobacco. She uses alcohol only on special social occasions which averages two to three times per month. She is up to date with her immunizations and received her annual influenza vaccine at her place of employment last month.

Current medication record   M.J. is presently treating an episode of tendonitis of the right elbow with ibuprofen 600 mg three times daily for the past 5 days. She originally tried 200 mg twice daily, but found no relief. The increased dosage of ibuprofen is providing satisfactory relief and she reports no gastrointestinal upset from this therapy.

Relevant past medical history   M.J. describes herself as being in excellent health with no chronic medical conditions. She has a history of exercise-induced asthma at age 7, but has not needed any drug therapy or medical care for the past 8 years.

Review of systems   A brief review of systems revealed no cardiovascular, renal, or gastrointestinal problems. As for her respiratory status, she reported only the cough and no shortness of breath or wheezing. M.J. is not pregnant.

Summary of the Assessment   The summary of my assessment of M.J. is that she is a healthy 23-year-old female who is bothered by coughing in the evening, which is disrupting her sleep and is felt to be a manifestation of her allergies to cat dander.

Drug therapy problem Her drug therapy problem is that she requires additional drug therapy to relieve the symptoms (cough) she is experiencing secondary to her animal allergies. M.J. agreed with this assessment.

Care plan Relief of symptoms associated with allergies to cat dander.

Goals of therapy We discussed goals of therapy and agreed that achieving a restful night of sleep tonight and for the next two nights without the constant coughing would be most desirable. During the day she is at work and leaves the cats alone in her apartment, so the cough is not a problem at work.

Therapeutic alternatives We discussed several alternatives including cough suppressants (codeine and dextromethorphan, which was not effective in the past) and antihistamines such as diphenhydramine, chlorpheniramine, and less sedating agents such as loratadine.

Pharmacotherapy M.J. was started on diphenhydramine HCl (Benadryl) 25 mg orally in the afternoon after work and 25 mg at bedtime. She agreed that if it caused her to feel drowsy, that might be beneficial in her case. She will also make her bedroom off limits to the cats in an attempt to minimize her exposure to allergens.

She will also continue taking 600 mg of ibuprofen three times each day for tendonitis.

Plan for follow-up evaluation I plan to follow-up and evaluate her new therapy next Tuesday and will evaluate effectiveness in terms of restful sleep and to make certain that she is not bothered with early morning drowsiness from her diphenhydramine therapy.

SUMMARY

The case presentation is a unique skill possessed by clinical practitioners. This skill will be necessary from the first patient cared for and can be mastered only through frequent practice. Presenting cases will benefit the practitioner by facilitating learning, seeking help, and sharing ideas. The simplicity of its structure encourages creativity and promotes effective practice dialogue.

EXERCISES

13-1 Present a patient case to a colleague for the purpose of soliciting help to resolve one of the drug therapy problems you have identified.

13-2 Prepare a written patient case presentation describing a patient who will be transferred to one of your colleagues for continued care.

13-3 Discuss the differences you would expect to find between a pharmacotherapy patient case presentation and a patient case presented by a medical student reporting his/her medical workup and physical examination. Be sure to comment on each of the major components of the case presentation format.

13-4 Discuss what you will do to prevent each one of the common problems encountered in patient case presentations. Explain how you will
  (a) prepare yourself;
  (b) state the purpose for your presentation;
  (c) describe the relationships between patient characteristics, medical conditions, and drug therapies;
  (d) provide evidence of effectiveness and safety;
  (e) acquire all the practice you will need.

REFERENCES

1. Billings, J.A., Stoeckle, J.D. *The Clinical Encounter: A Guide to the Medical Interview and Case Presentation.* St. Louis, MO: Medical Publishers of Mosby-Year Book Inc.; 1989, pp. 270–272.
2. Smith, R.C. *The Patient's Story: Integrated Patient-Doctor Interviewing.* Boston, MA: Little, Brown and Company; 1996.
3. Lipkin, M.J., Putman, S.M., Lazare, A. *The Medical Interview: Clinical Care, Education, and Research.* New York: Springer; 1995, p. 10.
4. Coulehan, J.L., Block, M.R. *The Medical Interview: Mastering Skills for Clinical Practice.* Philadelphia, PA: F.A. Davis Company; 2001.
5. Savett, L. *The Human Side of Medicine.* Westport, CT: Auburn House; 2002.

CHAPTER FOURTEEN

ESTABLISHING A NEW PHARMACEUTICAL CARE PRACTICE

Key Concepts

1. *The most important factor in building a successful pharmaceutical care practice is the preparedness of the practitioner.*

2. *Understanding the service you provide and articulating that service to patients and other practitioners is essential.*

3. *Find a supportive environment in which to practice.*

4. *Do not expect the practice site to change for you—teach them how to accommodate your new practice.*

5. *Recruit new patients through referrals, other patients, and collaborative practice agreements.*

6 *A network of qualified pharmaceutical care practitioners could be your most important asset.*

7 *Be realistic in your expectations. Commit 2 years to getting started.*

8 *Learn to write a business plan—your practice depends upon it.*

9 *Know how to charge for your service based on the resource-based relative value scale.*

10 *The best marketing scheme available is to provide high quality patient care.*

INTRODUCTION

The focus of this final chapter is different from the previous 13 chapters. This chapter is intended to introduce you to a number of the issues involved in establishing a pharmaceutical care practice. The focus is not the practitioner caring for one patient at a time as was the case in Chapters 1 through 13.

This chapter focuses on issues associated with establishing a practice. This chapter is not intended to provide you with the scope and detail you will need to become a good manager; that knowledge and experience should be gained from schools of management and experienced management personnel.

Pharmaceutical care is still new enough that there are relatively few practices that have been established long enough from which to learn. Therefore, it is necessary to learn from other patient care practitioners who have built successful practices, namely, nurse practitioners, chiropractors, physicians, dentists, and veterinarians. These practitioners have been building practices that are well managed and successful from both the professional and financial perspectives for many years. A number of resources are available from these practice areas.[1-5]

This chapter introduces a number of issues that are relevant when thinking about and initiating a new pharmaceutical care practice.

GUIDELINES FOR BUILDING A PATIENT CARE PRACTICE

Pharmaceutical care practice is a service that provides patient care. Guidelines that will affect the success of a practice as you begin to think about initiating a pharmaceutical care service will be presented.

These guidelines include the following:

1. Become a competent practitioner
2. Understand and describe your service
3. Identify or create a supportive practice environment
4. Accommodate the organization
5. Develop techniques to recruit patients
6. Be realistic about your expectations
7. Develop a business plan

Each of the guidelines is discussed below to stimulate thought about starting a new patient care practice.

Become a Competent Practitioner

The single most important variable in a new patient care practice is the quality of the practitioner providing the care. The success of the practice depends upon how knowledgeable and skilled the practitioner is and the level of commitment the practitioner has to patient care. In health care, the best practitioners are the busiest practitioners. Therefore, to assure your highest level of success in practice you want to gain experience with qualified colleagues until you are confident of your ability to function independently. The greatest advantage you can give yourself when starting a new practice is to ensure that you can provide care that meets the standards defined for practice. In any patient care service, the practitioner is the *product* that is marketed.

Understand and Describe Your Service

Pharmaceutical care practice is the first new patient care service to be introduced into the health care system in many years. Therefore, it will be new to everyone who comes in contact with you. You will have to describe this new service over and over again before physicians, nurses, and patients clearly understand what you will be doing. You should not get frustrated or interpret their questions as a lack of interest or support. Do not expect people to demand a service that they do not understand or have never experienced.

The most effective way to introduce new health care service is to provide it. This will show patients what they can expect and how they can benefit from the service. Realize that new behaviors have to be learned by everyone involved in the health care system and this will take time.

Identify a Supportive Practice Environment

The challenge of starting a business, especially a new patient care practice in an existing health care system, is a significant undertaking. Therefore, identify a practice setting that is conducive and friendly to your goal.

The major criteria to be considered in selecting your practice setting are whether patients feel comfortable and whether high quality pharmaceutical care can be provided in this setting. Be certain that the personnel with whom you work are supportive, friendly, and encouraging.

Accommodate the Organization

You will need to build your service within an existing organizational structure. Do not expect people to change to meet your needs—you are the *new* practitioner. The health care system has not accommodated a new practitioner very often or very recently, so do not expect it to change for you. Nurse practitioners and chiropractors have had to travel this same road. Some physicians may ignore you, nurses may prefer that you not be in their space, but neither of these reactions should be taken personally or interpreted as a negative reaction to pharmaceutical care. Physicians and nurses are busy, and they have important responsibilities. New personnel or new procedures interrupt their already complex schedule.

It will be necessary for you to understand the organization in which you practice well enough so you can teach the personnel (physicians, nurses, support personnel) what they need to do in order to accommodate your work. You will save everyone a significant amount of time if you think through what impact you will have on each person's routine and prepare those involved.

Expect to teach personnel and patients what you do over and over again. You and your service are new to the health care system—they may have no intuitive knowledge of the practice because it has never existed before. Patients and health care personnel do not know what to expect and this makes people uncomfortable and defensive. This is not a reflection on you or pharmaceutical care, but is related to the difficulty people have accommodating change. Physicians, nurses, and patients already have their own ideas of what a pharmacist does and how a pharmacist works within the health care system. Becoming a pharmaceutical care practitioner changes this. You will need to change their fixed idea of what you do and how you can contribute. This will take continual effort on your part. Remember that all behavior in health care is learned through experience. Therefore, providing the service to *show* others what is involved is much more effective than talking about the practice.

Develop Techniques to Recruit Patients

In a patient care service, the primary method for generating revenue is to provide care to patients. However in a new practice, a significant amount of work is required to recruit new patients. Obviously, each patient will need to learn what you have to offer, and the patient will have to learn how he/she can benefit from the service.

There is a natural tendency to want to print brochures, send mailings, or create posters to announce the service. Although these marketing approaches may help along the way, this is not the usual way a patient care service successfully expands. Patient care is too personal for these generic approaches, so the most effective way to expand your service is to provide the care and allow the patients themselves to market you through word of mouth and reputation. This is how most medical services become successful. You are the *product*, and your patients will be the most effective means for *selling* you to others. This takes some time, so be realistic in your expectations.

Physician referrals help to recruit patients at a faster rate if you are in a clinic or hospital setting. Physician referrals can introduce you to patients who are in need of the service in a more efficient manner. However, there are a number of issues you must be aware of with regard to physician referrals.

1. Referrals are a two-way street. Professionals function by depending upon each other. When a practitioner refers a patient to another, it is expected (the system depends) on that practitioner referring patients back to him/her. This is the only way a referral system is maintained.
2. Physicians will refer patients who are more severely ill, more complicated, and more challenging than the average patient. You will have to plan for this. The workload associated with referred patients is usually greater than patients who identify the need for the service themselves. Referrals will take more time and require more follow-up, on average.
3. Referrals can seldom be relied upon as the sole source for new patients. Referrals take some control out of your practice, and you must plan accordingly. Referrals are unpredictable. Therefore, it is important to recruit a steady, consistent clientele that is supplemented by referred

patients. For this reason, it is probably not a good idea to build an entire practice around referrals if you are a generalist practitioner. However, referrals can become more predictable and stable if you are in a practice situation that involves collaborative practice agreements or joint practices with specific physicians.[6] Collaborative agreements help to identify groups of patients that will be referred to you as a portion of their comprehensive care.

Recruiting patients is probably the most time and energy consuming activity required to establish a new practice. This activity can be made more manageable if you are successful at contracting for services to a specific patient population.

There are a number of additional mechanisms to recruit patients. One is to provide incentives to patients. This might include waiving a copayment for the service or offering a discount for the initial assessment. Or, you may be in a situation where you can provide care for a captive audience, such as all of the employees of your company, or a self-insured population.

When you begin your practice, it will be helpful if you establish a specific date on which you will begin. Establish hours for your service and commit to them. It is necessary for patients and colleagues to know where you will be so they can refer patients to you. You can begin by establishing *clinic hours* for 2–3 days a week, and as the service expands, add extra hours as needed.

Determine the number of patients you will need to maintain a viable practice and how long will it take to get there. The key to a successful practice is to add new patients continually so the practice can become financially viable over the long term. Providing care for numerous patients on a continuous basis requires an efficient and effective organization.

Identify a Network of Pharmaceutical Care Practitioners

It is commonly understood in practitioner circles that it is impossible to become a skilled practitioner on your own. You are going to need the help of colleagues. Identify qualified practitioners in your geographical area and schedule routine meetings to exchange information, questions, concerns, and experiences related to patient care. This network of practitioners may become your greatest asset.

Set Realistic Expectations

It takes time to build a practice, for many reasons: (1) you will not be very efficient at first; (2) patients need to learn what your practice is and what it can do for them; (3) you need to earn the trust of colleagues; and (4) you will need to learn how to make the system work for you.

Physicians, dentists, and chiropractors starting new practices take 2–3 years to build a clientele of significant size. Because pharmaceutical care is a new service in an existing health care system, you can expect that it may take even longer.

Develop a Business Plan

Establishing a new practice is similar to starting a business, and there is a specific, clearly delineated process involved. In addition to a number of legal steps that must be taken, there are a number of planning activities that must occur. Developing the business plan is one of the first steps in starting a new practice. It describes the service: the product, the market, the people, and the financial needs. The business plan is an important step because it helps the practitioner determine the feasibility and desirability of pursuing the steps necessary to start a practice. If it is necessary to seek outside financing for the new service, then the business plan is an important sales tool for raising capital from outside investors.

Most of today's medical and nursing practitioners have not had to take the time and energy to create a business plan because their *new* practices were extensions of existing group practices. However, because developing a pharmaceutical care practice is truly a new service, a business plan is required to improve the likelihood of success.

Business plans vary but contain a core structure that describes the service, the competition, the economic benchmarks, and the return on investment determinations. The list below represents the basic sections of a typical business plan for the new service.

1. Executive summary
2. General description of the service
3. Marketing plans
4. Operational plans
5. Management and organization
6. Structure and capitalization
7. Milestones
8. Financial plan

There are many references, consulting groups, and computer software programs that can help you construct your business plan, but the plan must be yours: you must write it and you must *own* it. It is often helpful to have a professional assist you once you have drafted your plan. However you must be able to describe your business plan to someone else within a moment's notice. Business plans represent a value proposition. Therefore, you need to consider what patients and/or colleagues value. The following outlines the major contents of a business plan to introduce a new service.[7] Most business plans include a 1-2 page executive summary describing the major components of the plan.

Executive summary

- Description of the service you will be offering
- Description of the problem you will be solving
- The market potential
- Why your service is the best answer to the problem
- Major milestones for growth of your service
- Financial summary

General description of the service

- Fundamental activities and nature of the service you offer
- The mission statement
- The problem you are addressing
- The objectives of your service
- Who is your client?
- Where will you offer the service?
- How is your service used?
- What are the unique features of the service?
- In what stage of development is the service? How ready is it for operation?

Marketing plans

- What are the factors that establish demand for your service?
- What are your relevant target markets?
- Which markets are of primary importance?
- What marketing strategies will be employed?
- How will you organize and implement your marketing plans?
- How will you make your service available to your clients?

- What is your pricing structure?
- What advertising and/or public relations campaign is needed?
- What is the impact of regulation and laws on your service?
- What are your forecasts of market share and growth?

Competition

- What is the relevant competition to your service?
- What are future sources of competition for your service?
- What impact will competition likely have?

Barriers to entry

- Do any legal, copyright, trademark, license barriers exist?
- Do you have consultants available in pharmaceutical care practice?
- What is the lead time to initiating the service?

Operational plans

- How will your service remain state-of-the-art?
- What continued development efforts are planned?
- What are the capital requirements to provide the service?
- What are the labor requirements to provide the service?
- What suppliers are required to support the service?

Management and operations

- What is the background of the key individuals in your organization?
- Who will be the key employees and/or support staff?
- Who will direct the service?
- What key advisors will be available?
- Develop an organizational chart
- Develop a policy statement of how support staff will be selected and trained

Structure and capitalization

- What legal form will this service company take?
- How much capital is needed?
- Describe the manner of financial participation or investment

Milestones

- Describe the first test market
- Calculate break-even performance
- Quantify expansion steps

Financial plan

- Describe the set of assumptions on which projections are based
- Project income statements for 5 years
- Project detailed cash flow statements for 2 years

The executive summary of your business plan is important because it serves as the primary document that others will evaluate. The content of the business plan serves to support what is presented in the executive summary. Business plans are similar to care plans in that both are proposals designed to achieve a specific set of goals. Your plan should clearly describe the value others are going to place upon your service. Be specific about the problem your service solves for people. Is it drug therapy problems? Is it minimizing confusion about drug therapies? Is it increasing confidence in the effectiveness and safety of medications?

Why does your customer, client, or patient have to have your service? What are the top three benefits of your service? What are the top three objections to the service? Market research can help identify what your intended clients want and what they may not want from your service. The time and energy spent in researching, planning, and writing a business plan is a valuable investment to help ensure the success of your new patient care service.

BECOMING FINANCIALLY VIABLE

The primary mechanism for a practitioner to generate revenue is to provide direct patient services. Therefore, the time you spend on other activities such as *managing* the practice will interfere with becoming financially viable. Successful practitioners delegate all activities other than patient care to someone else, so that their time is dedicated to seeing patients and generating revenue.

In order to be successful, you will need to provide care for a minimum of 10–15 patients per day. This activity represents a combination of new patients and established patients. A single practitioner with this volume of service would have 2400–3750 patient encounters annually, which represents a patient load of approximately 2000 patients at any time. This volume of patients is a full-time commitment to patient care.

Providing a financially viable service means providing people with the service they need, the way they want it. It means getting paid for that service. You will need a mechanism for billing. Patient care providers are reimbursed in very structured, predetermined ways. The most widely used approach to health services billing in the United States is the resource-based relative value scale (RBRVS). This approach is described in detail here.

The Resource-based Relative Value Scale

The method of payment based on the resource-based relative value scale became widely known and used in January of 1992 when it became the Medicare physician payment system throughout the United States.[9,10] The federal government now uses this system to pay for a broad range of patient care services. In 1993, the resource-based relative value scale was first developed and applied to pharmaceutical care practice.[11]

The basic principles underlying the RBRVS are well established.[9,10] Physicians and insurers have been using this system since the first relative value scale was developed by the California Medical Association in 1956. In a resource-based relative value scale, services are ranked according to the relative costs of the resources required to provide them.

> **Example** If Service A consumed twice as many resources (expertise, support personnel, time, supplies, overhead expense, and level of difficulty) as Service B, then Service A would have a relative value of two times that of Service A.

The data which led to Omnibus Budget Reconciliation Act (OBRA 89), the federal legislation which enacted the Medicare physician payment reform provisions, were generated by a Harvard University National Study. The study funded the development of RBRVS for almost 30 physician specialties. The American Medical Association (AMA) was intimately involved in this study to facilitate medicine's support of the new system. The AMA eventually accepted the results of the study and assisted in the development of a national system of payment for physician services based on a RBRVS system.[9,10]

This system is comprised of five levels of payment based on three documented key components: (1) the physician's documentation of the patient's medical history, (2) the physical examination findings, and (3) the complexity of the medical decision-making.

There are other factors which were built into the provision. For example, geographic differences were taken into account when calculating practice expenses, specialty differentials in payment for the same service was eliminated, and a process for determining the annual update in the conversion factor was defined. A tremendous amount of time, energy, research, and discussion went into the development of this system for physician payment. This system has been broadly applied to include payment for nonphysician practitioners' services, including

- physical and occupational therapists;
- physician assistants;
- nurse practitioners and clinical nurse specialists;
- certified registered nurse anesthetists;
- nurse midwives;
- clinical psychologists, and
- clinical social workers.

RBRVS applied to pharmaceutical care   In 1993, the RBRVS system was adapted to pharmaceutical care practice to determine both practitioner workload and reimbursement amounts.[11] The pharmaceutical care reimbursement grid was developed and is described in Table 14-1.

There are five levels of payment, similar to other RBRVS systems. The resources required, the complexity of the patient's case, and the levels of reimbursement are determined by three components:

- Number of medical conditions being managed with pharmacotherapy
- Number of drug therapy problems identified and resolved
- Number of medications involved

Across the top of the grid are displayed the five *levels of payment*. Payment by the resource-based relative value scale is calculated at one of these levels. The payment level in this system is based on documented patient need and is calculated to be at the lowest level where all the key components are met. The levels of need vary from *straightforward* at Level 1 to the *highest complexity* at Level 5. The quantitative criteria are described on the grid.

Example   When a patient is taking two medications, has no drug therapy problems, and one medical condition, the encounter is designated as Level 1.

Table 14-1 The pharmaceutical care reimbursement grid based on RBRVS

Key components	Level #1[a] (0.4)[b] 99201[c]	Level #2 (1.0) 99202	Level #3 (1.8) 99203	Level #4 (2.5) 99204	Level #5 (3.0) 99205
Assessment of drug-related needs	*Problem-focused* 0–1 Medication	*Expanded problem* 1–2 Medications	*Detailed* 3–4 Medications	*Expanded detailed* 5–8 Medications	*Comprehensive* ≥9 Medications
Identification drug therapy problems	*Problem-focused* 0 Drug therapy problems	*Expanded problem[d]* 1 Drug therapy problem	*Detailed* 2 Drug therapy problems	*Expanded detailed[d]* 3 Drug Therapy problems	*Comprehensive* ≥4 Drug therapy problems
Care planning & follow-up evaluation	*Straightforward* 1 Medical condition	*Straightforward* 1 Medical condition	*Low complexity* 2 Medical conditions	*Moderate complexity* 3 Medical conditions	*High complexity* ≥4 Medical conditions
Amount	$	$$	$$$	$$$$	$$$$$

[a]Service level.
[b]Resource-based relative value unit.
[c]An example of a current procedural terminology (CPT) billing code for payment level calculation.
[d]Additional patient information required.

Remember, the case is designated at the lowest level where *all three criteria* are met. The variables that go into the calculation of the level of patient need are presented down the left hand side of the grid in Table 14-1. Let us discuss how these variables integrate to create the level of patient need.

> **Example** When a patient has four medical conditions that require six medications and who had two drug therapy problems that were identified and resolved, the encounter is designated as Level 3.

One of the strengths of the resource-based relative value scale is that it is self-auditing. This scale always yields a patient need at the lowest level of the three documented criteria. This internal logic promotes comprehensive documentation, yet rewards efficiency.

> **Example** If the practitioner documents that a patient has seven medical conditions and is taking nine drugs, and one drug therapy problem is identified and resolved, then the patient's needs are designated at Level 2.

> If the practitioner documents a patient's needs to be two medical conditions and two drug therapy problems involving two prescription medications, the patient's needs would be Level 2. However, if this same patient also was taking daily aspirin to prevent a myocardial infarction and the practitioner documented this additional preventive pharmacotherapy, then the patient's needs would be increased to Level 3.

Although a different *intensity* of work is provided by the pharmaceutical care practitioner at each of the five reimbursement levels, the nature of the work is the same at *all* levels. The *work* includes the following:

- Assessment of drug-related needs
- Identification of drug therapy problems
- The nature of the risks reflected in care planning and follow-up evaluation.

We will discuss each of the components of the work. This work and the relative resources required to provide the service are what creates the five levels of care.

Determining the assessment of drug-related needs The resource-based relative value scale recognizes five different levels of work. A major criterion determining the different levels is the number of medications the patient is taking. This affects the amount of information necessary to provide pharmaceutical care and the amount of data integration required. The most straightforward workup is a *problem-focused workup* and involves a single form of drug therapy. The next level is an *expanded problem-focused workup* and is appropriate when one or two medications are required. With three or four active medications, the practitioner must conduct a *detailed workup*, with five to eight, an *expanded detailed workup*. Finally, when a patient requires nine or more medications *a comprehensive workup* of drug therapy is required.

This system is based on the documented patient need as determined by each patient's diseases, drug therapy problems, and medications. It is not specific to any particular disease state or drug product. The five levels of service encompass the wide variation in skill, effort, time, responsibility, and knowledge required for the prevention and resolution of drug therapy problems. In the medical system of RVRBS the key components in selecting the appropriate level are history, examination, and medical decision-making (diagnosis).[10,12] In the pharmaceutical care system of RBRVS the key components in selecting the appropriate level is the number of medical conditions being managed with drug therapies, the number of drug therapy problems resolved, and the number of medications involved in both.[11] The specific values for number of medical conditions, drug therapy problems, and drugs for each level of service on the pharmaceutical care reimbursement grid were determined based upon the findings from the Minnesota Pharmaceutical Care Project.[11]

> **Example** Examine a case involving a 52-year-old female patient who was being treated with sertraline (Zoloft) for major depression, was managing her hypothyroidism with levothyroxine (Synthroid), had long-standing hypertension controlled with metoprolol and hydrochlorothiazide, and was also taking aspirin daily to prevent a stroke or heart attack. If the practitioner identified and resolved two drug therapy problems for this patient (dose of sertraline was too low to provide effective control of depressive symptoms, and patient required potassium supplements to prevent hypokalemia), then this would represent a Level 3. This patient's needs were determined based on four medical conditions (treatment of depression, hypothyroidism, hypertension, and prevention of MI/stroke), six medications (sertraline, levothyroxine, metoprolol, hydrochlorothiazide, potassium chloride, aspirin), and two drug therapy problems. Note that if the practitioner had documented that this patient was hypokalemic, the case would contain five medical conditions but would not change the RBRVS level.

If the practitioner did not decide that this same patient needed daily potassium supplementation, then the case would represent Level 2 (four medical conditions, five medications, one drug therapy problem).

If at the next follow-up visit, the practitioner evaluated the patient's hypertension and depression and found them both to be stable, but did decide that the patient required additional drug therapy in the form of daily potassium chloride supplements to treat hypokalemia, then at this later visit the case would represent Level 2 (three medical conditions evaluated, involving four medications, and one drug therapy problem).

Examine this same patient at her third follow-up evaluation, if the practitioner documents that her depression and hypertension are both stable, her preventive aspirin continues to be effective, her hypokalemia is improved, and she has no drug therapy problems at this time, it would be Level 1 (four medical conditions, five medications, and no drug therapy problems).

Determining complexity: number of drug therapy problems   The complexity of the assessment process follows the same descriptive categories as presented above for the levels of workup. However, the variable of interest is the number of drug therapy problems identified and resolved. Each drug therapy problem requires a sophisticated decision-making process for its identification and resolution (see Chapter 6–7).

Determining the nature of the risks reflected in care planning and follow-up evaluation   The level of risk associated with the care of the patient is determined by the number of active medical conditions or illnesses being managed with drug therapies. Clearly, number and type of medications as well as number and type of drug therapy problems also represent risk, but these contribute in their own way to the level of reimbursement. Therefore, this variable depends on the number of active medical problems experienced by the patient and requiring pharmacotherapy.

Each medical condition will require the practitioner establish goals of therapy and establish an appropriate care plan with the patient to accomplish the goals. In addition, it will be necessary to evaluate the outcomes at a follow-up visit.

Time: determining the amount of face-to-face time spent with the patient   Time is not a major criterion used in the RBRVS. Whenever time is described within the RBRVS system, it is considered to be an average of the face-to-face time required to provide that level of services by the average practitioner.

Example If the RBRVS estimate for Level 2 was 15 min, and you can provide that level of service in 10–12 minutes, it reflects your efficiency. If that same level of service requires 18–25 min of face-to-face time, this also reflects on your efficiency.

In some situations, time estimates are useful because practitioners can document special situations when excess time was required and thereby increase the service level by one. In these unusual circumstances, a *modifier* is used and additional documentation is necessary.[10] The specific times associated with each level of payment are averages representing a range of times which may be higher or lower depending on actual practice circumstances and the skill level of the practitioner.

It is important to note that time refers only to *face-to-face* time. Face-to-face time is defined as that time the practitioner spends with the patient and/or family. This includes the time in which the practitioner performs such tasks as completing a Pharmacotherapy Workup, making an assessment, identifying drug therapy problems, preparing a care plan, providing the patient with individualized information, and any support personnel time spent.

Practitioners will also spend time doing work before and after the face-to-face encounter with the patient, performing such tasks as reviewing records and tests, arranging for follow-up services, and communicating further with other professionals. This time is not included in the face-to-face time estimate component of the RBRVS.

Other grid notation Across the top of the pharmaceutical care reimbursement grid in Table 14-1 you will see two other numbers (b, c). The number in parenthesis (e.g., in Level 1 the number is 0.4) represents the relative amount of resources required to provide care at this level of complexity. Level 1 requires 40% of the resources required at Level 2. Level 5 requires 300% more resources than does providing care at Level 2. These *relative* values were calculated based on estimates from the first pharmaceutical care practices.[11] Validation from additional pharmaceutical care practices will be necessary.

The last number in the level of payment box in Table 14-1 represents an example of a current procedural terminology (CPT) billing code which was created in a format consistent with the other health care reimbursement systems in place.[12] This number is a temporary assignment and is for reference only, because federal recognition of the pharmaceutical care practitioner's work is still being established.

Calculating the reimbursement amount The reimbursement dollar amount is calculated based on the variables described above, and reflects the resources required to provide documented care at each level. Note that Level 2 involves patients with one drug therapy problem, one medical condition, and/or one medication and the assigned relative value is also one. This represents *unity* in the RBRVS, therefore all reimbursement amounts are relative to Level 2.

The actual dollar amount assigned to Level 2 is the sum of all the resources used to deliver care at this level. The data for calculating this amount is presently unique to each practice site until enough practices are established to develop a national database.

RBRVS as a workload measurement tool The RBRVS has been functioning since 1993 and has been used to generate charges for care delivered to over 20,000 patients. In addition to a billing structure, the system functions as a workload measurement tool. Because each level of care demands and consumes different amounts of resources, it is important to be aware of the distribution of patients in a practice. Figure 14-1 shows the data that reflect the complexity distribution of all 26,238 encounters for the 5136 patients in ambulatory care settings who received pharmaceutical care between 1996 and 2002 (see Chapter 2 for a detailed description of the study sample).

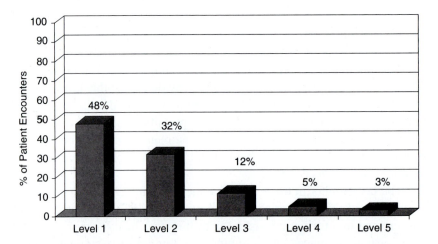

Figure 14-1 Workload based on patient complexity in the resource-based relative value scale. All documented pharmaceutical care encounters ($n = 26,238$) from sample patients ($n = 5136$) described in Chapter 2.

It is important to realize that the majority of patients seen in a generalist practice are Levels 1, 2, and 3. It should be emphasized here that a patient with no drug therapy problems still requires an assessment by the pharmaceutical care practitioner to ensure that all goals of therapy continue to be met and that positive outcomes are achieved. Its corollary is the dentist who sees patients every 6 months to assure good oral hygiene is being maintained and that no dental problems have developed.

Meeting reimbursement objectives   The RBRVS meets all of the reimbursement criteria for pharmaceutical care practice. It allows payment for all of the practitioner's direct patient care services. The patient is the focus of the payment system. This approach is completely consistent with the philosophy and practice of pharmaceutical care, as can be seen by our ability to adapt each aspect of the RBRVS to the practice vocabulary. Finally, the RBRVS is self-auditing consistent with how care providers are reimbursed for patient care.

Payment for pharmaceutical care services will be necessary to sustain practices in the future. It will be important to establish new practices as quickly and successfully as possible. There has been an immense void created in our health care system by the rapid proliferation of pharmaceuticals coupled with the lack of a rational approach to their use.

SUMMARY

Establishing a new pharmaceutical care practice may not be the priority of every new practitioner, however it is an important step in developing pharmaceutical care as a new service within the health care system. You will be well positioned to start a new practice when you become competent as a practitioner, understand and articulate the service to others, identify a supportive practice environment, accommodate the existing organization, develop techniques to recruit patients, build a network of qualified pharmaceutical care practitioners, set realistic expectations, and develop a business plan. Too many patients are suffering needlessly due to a lack of effective drug therapy, unintended adverse effects, lack of follow-up, and confusing instructions. Pharmaceutical care practice is a solution to this health care problem.

Pharmaceutical care practice is entering its second decade. Many patients have already benefited from pharmaceutical care services provided by the first generation of practitioners. Pharmaceutical care practice delineated clear and direct patient care responsibilities. The early successes of pharmaceutical care practices are due to the correctness of its principles and clarity of its purpose.

These principles and clarity of purpose should provide clear direction for those responsible for the preparation of the next generation of pharmaceutical care practitioners as well as clear roles for future pharmacy leaders.

The expansion of pharmaceutical care as a patient care service will require the development of new practices across the country and around the world. Patients need ready access to this service. This will not be accomplished through advertising campaigns or public relations programs. Success will require new practitioners who are ready to commit the energy required to initiate new practices, one patient at a time.

Expanding the availability of pharmaceutical care to patients in need is a priority of all practitioners, and establishing new practices is an important step in making this a reality.

EXERCISES

14-1 Describe the value of a network of pharmaceutical care practitioner colleagues when you are establishing a new pharmaceutical care practice.

14-2 What are three behaviors you can engage in to demonstrate that you are actively accommodating the existing organizational structure as you establish a new pharmaceutical care service?

14-3 Construct a draft of a business plan for a new pharmaceutical care practice to be established in an ambulatory care clinic. Include an executive summary, general description of the service, operational plans, milestones, and a financial plan. Have a colleague review it.

14-4 Calculate how many patients you will have to care for each working day to earn the level of income you desire, assuming the following parameters:
  (a) One-half of all the gross revenue you generate can be counted as salary and benefits for you.
  (b) Each patient encounter will generate (on average) $60.00 in gross revenue.

How soon would you expect to build a practice of this size?

REFERENCES

1. Bradford, V. *The Total Service Medical Practice: 17 Steps to Satisfying Your Internal and External Customers.* Chicago: Irwin Professional Publishing; 1997.
2. Joseph, S.R. *Marketing the Physician Practice.* Chicago, IL: American Medical Association; 2000. Chapter 3: Developing a Marketing Plan, pp. 33–41.

3. Koch, W.H. *Chiropractic—The Superior Alternative*. Calgary, AB, Canada: Bayeux Arts Inc.; 1995.
4. Silker, E.L., Riewer, D.M. *Dentistry: Building Your Million Dollar Solo Practice*. Lakeshore, MN: Silk Pages Publishing; 1995.
5. Nicoleti, B., *Five Strategies for a More Vital Practice*. Jan 2004, www.aafp.org/fpm. Accessed 3/5/04.
6. McDonough, R.P., Doucette, W.R. Dynamics of pharmaceutical care: developing collaborative working relations between pharmacists and physicians. *J Am Pharm Assoc* 2001; 41(5):682–692.
7. Schaffer, C.A. *A Guide to Starting a Business in Minnesota*. St. Paul, MN: Minnesota Department of Trade and Economic Development; 2001.
8. Kapron, J.C. Biz Plan Builder® Express: A Guide to Creating a Business Plan with Biz Plan Builder®. JIAN Tools for Sale, Inc. Thompson, Australia. 2004; Chapter 1: Business Plan Basics, pp. 1–13.
9. AMA, *American Medical Association. Medicare Physician Payment Reform: The Physicians' Guide*, vol. 1. Chicago, IL: American Medical Association; 1992.
10. Gallagher, P.E. (ed), AMA, *American Medical Association: Medicare RBRVS: The Physicians' Guide 2000*. Chicago, IL: American Medical Association; 2000, p. 81.
11. Cipolle, R., Strand, L.M., Morley, P.C. *Pharmaceutical Care Practice*. New York: McGraw Hill; 1998.
12. Kirschner, C.G., Burkett, R.C., Coy, J.A., Edwards, N.K., Kotowicz, G.M., Leoni, G., Malone, Y., McNamara, M.R., Mosley, B.R., O'Hara, K.E., Riesbeck, M.A. AMA, *American Medical Association. Physicians' Current Procedural Terminology: CPT '94*. Chicago, IL: American Medical Association; 1994, p. 3.

STANDARDS OF PRACTICE FOR PHARMACEUTICAL CARE

Standards of practice for pharmaceutical care are:

- Standards of care: A set of expectations of the performance of an *individual* practitioner
- Professional standards: A set of expectations for a *community* of practitioners

STANDARDS OF CARE FOR PHARMACEUTICAL CARE PRACTITIONERS

Category	Standard
I. Assessment	1. The practitioner collects relevant patient-specific information to use in decision-making concerning all drug therapies.
	2. The practitioner analyzes the assessment data to determine if the patient's drug-related needs are being met, that all the patient's medications are appropriately indicated, the most effective available, the safest possible, and the patient is able and willing to take the medication as intended.
	3. Identification of drug therapy problems: The practitioner analyzes the assessment data to determine if any drug therapy problems are present.

(Continued)

Category	Standard
II. Care plan development	4. The practitioner identifies goals of therapy that are individualized to the patient.
	5. The practitioner develops a care plan that includes interventions to: resolve drug therapy problems, achieve goals of therapy, and prevent drug therapy problems.
	6. The practitioner develops a schedule to follow-up and evaluate the effectiveness of drug therapies and assesses any adverse events experienced by the patient.
III. Follow-up evaluation	7. The practitioner evaluates the patient's actual outcomes and determines the patient's progress toward the achievement of the goals of therapy, determines if any safety or compliance issues are present, and assesses whether any new drug therapy problems have developed.

Standard of Care 1: Collection of Patient-specific Information

The practitioner collects relevant patient-specific information to use in decision-making concerning all drug therapies.

Measurement criteria

1. Pertinent data are collected using appropriate interview techniques.
2. Data collection involves the patient, family and care-givers, and health care providers when appropriate.
3. The medication experience is elicited by the practitioner and incorporated as the context for decision-making.
4. The data are used to develop a pharmacologically relevant description of the patient and the patient's drug-related needs.
5. The relevance and significance of the data collected are determined by the patient's present conditions, illnesses, wants, and needs.
6. The medication history is complete and accurate.
7. The current medication record is complete and accurate.
8. The data collection process is systematic and ongoing.
9. Only data that are required and used by the practitioner are elicited from the patient.
10. Relevant data are documented in a retrievable form.
11. All data elicitation and documentation is conducted in a manner that ensures patient confidentiality.

Standard of Care 2:
Assessment of Drug-related Needs

The practitioner analyzes the assessment data to determine if the patient's drug-related needs are being met, that all the patient's medications are appropriately indicated, the most effective available, the safest possible, and the patient is able and willing to take the medication as intended.

Measurement criteria

1. The patient-specific data collected in the assessment are used to decide if all of the patient's medications are appropriately indicated.
2. The data collected are used to decide if the patient needs additional medications that are not presently being taken.
3. The data collected are used to decide if all of the patient's medications are the most effective products available for the conditions.
4. The data collected are used to decide if all of the patient's medications are dosed appropriately to achieve the goals of therapy.
5. The data collected are used to decide if any of the patient's medications are causing adverse effects.
6. The data collected are used to decide if any of the patient's medications are dosed excessively and causing toxicities.
7. The patient's behavior is assessed to determine if all his or her medications are being taken appropriately in order to achieve the goals of therapy.

Standard of Care 3:
Identification of Drug Therapy Problems

The practitioner analyzes the assessment data to determine if any drug therapy problems are present.

Measurement criteria

1. Drug therapy problems are identified from the assessment findings.
2. Drug therapy problems are validated with the patient, his/her family, care-givers, and/or health care providers, when necessary.
3. Drug therapy problems are expressed so that the medical condition and the drug therapy involved are explicitly stated and the relationship or cause of the problem is described.

4. Drug therapy problems are prioritized, and those that will be resolved first are selected.
5. Drug therapy problems are documented in a manner that facilitates the determination of goals of therapy within the care plan.

Standard of Care 4:
Development of Goals of Therapy

The practitioner identifies goals of therapy that are individualized to the patient.

Measurement criteria

1. Goals of therapy are established for each indication for drug therapy.
2. Desired goals of therapy are described in terms of the observable or measurable clinical and/or laboratory parameters to be used to evaluate effectiveness of drug therapy.
3. Goals of therapy are mutually negotiated with the patient and health care providers when appropriate.
4. Goals of therapy are realistic in relation to the patient's present and potential capabilities.
5. Goals of therapy are attainable in relation to resources available to the patient.
6. Goals of therapy include a timeframe for achievement.

Standard of Care 5:
Statement of Interventions

The practitioner develops a plan of care that includes interventions to: resolve drug therapy problems, achieve goals of therapy, and prevent drug therapy problems.

Measurement criteria

1. Each intervention is individualized to the patient's conditions, needs, and drug therapy problems.
2. All appropriate therapeutic alternatives to resolve drug therapy problems are considered, and the best are selected.
3. The plan is developed in collaboration with the patient, his/her family and/or care-givers, and health care providers, when appropriate.
4. All interventions are documented.
5. The plan provides for continuity of care by including a schedule for continuous follow-up evaluation.

Standard of Care 6:
Establishing a Schedule for Follow-up Evaluations

The practitioner develops a schedule to follow-up and evaluate the effectiveness of the outcomes from drug therapies and assess any adverse events experienced by the patient.

Measurement criteria

1. The clinical and laboratory parameters to evaluate effectiveness are established, and a timeframe for collecting the relevant information is selected.
2. The clinical and laboratory parameters that reflect the safety of the patient's medications are selected, and a timeframe for collecting the relevant information is determined.
3. A schedule for the follow-up evaluation is established with the patient.
4. The plan for follow-up evaluation is documented.

Standard of Care 7: Follow-up Evaluation

The practitioner evaluates the patient's actual outcomes and determines the patient's progress toward the achievement of the goals of therapy, determines if any safety or compliance issues are present, and assesses whether any new drug therapy problems have developed.

Measurement criteria

1. The patient's actual outcomes from drug therapies and other interventions are documented.
2. The effectiveness of drug therapies is evaluated, and the patient's status is determined by comparing the outcomes within the expected timeframe to achieve the goals of therapy.
3. The safety of the drug therapy is evaluated.
4. Patient compliance is evaluated.
5. The care plan is revised, as needed.
6. Revisions in the care plan are documented.
7. Evaluation is systematic and ongoing until all goals of therapy are achieved.
8. The patient, family and/or care-givers, and health care providers are involved in the evaluation process, when appropriate.

THE STANDARDS FOR PROFESSIONAL BEHAVIOR

Category	Standard
Quality of care	The practitioner evaluates his/her own practice in relation to professional practice standards and relevant statutes and regulations.
Ethics	The practitioner's decisions and actions on behalf of patients are determined in an ethical manner.
Collegiality	The pharmaceutical care practitioner contributes to the professional development of peers, colleagues, students, and others.
Collaboration	The practitioner collaborates with the patient, family and/or care-givers, and health care providers in providing patient care.
Education	The practitioner acquires and maintains current knowledge in pharmacology, pharmacotherapy, and pharmaceutical care practice.
Research	The practitioner routinely uses research findings in practice and contributes to research findings when appropriate.
Resource allocation	The practitioner considers factors related to effectiveness, safety, and cost in planning and delivering patient care.

Standard I: Quality of Care

The practitioner evaluates his/her own practice in relation to professional practice standards and relevant statutes and regulations.

Measurement criteria

1. The pharmaceutical care practitioner uses evidence from the literature to evaluate his/her performance in practice.
2. The pharmaceutical care practitioner seeks peer review on a continual and frequent basis.
3. The pharmaceutical care practitioner utilizes data generated from his/her practice to critically self-evaluate performance.

Standard II: Ethics

The practitioner's decisions and actions on behalf of patients are determined in an ethical manner.

Measurement criteria

1. The practitioner maintains patient confidentiality.
2. The practitioner acts as a patient advocate.
3. The practitioner delivers care in a nonjudgmental and nondiscriminatory manner that is sensitive to patient diversity.
4. The practitioner delivers care in a manner that preserves/protects patient autonomy, dignity, and rights.
5. The practitioner seeks available resources to help formulate ethical decisions.

Standard III: Collegiality

The pharmaceutical care practitioner contributes to the professional development of peers, colleagues, and others.

Measurement criteria

1. The practitioner offers professional assistance to other practitioners whenever asked.
2. The practitioner promotes relationships with patients, physicians, nurses and other health care providers.

Standard IV: Collaboration

The practitioner collaborates with the patient, significant others, and health care providers in providing patient care.

Measurement criteria

1. The patient is seen as the ultimate decision maker, and the practitioner collaborates accordingly.
2. The practitioner collaborates with the patient's health care providers whenever it is in the best interest of the patient.

Standard V: Education

The practitioner acquires and maintains current knowledge in pharmacology, pharmacotherapy, and pharmaceutical care practice.

Measurement criteria

1. The practitioner uses the skills of reflectivity to identify areas where knowledge needs to be supplemented.
2. The practitioner continually updates knowledge with publications, professional journal subscriptions, current texts, practitioner interactions, and continuing education programs.

Standard VI: Research

The practitioner routinely uses research findings in practice and contributes to research findings when appropriate.

Measurement criteria

1. The practitioner uses research as the basis for practice.
2. The pharmaceutical care practitioner systematically reviews the literature to identify knowledge, skills, techniques, and products that are helpful in practice and implements them in a timely manner.
3. The practitioner approaches his/her practice with a perspective to conduct applied research in practice when appropriate.

Standard VII: Resource Allocation

The practitioner considers factors related to effectiveness, safety, and cost in planning and delivering patient care.

Measurement criteria

1. The pharmaceutical care practitioner is sensitive to the financial needs and resource limitations of the patient, the health care providers, and the institutions with which he/she interacts.
2. Decisions are made by the pharmaceutical care practitioner to conserve resources and maximize the value of those resources consumed in practice.

GLOSSARY

advocacy (patient)
- The willingness to assume an active role in obtaining resources or resolving problems on behalf of a patient
- May require an intervention on the part of a health care professional for the benefit of a patient

assessment
- A systematic review and appraisal of the patient's drug-related needs
- Completed for the purpose of: assuring that all the patient's drug therapy is *appropriately indicated*, the *most effective* available and the *safest* possible; assuring that the patient is able and willing to *comply* with the pharmacotherapeutic regimen, and identifying drug therapy problems
- Includes the decision making processes of the Pharmacotherapy Workup
- One of three steps in the patient care process in the practice of pharmaceutical care (the *care plan* and the *follow-up evaluation* complete the process)

beneficence
- Doing what is best for the patient
- One of the primary ethical principles that underlies the practice of pharmaceutical care

care plan
- A detailed schedule outlining the practitioner's and the patient's activities and responsibilities; designed to achieve goals of therapy, and resolve and prevent drug therapy problems
- Organized according to medical condition or indication for drug therapy
- Includes (1) a statement of the goals of therapy, (2) the interventions by the practitioner and the actions to be taken by the patient to resolve any drug therapy problems, meet the goals of therapy, and prevent drug therapy problems, and (3) a schedule for the follow-up evaluation

caring

- A state of responsiveness to others which entails the willingness to become personally involved
- The commitment to alleviate another person's vulnerability and suffering
- Considered to be the cornerstone of the therapeutic relationship and a principle component of the philosophy of pharmaceutical care practice
- Consists of three activities that the practitioner must accomplish: (1) assess the patient's needs, (2) obtain the resources required to meet these needs, (3) determine if the help provided has produced positive or negative outcomes.

clinical pharmacy

- An emphasis in the profession of pharmacy from the mid-1960s to the present which moved the focus from drug product to patient-oriented services including consultations
- Includes a number of different services such as individualized (pharmacokinetic) dosing services, and drug utilization review, which are primarily provided in the institutional setting
- The majority of the services are provided to/for physicians or at the request of physicians or are directed toward institutional policies and procedures
- ACCP Definition (Draft): A health science discipline that embodies the application and development, by pharmacists, of scientific principles of pharmacology, toxicology, therapeutics, clinical pharmacokinetics, pharmacoeconomics, pharmacogenomics, and other life science for the care of patients

clinically competent

- A practitioner who is legally and ethically informed and is able to draw upon appropriate pharmaceutical knowledge while problem solving to meet the patient's needs

compliance

- The ability and willingness of a patient to adhere to a pharmacotherapeutic regimen agreed upon between patient and practitioner
- The terms adherence and concordance are also used
- The term is used here specifically to mean compliance with a dosage regimen, not compliance with the orders of a paternalistic or authoritarian figure

confidentiality (patient)

- The act of protecting a patient's personal information from public view
- Keeping private all aspects of a patient's care in the manner deemed acceptable to the patient and prescribed by law (see Health Insurance Portability and Accountability Act (HIPAA), April 14, 2003)
- One of the ethical principles that underlies the practice of pharmaceutical care

conflict of interest
- Personal, financial, or political interests that undermine an individual's ability to meet or fulfill primary professional, ethical, or legal obligations

contraindication
- A condition or factor that renders the use of a drug product in the care of a specific patient improper or undesirable
- A reason or explanation, such as a symptom or condition, that makes a particular treatment or procedure inadvisable

current medication record
- Organized information describing all of the drug therapies a patient is presently taking or receiving
- Includes the indication for the medication, the specific drug product, dosage regimen, duration of therapy, and clinical results to date
- Includes prescription products, nonprescription agents, alternative products, vitamins, nutritional supplements, herbal remedies, and any other product the patient is taking that is intended to have therapeutic effects

diagnosis
- The process of determining the nature of a medical disease and distinguishing one disease from another
- Identification of a disease by considering the patient's signs and symptoms, history, laboratory findings, and physical examination when necessary

disease
- Specific illness or medical disorder characterized by a recognizable set of signs and symptoms
- A pathological, objectified condition of the body that presents a group of physiologically- and biologically-defined symptoms.
- Any abnormality or failure to function, except those which result directly from physical injury

dosage
- The total amount of active medication that a patient takes over a specified period of time
- Includes the dose of the medication, the method of administration, the frequency, and the duration of treatment

dose
- The amount of active ingredient that the patient takes each time he or she self-administers the drug product
- The amount of drug administered to the patient as a single event

dosing interval
- The amount of time between administered doses (eg. every 8 hours)
- Frequency of doses over a specified period of time (eg. 3 times a day)

drug
- Any substance or product used by or administered to a patient for therapeutic, preventive, or diagnostic purposes.

drug-related morbidity
- The incidence and prevalence of disease and illness or harm associated with drug therapy
- One aspect of the social need addressed in the philosophy of pharmaceutical care practice

drug-related mortality
- The incidence and prevalence of death associated with drug therapy
- One aspect of the social need addressed in the philosophy of pharmaceutical care practice

drug-related need
- The health care needs of a patient related to drug therapy for which the pharmaceutical care practitioner can offer professional assistance
- Includes (1) the appropriate use of the medication for each medical condition; (2) the most effective product for each indication; (3) the safest drug regimen possible and; (4) the willingness and ability of the patient to comply with the instructions for taking a medication

drug therapy
- Includes the drug product and the dosage regimen being taken by a patient for a therapeutic indication
- Used synonymously with pharmacotherapy

drug therapy problem
- Any undesirable event experienced by a patient which involves, or is suspected to involve, drug therapy and that interferes with achieving the desired goals of therapy
- Stated to include a description of the patient's condition or problem, the drug therapy involved, and the association between the two
- A problem that is categorized in the following way:
  - A. inappropriate *indication* for use
    1. patient needs additional drug therapy
    2. patient is taking unnecessary drug therapy
  - B. *ineffective* drug therapy
    3. patient is taking an ineffective drug product
    4. patient is taking too low of a dosage
  - C. *unsafe* drug therapy
    5. patient is experiencing an adverse drug reaction
    6. patient is taking too high of a dosage
  - D. inappropriate *compliance*
    7. patient is unable or unwilling to take the drug therapy as intended

effectiveness (of drug therapy)
- Ability of the drug therapy to produce the desired or intended beneficial result (outcome) in a specific patient

efficacy
- The evidence that a drug can produce a beneficial effect in a population of patients.

ethical dilemma
- The conflict that results from two different resolutions to a situation, both of which are ethical
- Result of a clinical situation that involves two individuals with different values, different levels of knowledge, expectations, and desires
- Used synonymously with ethical problem and ethical issue

ethical principles
- Concepts that describe the moral standards applied in patient care
- Form the foundation of the philosophy of pharmaceutical care practice
- Include beneficence, non-maleficence, veracity, justice, fidelity, autonomy, and confidentiality

ethics
- A set of moral principles or values that help to establish right from wrong encompassed in the standards of professional behavior for a practitioner
- Character or ideals governing an individual or profession

evaluation (follow-up)
- Patient encounters at planned intervals to determine outcomes of drug therapy
- Purpose is to record actual patient outcomes resulting from pharmacotherapy, evaluate progress of the patient toward achieving goals of therapy, determine if previous drug therapy problems have been resolved, and assess whether new drug therapy problems have developed
- The third component of the patient care process in the practice of pharmaceutical care (the other two are *assessment* and *care plan*)

expired
- One of the standard terms for describing the outcome status of a patient's medical condition being treated with pharmacotherapy
- Patient died while receiving drug therapy

failure
- One of the standard terms for describing the outcome status of a patient's medical condition being treated with pharmacotherapy
- The goals of therapy have not been achieved despite adequate dosages and adequate duration of therapy. Discontinuation of the present medication and initiation of new drug therapy is required

fidelity
- The act of being faithful and keeping promises
- One of the primary ethical principles that underlies the practice of pharmaceutical care

generalist
- A practitioner who provides continuing, comprehensive, and coordinated care to a population of patients undifferentiated by gender, disease, drug treatment, or organ system

goals of therapy
- The desired endpoint for pharmacotherapy
- Expressed as: prevention of a disease or illness, curing a disease, the reduction or elimination of signs and symptoms, slowing the progression of a disease, the normalization of laboratory values, or a way to facilitate the diagnostic process
- Includes clinical *parameters* (signs and symptoms) and/or laboratory *values* which are observable, measurable, and realistic, a desired value or observable change in the parameter, and a specific *timeframe*

illness
- The patient's lived experience of a disease or condition
- May be considered as a "process," often occurring over a protracted period of time
- The experience of illness encompasses physical, social, psychological, and cultural factors

improved
- One of the standard terms for describing the outcome status of a patient's medical condition being treated with pharmacotherapy
- Adequate progress is being made toward achieving the goals of therapy at this point in time. The same drug therapy will be continued

incidence
- The number of new cases or occurances of illness arising in a population over an established period of time

indication (for drug therapy)
- Reason for the use of drug therapy for the treatment, prevention, or diagnosis of a condition (illness, symptom) in a specific patient
- A sign or symptom to suggest the necessity or advisability to initiate pharmacotherapy

justice
- Fair, equitable, and appropriate treatment in light of what is due or owed to persons
- One of the primary ethical principles that underlies the practice of pharmaceutical care

medication
- A drug product being used for therapeutic, preventive, or diagnostic purposes by a patient

medication experience
- The sum of all the events in a patient's lifetime that relate to drug therapy
- The patient's personal experience with medications
- The lived experience that includes a patient's attitudes, beliefs, preferences, concerns, expectations and medication taking behavior
- Includes the patient's expression of the experience, the patient's medication history, and the patient's current medication record

medication history
- A record of past uses of medications and preventive pharmacotherapies
- Includes prescription medications, nonprescription products, alternative therapies, nutritional supplements, and all other agents used by the patient for therapeutic purposes
- Includes immunizations, social drug use, medication allergies and adverse reactions, alerts, special needs, and a history of relevant medication use

medication taking behavior
- The decisions a patient makes and acts upon related to the use of drug products and dosage regimens observed as patient compliance
- Is influenced by the patient's beliefs, attitudes, preferences, and wants, and experiences related to drug therapy

morality
- Used synonymously with ethics (see *ethics*)

non-maleficence
- Above all, do no harm
- One of the primary ethical principles that underlies the practice of pharmaceutical care

onset of action
- Amount of time from the administration of the medication to the first evidence of its pharmacological effect

outcomes, patient
- The *actual* results of interventions involving drug therapies
- Can have characteristics that are economic (i.e., cost), social/behavioral (i.e., patient preferences), or physiological and clinical (i.e., laboratory values, signs and symptoms)

outcome status
- The primary clinical decision made at a follow-up evaluation for each medical condition being managed with drug therapy
- Characterizes the effectiveness of the patient's drug therapy over time

- Is described with a standard set of definitions for medical conditions that are resolved, stable, improved, partially improved, unimproved, worsened, failure, and expired

partially improved
- One of the standard terms for describing the outcome status of a patient's medical condition being treated with pharmacotherapy
- Some measurable progress is being made toward achieving the desired goals of therapy, but adjustments in drug therapy are required. Usually dosage changes or the addition of additive or synergistic therapies is required

paternalistic (approach to patient care)
- An approach in which an authority figure undertakes to regulate the conduct of those in his/her control in matters affecting them as individuals as well as in their relations to that authority and to each other
- Characterized by practitioners making decisions with little regard to the patient's wishes
- An authoritarian approach which is inconsistent with the practice of pharmaceutical care

patient
- An individual who receives or requires health care services
- A person who possesses a unique set of needs, values, and beliefs that are brought to an interaction with a health care practitioner
- Sometimes described as client, consumer, or customer

patient-centered
- Care that places the patient's needs as the focus of the clinician's work
- Care that maintains the patient as a "holistic" being and does not fragment the patient into disease groups, organ systems, or drug categories
- A cornerstone of the philosophy of pharmaceutical care practice

patient care process
- A standard set of activities undertaken by all patient care practitioners
- The systematic activities that occur when a practitioner provides pharmaceutical care to a patient, consisting of the assessment, care plan, and follow-up evaluation
- A process that allows the practitioner to make rational, well-reasoned, and evidence-based decisions

pharmaceutical care
- A patient-centered practice in which the practitioner assumes responsibility for a patient's drug-related needs and is held accountable for this commitment
- A health care professional practice designed to meet the patient's drug-related needs by identifying, resolving, and preventing drug therapy problems

pharmacotherapy
- Includes the drug product and the dosage regimen being taken by a patient for an indication

- Used synonymously with drug therapy
- The use of drugs to treat or prevent human disease

Pharmacotherapy Workup

- A rational decision making process used in pharmaceutical care practice
- The practitioner's clinical decisions involved in assessing a patient's drug-related needs, identifying drug therapy problems, establishing goals of therapy, selecting interventions, and evaluating outcomes
- Description of the thought processes, hypotheses, established relationships, decisions, and resolved problems in providing pharmaceutical care

practice

- The creative application of knowledge, guided by a common philosophy and patient care process, to the resolution of specific problems in a manner and at a standard accepted by society
- The experiences a practitioner encounters in the process of caring for patients

practice philosophy

- A set of values that guides behaviors associated with a professional practice
- Aids the practitioner in making clinical, ethical, and management decisions and is used by a practitioner to determine what is important and to set priorities.
- Indicates what should be done at all times, and applies to all practitioners in a professional practice
- Guides how a practitioner practices, day in and day out
- The philosophy of practice for pharmaceutical care includes meeting the social obligation to minimize drug-related morbidity and mortality, accepting direct responsibility to identify, resolve, and prevent drug therapy problems, and applying the caring paradigm in a patient-centered manner

practitioner

- An individual who possesses a unique body of knowledge, skills, and values and uses this to meet the health care needs of a patient
- Subscribes to a specific philosophy of practice and way of practicing (patient care process) that is consistent with other members of the profession
- An individual who practices based upon specific standards of care and standards for professional behavior and holds him/herself as well as colleagues, to these standards
- Used synonymously with clinician

prevalence

- The number of all cases or occurances during a particular period of time

preventive

- Measures intended to thwart or ward off illness or disease, includes drug therapies and interventions to reduce the risk of drug therapy problems and/or medical conditions from developing

profession
- A vocation requiring training in the arts or sciences and advanced studies in a specialized field
- A body of qualified persons in a specific occupation or field
- Embodies the following attributes: (1) service above self interest; (2) application of specialized knowledge; (3) skills in the service of humanity; (4) an ethical code; (5) a fiduciary practitioner-client relationship; (6) registration or state certification, which embodies standards of training and practice in some statutory form; (7) regulation of advertising services; and (8) independence from external control

professional ethics
- A set of moral principles and values defined by the philosophy of practice
- Prescriptive, appropriate behavior for practitioners

reflective practitioner
- The practitioner who engages in active, deliberate, and conscious activity to become aware, critically analyze, and learn from practice experiences in order to improve clinical competence and patient relationships

resolved
- One of the standard terms for describing the outcome status of a patient's medical condition being treated with pharmacotherapy
- Goals of therapy have been achieved. Drug therapy has been completed or can now be discontinued. Usually associated with therapy for an acute disorder

specialist
- A practitioner who identifies, resolves, and prevents problems that are more complex than those addressed by the generalist
- Uses the same patient care process as the generalist to facilitate communication between the two practitioners
- Usually sees patients on a referral or consulting basis
- In the medical fields, is associated with a specific area of practice such as nephrology, pulmonary, medicine, cardiology, neurology, urology, gastroenterology and infectious diseases

safety (of the patient)
- Extent to which a patient is free from side effects, toxicity, or other undesirable pharmacological actions that a drug is known to exhibit at the doses used to treat patients

stable
- One of the standard terms for describing the outcome status of a patient's medical condition being treated with pharmacotherapy
- Goals of therapy have been achieved. The same drug therapy will be continued. Usually associated with therapy for chronic disorders

standards for professional behavior
- Authoritative statements in which a profession describes the responsibilities for which its practitioners are held accountable

- Practitioner's accountability to the public
- Includes guidelines for: quality of care, ethics, collegiality, collaboration, education research, and resource allocation

standards of care

- The level at which a practitioner is expected to provide care to a patient
- The set of behaviors each patient has a right to expect from a practitioner claiming to provide care in a particular profession
- The set of behaviors that is subject to evaluation by peers, regulators, and the public
- Includes guidelines for: assessment, drug therapy problem identification, care plan development, and follow-up evaluation

strength (of a product)

- The amount of active ingredient available in each dosage form (eg. 750 mg per tablet)

therapeutic relationship

- A partnership or alliance between the practitioner and the patient formed for the purpose of optimizing the patient's medication experience
- Characterized by: *trust, empathy, respect, authenticity*, and *responsiveness.*

unimproved

- One of the standard terms for describing the outcome status of a patient's medical condition being treated with pharmacotherapy
- No measurable progress in achieving goals of therapy can be demonstrated at this time. It is judged that more time is needed to produce adequate response. No changes will be made. The same drug therapy will be continued at this time

worsened

- One of the standard terms for describing the outcome status of a patient's medical condition being treated with pharmacotherapy
- There has been a decline in health status while receiving the current drug regimen. Some adjustments in drug product selection and/or drug dosage are required

PHARMACOTHERAPY
WORKUP NOTES

Pharmacotherapy Workup© **NOTES**	**ASSESSMENT**				

<table>
<tr><td rowspan="7">CONTACT INFORMATION</td><td colspan="5">Name</td></tr>
<tr><td colspan="2">Address</td><td>City</td><td>State</td><td>Postal Code</td></tr>
<tr><td>Telephone (h)</td><td>(w)</td><td>(cell)</td><td colspan="2">e-mail</td></tr>
<tr><td colspan="3">Pharmacy Name</td><td colspan="2">Clinic Name</td></tr>
<tr><td colspan="3">(tel)</td><td colspan="2">(tel)</td></tr>
</table>

<table>
<tr><td rowspan="7">DEMOGRAPHICS</td><td>Age</td><td>Date of Birth</td><td colspan="2">Gender: M/F</td></tr>
<tr><td>Weight</td><td>Height</td><td colspan="2">Lean Body Weight</td></tr>
<tr><td>Pregnancy status: Y/N</td><td>Breast Feeding: Y/N</td><td colspan="2">Due Date</td></tr>
<tr><td colspan="4">Occupation</td></tr>
<tr><td colspan="4">Living Arrangements/Family</td></tr>
<tr><td colspan="4">Health Insurance (coverage issues):</td></tr>
</table>

REASON FOR THE ENCOUNTER

<table>
<tr><td rowspan="12">MEDICATION EXPERIENCE</td><td rowspan="2">What is the patient's general attitude toward taking medication?</td><td colspan="2">Needs attention in care plan</td></tr>
<tr><td>Y</td><td>N</td></tr>
<tr><td rowspan="2">What does the patient want/expect from his/her drug therapy?</td><td colspan="2">Needs attention in care plan</td></tr>
<tr><td>Y</td><td>N</td></tr>
<tr><td rowspan="2">What concerns does the patient have with his/her medications?</td><td colspan="2">Needs attention in care plan</td></tr>
<tr><td>Y</td><td>N</td></tr>
<tr><td rowspan="2">To what extent does the patient understand his/her medications?</td><td colspan="2">Needs attention in care plan</td></tr>
<tr><td>Y</td><td>N</td></tr>
<tr><td rowspan="2">Are there cultural, religious, or ethical issues that influence the patient's willingness to take medications?</td><td colspan="2">Needs attention in care plan</td></tr>
<tr><td>Y</td><td>N</td></tr>
<tr><td rowspan="2">Describe the patient's medication taking behavior</td><td colspan="2">Needs attention in care plan</td></tr>
<tr><td>Y</td><td>N</td></tr>
</table>

	Birth	1 mo	2 mos	4 mos	6 mos	12 mos	15 mos	18 mos	24 mos	4–6 yrs	11–12 yrs	13–18 yrs
Hepatitis B	Dose 1		Dose 2			Dose 3						
Diphtheria, Tetanus, Pertussis			1	2	3		4					
Haemonphilus influenzae Type b			1	2	3	4						
Polio-inactivated			1	2			3			4		
Measles, Mumps, Rubella						1				2		
Varicella (chicken pox)												
Pneumococcal			1	2	3	4						
Hepatitis A (children in high risk regions)									Hepatitis A Series			
Influenza (children ≥ 6 with asthma, diabetes, HIV, sickle cell, cardiac disease)					Yearly							

☐ Current on all childhood immunizations

	19–49 Years	50–64 Years	65 Years & older
Tetanus, Diphtheria (Td)	1 booster every 10 years	1 booster every 10 years	1 booster every 10 years
Influenza	1 dose annually for persons with medical or occupational indications or household contacts of persons with indications	1 annual dose	1 annual dose
Pneumococcal (polysaccharide)	1 dose for persons with medical or other indications (1 dose revaccination for immunosuppressive conditions)	1 dose for person with medical or other indications (1 dose revaccination for immunosuppressive conditions)	1 dose for unvaccinated persons 1 dose revaccination

☐ Current on all adult immunizations

*see http:///www.cdc.gov/nip for more information

Substance	History of Use	Substance	History of Use
Tobacco ☐ No tobacco use	☐ 0–1 packs per day ☐ >1 packs per day ☐ previous history of smoking ☐ attempts to quit	Alcohol ☐ No alcohol use	☐ < 2 drinks per week ☐ 2–6 drinks per week ☐ > 6 drinks per week ☐ history of alcohol dependence
Caffeine ☐ No caffeine use	☐ < 2 cups per day ☐ 2–6 cups per day ☐ > 6 cups per day ☐ history of caffeine dependence	Other recreational drug use	

CHILDHOOD IMMUNIZATIONS*

ADULT IMMUNIZATIONS*

SOCIAL DRUG USE

ALLERGIES & ALERTS

Medication Allergies (drug, timing, reaction—rash, shock, asthma, nausea, anemia)

Adverse reactions to drugs in the past

Other Alerts/Health Aids/Special Needs (sight, hearing, mobility, literacy, disability)

CURRENT MEDICAL CONDITIONS AND MEDICATIONS

INDICATION	DRUG PRODUCT	DOSAGE REGIMEN dose, route, frequency, duration	START DATE	RESPONSE effectiveness/safety

PAST DRUG THERAPIES

INDICATION	DRUG THERAPY	RESPONSE	DATE

PAST MEDICAL HISTORY (RELEVANT ILLNESSES, HOSPITALIZATIONS, SURGICAL PROCEDURES, INJURIES, PREGNANCIES, DELIVERIES)

NUTRITIONAL STATUS (NOTE DAILY INTAKE OF CALORIES, CALCIUM, SODIUM, CHOLESTEROL, FIBER, POTASSIUM, VITAMIN K)			
calories	K^+	cholesterol	Vitamin K
calcium	Na^+	fiber	

OTHER FOOD OR DIETARY RESTRICTIONS / NEEDS

Vital signs: BP _____/_____   HR _____bpm   Resp Rate _____   Temp____

		y/n			y/n
REVIEW OF SYSTEMS	General Systems	Poor appetite	GU/Reproductive	Dysmenorrhea/ menstrual bleeding
		Weight change		Incontinence
		Pain		Impotence
		Headache		Decreased sexual drive
		Dizziness (vertigo)		
	EENT	Change in vision		Vaginal discharge or itching
		Loss of hearing		Hot flashes
		Ringing in the ears (tinnitus)	Kidney/Urinary	Urinary frequency
		Bloody nose (epistaxis)		Bloody urine (hematuria)
		Allergic rhinitis		Renal dysfunction
		Glaucoma	Hematopoietic Symptoms	Excessive bruising
		Bloody sputum (hemoptysis)		Bleeding
	Cardiovascular	Chest pain		Anemia
		Hyperlipidemia	Musculoskeletal	Back pain
		Hypertension		Arthritis pain (osteo/rheumatoid)
		Myocardial Infarction		Tendonitis
		Orthostatic hypotension		Painful muscles
	Pulmonary	Asthma	Neuropsychiatric	Numb, tingling sensation in extremities (parasthesia)
		Shortness of breath		
		Wheezing		Tremor
	Gastrointestinal	Heartburn		Loss of balance
		Abdominal pain		Depression
		Nausea		Suicidal
		Vomiting		Anxiety, nervousness
		Diarrhea		Inability to concentrate
		Constipation		Seizure
	Skin	Eczema/Psoriasis		Stroke/TIA
		Itching (pruritis)		Memory loss
		Rash	Infectious Disease	HIV/AIDS
	Endocrine Systems	Diabetes		Malaria
		Hypothyroidism		Syphilis
		Menopausal Symptoms		Gonorrhea
	Hepatic	Cirrhosis		Herpes
		Hepatitis		Chlamydia
	Nutrition/Fluid/ Electrolytes	Dehydration		Tuberculosis
		Edema		
		Potassium deficiency		

DRUG THERAPY PROBLEMS TO BE RESOLVED

MEDICAL CONDITION AND DRUG THERAPY INVOLVED	INDICATION
	Unnecessary Drug Therapy __No medical indication __Duplicate therapy __Nondrug therapy indicated __Treating avoidable ADR __Addictive/recreational **Needs Additional Drug Therapy** __Untreated condition __Preventive/prophylactic __Synergistic/potentiating
MEDICAL CONDITION AND DRUG THERAPY INVOLVED	EFFECTIVENESS
	Needs Different Drug Product __More effective drug available __Condition refractory to drug __Dosage form inappropriate __Not effective for condition **Dosage Too Low** __Wrong dose __Frequency inappropriate __Drug interaction __Duration inappropriate
MEDICAL CONDITION AND DRUG THERAPY INVOLVED	SAFETY
	Adverse Drug Reaction __Undesirable effect __Unsafe drug for patient __Drug interaction __Dosage administered or changed too rapidly __Allergic reaction __Contraindications present **Dosage Too High** __Wrong dose __Frequency inappropriate __Duration inappropriate __Drug interaction __Incorrect administration
MEDICAL CONDITION AND DRUG THERAPY INVOLVED	COMPLIANCE
	Noncompliance __Directions not understood __Patient prefers not to take __Patient forgets to take __Drug product too expensive __Cannot swallow/administer __Drug product not available

(Left margin vertical label: DRUG THERAPY PROBLEMS)

___No Drug Therapy Problem(s) at this time

Pharmacotherapy Workup© NOTES   CARE PLAN

INDICATION _____
(Description and history of the present illness or medical condition including previous approaches to treatment and responses)

GOALS OF THERAPY (improvement or normalization of signs/symptoms/laboratory tests or reduction of risk)
1.

2.

DRUG THERAPY PROBLEMS to be resolved

☐ None at this time

Therapeutic Alternatives (to resolve the drug therapy problem)
1.

2.

PHARMACOTHERAPY PLAN (Includes current drug therapies and changes)

MEDICATIONS (DRUG PRODUCTS)	DOSAGE INSTRUCTIONS (DOSE, ROUTE, FREQUENCY, DURATION)	NOTES CHANGES

Other interventions to optimize drug therapy

SCHEDULE FOR NEXT FOLLOW-UP EVALUATION:

Medical Condition: _____

	Outcome Parameter	Pretreatment Baseline (Date)	First Follow-up (Date)	Second Follow-up (Date)
EFFECTIVENESS	Sign/symptom			
	Sign/symptom			
	Lab value			
	Lab value			
SAFETY	Sign/symptoms			
	Signs/symptoms			
	Lab value			
	Lab value			
	Other			
STATUS	STATUS **Initial:** goals being established, initiate new therapy **Resolved:** goals achieved, therapy completed **Stable:** goals achieved, continue same therapy **Improved:** adequate progress being made, continue same therapy **Partial Improvement:** progress being made, adjustments in therapy required **Unimproved:** no progress yet, continue same therapy **Worsened:** decline in health, adjust therapy **Failure:** goals not achieved, discontinue current therapy and replace with different therapy			
	New Drug Therapy Problems Identified		☐ none at this time ☐ documented	☐ none at this time ☐ documented

Date	Schedule for next follow-up	Comments

Signature_____ Date_____

Parameters commonly used to evaluate effectiveness and/or safety of drug therapy

Parameter	Goals of therapy (normal values)	Clinical use
Blood pressure	Goals of therapy include: systolic blood pressure of 110–140 mmHg diastolic blood pressure of 75–85 mmHg <130/80 with diabetes or kidney disease	Used to evaluate effectiveness and safety of antihypertensive drug therapies such as diuretics, beta blockers, angiotensin-converting enzyme (ACE) inhibitors, angiotensin II receptors blockers, aldosterone antagonists, calcium blockers.
Total cholesterol	Goal of therapy < 200 mg/dL (SI < 5.17 mmol/L)	Represents all of the different kinds of cholesterol in the blood and includes high-density lipids (HDL), low-density lipids (LDL), and triglycerides (TG).
LDL Low-density lipoprotein	Goal of therapy varies depending on other risk factors including cigarette smoking, hypertension, HDL < 40 mg/dL, family history of coronary heart disease (CHD) and male >45 or female >55. • without other risk factors <160 mg/dL (SI <4.1 mmol/L) • with 2 risk factors <130 mg/dL (SI <3.4 mmol/L) • with CHD and ≥2 risk factors <100 mg/dL (SI <2.6 mmol/L)	Used to evaluate the effectiveness of lipid lowering drug therapies including atorvastatin (Lipitor), fluvastatin (Lescol), lovastatin (Mevacor), pravastatin (Pravachol), simvastatin (Zocor) nicotinic acid (Niacin) gemfibrozil (Lopid), clofibrate (Atromid-S) colestipol (Colestid), cholestyramine (Questran)
HDL High-density lipoprotein	Goals of therapy > 40 mg/dL (SI>1.04 mmol/L)	HDL removes excess cholesterol from peripheral tissues and is considered "good" cholesterol. Elevated HDL levels are associated with decreased risk for coronary heart disease.
Triglycerides	<160 mg/dL <1.8 mmol/L	Elevated triglycerides considered an independent risk factor for coronary heart disease.
Glucose	Goal of therapy includes: preprandial blood glucose of 80–120 mg/dL bedtime blood glucose of 100–140 mg/dL Fasting plasma glucose of >126 mg/dL on two occasions is consistent with the diagnosis of diabetes mellitus	Used to evaluate drug therapy to manage hyperglycemia associated with diabetes mellitus including insulin (Humulin) (Novolin), glipizide (Glutcotrol), glyburide (Diabeta) (Mircronase), pioglitazone (Actos), rosiglitazone (Avandia)

(Continued)

Parameters commonly used to evaluate effectiveness and/or safety of drug therapy (*Continued*)

Parameter	Goals of therapy (normal values)	Clinical use
HbA_{1c} Hemoglobin A_{1c}	Goal of therapy <7% Normal range 4–6%	Used to evaluate the effectiveness of glucose control in patients with diabetes. Reflects the blood glucose control over the past 2–3 months.
TSH Thyroid stimulating hormone	Goals of therapy include the reduction of TSH levels to the normal range of 0.3–5 µU/mL (SI 0.3–5 mU/L)	Used to evaluate the effectiveness of thyroid replacement therapy to manage hypothyroidism. levothyroxine (Synthroid). Elevated TSH levels are indicative of hypothyroidism.
INR International normalized ratio	Goal of therapy varies with the indication. INR 2.0–3.0 for atrial fibrillation, deep vein thrombosis, pulmonary emboli INR 2.5–3.5 for mechanical prosthetic values	Used to evaluate the effectives and safety of anticoagulant therapy. Used to determine dosage adjustments for warfarin (Coumadin) therapy.
K^+ Serum potassium	Goal of therapy is to maintain serum potassium within the normal range of 3.5–5.0 meq/L (SI 3.5–5.0 mmol/L)	Used to evaluate and prevent cardiac toxicity associated with hypokalemia caused by diuretics, diarrhea/vomiting. Can aggravate digoxin (Lanoxin) toxicity. Hyperkalemia associated with renal dysfunction, ACE inhibitors including captopril (Capoten), enalapril (Vasotec), lisinopril (Prinivil) (Zestril), ramipril (Altace)
Creatinine serum creatinine (SCr) creatinine clearance (CrCl)	Creatinine normal range 0.6–1.3 mg/dL (SI 53–115 µmol/L) Creatinine Clearance normal range 80–100 mL/min Drug dosage adjustments often required when CrCl is <30 mL/min	Used as a guideline to determine appropriate dosage of medications which are dependent on renal function for elimination. Used to determine if drug therapy is causing nephrotoxicity or if drugs are accumulating to unsafe levels due to decreasing renal function.
ALT Alanine aminotransferase	Normal values male 10–40 U/L, female 8–35 U/L	Used to evaluate liver damage caused by medications such as simvastatin (Zocor), pravastatin, Lovastatin (Mevacor), Atorvastatin (Lipitor) (Pravachol), fluvastatin (Lescol), carbamazepine, phenytoin, acetaminophen
AST Aspartate aminotransferase	male 20–40 U/L, female 15–30 U/L	If elevated 2–3 times drug-induced hepatic damage to be suspected

PHARMACOTHERAPY PATIENT CASE PRESENTATION

Assessment

Brief description of the patient (age, gender, appearance)

Primary reason for the patient encounter or visit

Additional patient background/demographics

The medication experience as reported by the patient (wants, expectations, concerns, understanding, preferences, attitudes, and beliefs that determine the patient's medication taking behavior)

Comprehensive medication history (allergies, alerts, social drug use, and immunization status)

Current medication record: description of all medical conditions being managed with pharmacotherapy with the following associations made:
Indication–Drug product–Dosage regimen–Result to date

Relevant past medical history: outcomes of past medication use

Review of systems

Identification of drug therapy problems: description of the drug therapy problem, medications involved, and causal relationships

Prioritization of multiple drug therapy problems

Summary of the assessment

(Continued)

The Care Plan (for each indication)

Goals of therapy

Clinical and laboratory parameters used to define the goal of therapy

    Observable, measurable value and timeline for each

How you plan to resolve the patient's drug therapy problems

    Therapeutic alternative approaches considered

    Rationale for your product and dosage selections

How you plan to achieve the goals of therapy

Nonpharmacologic interventions

Prevention of drug therapy problems

Schedule for follow-up evaluation

Follow-up Evaluation

Clinical and/or laboratory evidence of effectiveness of drug therapies for each
  indication

Clinical and/or laboratory evidence of safety of every drug regimen

Evidence of compliance

Evaluation of outcome status

Changes required in drug therapies

Schedule for future evaluations

Summary of Case

INDEX

Page numbers followed by italic *f* or *t* denote figures or tables, respectively.